P9-DUO-793

PROGRESS IN BRAIN RESEARCH

VOLUME 38

TOPICS IN NEUROENDOCRINOLOGY

PROGRESS IN BRAIN RESEARCH

ADVISORY BOARD

W. Bargmann	Kiel
H. T. Chang	Shanghai
E. De Robertis	Buenos Aires
J. C. Eccles	Buffalo
J. D. French	Los Angeles
H. Hydén	Göteborg
J. Ariëns Kappers	Amsterdam
S. A. Sarkisov	Moscow
J. P. Schadé	Amsterdam
F. O. Schmitt	Brookline (Mass.)
T. Tokizane	Tokyo
J. Z. Young	London

PROGRESS IN BRAIN RESEARCH

VOLUME 38

TOPICS IN NEUROENDOCRINOLOGY

EDITED BY

J. ARIËNS KAPPERS

AND

J. P. SCHADÉ

Central Institute for Brain Research, Amsterdam (The Netherlands)

ELSEVIER SCIENTIFIC PUBLISHING COMPANY

AMSTERDAM / LONDON / NEW YORK

1972

291250

ELSEVIER SCIENTIFIC PUBLISHING COMPANY
335 JAN VAN GALENSTRAAT,
P.O. BOX 211, AMSTERDAM, THE NETHERLANDS

AMERICAN ELSEVIER PUBLISHING COMPANY, INC.
52 VANDERBILT AVENUE, NEW YORK, N.Y. 10017

Science

LIBRARY OF CONGRESS CARD NUMBER 70-190681

ISBN 0-444-41049-X

WITH 88 ILLUSTRATIONS AND 15 TABLES

COPYRIGHT © 1972 BY ELSEVIER SCIENTIFIC PUBLISHING COMPANY, AMSTERDAM

ALL RIGHTS RESERVED.
NO PART OF THIS PUBLICATION MAY BE REPRODUCED, STORED IN A RETRIEVAL SYSTEM,
OR TRANSMITTED IN ANY FORM OR BY ANY MEANS, ELECTRONIC, MECHANICAL, PHOTO-
COPYING, RECORDING, OR OTHERWISE, WITHOUT THE PRIOR WRITTEN PERMISSION OF
THE PUBLISHER, ELSEVIER SCIENTIFIC PUBLISHING COMPANY,
JAN VAN GALENSTRAAT 335, AMSTERDAM

PRINTED IN THE NETHERLANDS

List of Contributors

H. A. BERN, Department of Zoology and its Cancer Research Genetics Laboratory, University of California, Berkeley, Calif. (U.S.A.).

L. BISANTI, Department of Anatomy, Università Cattolica del S. Cuore, Rome (Italy).

C. CAVALLOTTI, Department of Anatomy, Università Cattolica del S. Cuore, Rome (Italy).

D. DE WIED, Rudolf Magnus Institute for Pharmacology, Medical Faculty, University of Utrecht, Utrecht (The Netherlands).

B. T. DONOVAN, Institute of Psychiatry, De Crespigny Park, London (Great Britain).

J. J. DREIFUSS, Département de Physiologie de l'Université, Ecole de Médecine, Genève (Switzerland).

A. L. R. FINDLAY, Physiological Laboratory, Cambridge (Great Britain).

W. F. GANONG, Department of Physiology, University of California, San Francisco, San Francisco, Calif. (U.S.A.).

J. D. GRAU, Laboratoire de Radioimmunologie, Institut de Médecine de l'Université, Liège (Belgium).

M. B. TER HAAR, Department of Human Anatomy, University of Oxford, Oxford (Great Britain).

M. A. HAGE, Department of Anatomy, Medical Faculty Rotterdam, Rotterdam (The Netherlands).

B. HALÁSZ, 2nd Department of Anatomy, University Medical School, Budapest (Hungary).

J. N. HAYWARD, Departments of Anatomy and Neurology, School of Medicine, University of California, Los Angeles, Calif. (U.S.A.).

W. DE JONG, Rudolf Magnus Institut for Pharmacology, Medical Faculty, University of Utrecht, Utrecht (The Netherlands).

J. F. JONGKIND, Central Institute for Brain Research, Amsterdam (The Netherlands).

SIR FRANCIS KNOWLES, Department of Anatomy, King's College, Strand, London (Great Britain).

T. C. LEE, Rudolf Magnus Institute for Pharmacology, Medical Faculty, University of Utrecht, Utrecht (The Netherlands).

J. J. LEGROS, Laboratoire de Radioimmunologie, Institut de Médecine de l'Université, Liège (Belgium).

P. C. B. MACKINNON, Department of Human Anatomy, University of Oxford, Oxford (Great Britain).

J. MOLL, Department of Anatomy, Medical Faculty Rotterdam, Rotterdam (The Netherlands).

J. J. NORDMANN, Laboratoire de Radioimmunologie, Institut de Médecine de l'Université, Liège (Belgium).

M. PALKOVITS, Rudolf Magnus Institute for Pharmacology, Medical Faculty, University of Utrecht, Utrecht (The Netherlands).

E. PAPAIKONOMOU, Department of Pharmacology, Free University, Medical Faculty, Amsterdam (The Netherlands).

G. P. VAN REES, Department of Pharmacology, University of Leiden, Leiden (The Netherlands).

M. W. RIBBE, Department of Anatomy, Medical Faculty Rotterdam, Rotterdam (The Netherlands).

J. P. SCHADÉ, Central Institute for Brain Research, Amsterdam (The Netherlands).

B. SCHARRER, Department of Anatomy, Albert Einstein College of Medicine, Bronx, N.Y. (U.S.A.).

J. C. SLOPER, Department of Experimental Pathology, Charing Cross Hospital Medical School, Fulham (Great Britain).

P. G. SMELIK, Department of Pharmacology, Free University, Amsterdam (The Netherlands).

D. F. SWAAB, Central Institute for Brain Research, Amsterdam (The Netherlands).

B. VAN DER WAL, Rudolf Magnus Institute for Pharmacology, Medical Faculty, University of Utrecht, Utrecht (The Netherlands).

H. VAN WILGENBURG, Central Institute for Brain Research, Amsterdam (The Netherlands).

H. ZIMMERMANN, Fachbereich Biologie, Universität Regensburg, Regensburg (G.F.R.).

Contents

Introduction

For the VIIth Summer School for Brain Research, organized by the Netherlands Central Institute for Brain Research, Amsterdam, the topic Neuroendocrinology was chosen, partly because this is a rather complicated interdisciplinary subject which is rarely taught at any University as a theme in its own right, and partly because not a few workers at the Institute are especially interested in this field.

It is, perhaps, not entirely out of place to say a few words about this topic by way of general introduction giving a definition of the concept "neuroendocrinology" and, very briefly and schematically, some broad outlines concerning the nature of neuroendocrinological connections and the chemical agents involved. In the first paper, Professor Scharrer will give much more detailed information on these latter subjects.

As for a definition one may say that neuroendocrinology is that branch of the Neurosciences investigating the morphological and functional connections between the central nervous system and the endocrine systems. It is evident that several different disciplines such as anatomy, physiology, biochemistry and pharmacology should cooperate in elucidating these connections, their details as well as their more general implications which are also of great clinical importance.

The definition given indicates that neuroendocrinology is concerned with the functional interdependence between those two systems of the organism, the central nervous system and the endocrine apparatus, which are of the utmost importance for the functional coordination and integration of its many parts. The systems mentioned do not only ensure homeostasis by dealing adequately with the many and various stimuli, both from the milieu externe and interne, with which the organism has to cope at any moment during its existence, but they also ensure its growth and development, its reproduction and its faculties of communication.

The definition, moreover, includes that the central nervous system regulates the function of the different endocrine systems while, on the other hand, these systems influence the function of the nervous system. Endocrine systems often consist of chains constituted of several endocrine centres or organs which are functionally interrelated, the last organ of this chain or axis exerting the final effect on specific target or receptor cells.

Accepting that the central nervous system contains the primary centres involved in neuroendocrinological relationship, the pathways leading from this system to endocrine organs can be termed efferent pathways. They will be dealt with later. Afferent pathways, then, are those along which the products of the peripheral endocrine organs, hormones, are transported to the central nervous system. These latter pathways will mainly, although perhaps not exclusively, consist of blood vascular channels. Such hormones do not only regulate the function of centres, situated in the central nervous system and primarily involved in neuroendocrinological regulation, by way of their feedback activity. Hormones, produced in one endocrine organ, can also regulate the function of other peripheral endocrine organs by way of short feedback vascular connections. It should, moreover, be realized that hormones produced in peripheral endocrine organs do not only exert, in the central nervous system, an either excitatory or inhibitory influence on the centres from which the efferent pathways originate, but also on other neural centres such as, for instance, on those involved in behavioural mechanisms concomitant with neuroendocrinological events.

Most of the papers in this volume are especially concerned with the efferent links in neuroendocrinological relationship, dealing with the neural centres in which effector substances are produced, the nature and origin of these products, the pathways along which they are transported to their target cells, the way in which they are released, and their mode of action on endocrine and non-endocrine effector cells. It goes without saying that the field of neuroendocrinology is so large and deep that it was impossible to dig it up entirely in the single short week during which the Summer School was held.

We shall now deal briefly with the efferent connections. The primary neural centres from which they originate are all situated in parts of the brain and of the spinal cord which belong to the central part of the autonomic nervous system which is involved in the functional regulation of organs in general. Thus, these primary centres are to be found in the hypothalamus, that most important integration centre of autonomic functions, and in parasympathetic and orthosympathetic nuclei of the brain stem and cord.

The nature of the neurochemical effector substances and the pathways along which they are transported from the central nervous system to the endocrine effector organs vary a great deal. Giving first some examples of neural pathways originating from the spinal cord and brain stem, it is, for instance, known that the function of the adrenal medulla is regulated by preganglionic orthosympathetic nerve fibres originating in the intermediate lateral nucleus of the cord and coursing in the splanchnic nerves. The function of the pinealocytes in the mammalian pineal gland, an endocrine organ of neural origin, is, however, regulated by postganglionic noradrenergic orthosympathetic fibres and, as has been recently found, by postganglionic cholinergic parasympathetic fibres. The first type of fibres mentioned originates in the superior cervical ganglia and the second type from intramural pineal parasympathetic nerve cells. The central orthosympathetic preganglionic cells innervating the superior cervical ganglia are situated in the rostral part of the intermediate lateral nucleus in the cord while the parasympathetic preganglionic cells innervating the intramural pineal nerve cells lie in one of the parasympathetic nuclei of the brain stem. So far, it is not exactly known in which one.

More examples of endocrine organs, innervated by peripheral autonomic nerve fibres, could be given. The mode of impulse transmission between the endings of these fibres and their target cells varies. The neurochemical mediator substance, released at these endings, is not consistently transmitted to the effector cells by conventional synaptic junctions. A less well-directed and slower transmission of the stimulus is often realized in case the nerve terminals lie at some distance from the receptor cells.

Then, the neurohumor, once released, diffuses slowly in the organ along perivascular or wide intercellular spaces, as is true in the pineal gland, or in stromal tissue. From the above it appears that neural centres in the spinal cord and the brain stem, belonging to the central autonomic nervous system, send impulses regulating the function of endocrine organs along neural pathways belonging exclusively to the peripheral autonomic system, either directly by preganglionic fibres or by both, preganglionic and postganglionic fibres. The neurochemical transmitter substances involved belong to the category of the neurohumors. In mammals, centres producing neurohormones are, so far, not known to occur in the brain stem and the spinal cord. Such a centre is, however, present in the caudal end of the spinal cord of lower vertebrates as will be shown by Professor Bern in his paper.

The way in which neural centres in the hypothalamus are linked to endocrine organs by efferent pathways is much more complicated while, moreover, the nature of the neurochemical mediator substances involved is more varied. Neural centres in the hypothalamus produce neurohumors, although of a somewhat special kind, as well as neurohormones which are transported to their endocrine target cells along pathways which may consist of more than one link, these links being sometimes of a different nature.

The term "neurohormones" applies to all chemical mediators which are produced by neurosecretory cells, this production being the principal if not the only task of this cell type. Neurosecretory cells show morphological and physiological features characteristic of both, nerve cells and secretory cells. Neurohormones finally reach their target cells by vascular pathways. The term "neurohormones" does not imply anything about the chemical composition of these substances. They may, for instance, be of a proteinaceous or of an aminergic nature. For their definition as neurohormones it is only of importance that they are produced by neuro(secretory) cells and reach their target cells finally along vascular pathways. That this definition sometimes causes difficulties will be clear, especially when aminergic neurohormones are concerned.

As I am sure that Professor Scharrer will go deeper into this question, I will only mention here that three different kinds of "neurohormones" can be distinguished:

(1) Neurohormones of which the polypeptide nature has been well-established for some time: vasopressin and oxytocin. These neurohormones are produced in the hypothalamic magnocellular supraoptic and paraventricular nuclei. The axons of the cells constituting these nuclei form the supraoptico-paraventriculo-hypophysial tract. Most, but not all fibres of this tract end in the infundibular process of the neurohypophysis.

(2) Neurohormones of which the proteinaceous chemical composition, at least of part of them, has been established quite recently. These are the so-called releasing, or better regulating (B. Scharrer) or hypophysiotropic factors. These neurohormones are produced in the parvocellular arcuate and tuberal hypothalamic nuclei situated in the baso-medial part of the hypothalamus. The axons of these cells form the tubero-infundibular tract. Their terminals are situated in the median eminence.

4

(3) Aminergic neurohormone(s) which is probably produced by nerve cells lying in the arcuate nucleus of the hypothalamus. Their axons join the tubero-infundibular tract to end in the median eminence. The question whether the aminergic compound (*e.g.*, dopamine) produced in this third neuronal system should be termed either a neurohormone or a neurohumor depends on the different opinions existing on its target, and, in connection therewith, on the pathway along which this target is reached (see below).

The neurohormones mentioned are transported along the axons of the hypothalamic nerve cells in which they are produced to the axon terminals in which they are stored and from which they are released. In mammals, axons along which neurohormones are transported do not leave the central nervous system. They end either in the infundibular process of the neurohypophysis or in the median eminence. Here, the axon terminals are in close contact with the outer basement membrane of perivascular spaces surrounding capillary plexuses. Together with these plexuses the axon terminals form a so-called "neurohemal organ".

The neurohormones stored in the axon terminals of the supraoptico-paraventriculo-hypophysial tract fibres, present in the infundibular process of the neurohypophysis as mentioned sub (1), are depleted into capillaries which drain directly into the systemic circulation by which these neurohormones finally reach their target or receptor cells which are not necessarily endocrine cells exclusively. The neurohormones mentioned sub (2) which are stored in axon terminals situated in the median eminence are depleted into the primary capillary plexus of the hypophysial portal system by which they are conveyed, probably exclusively, to their different and specific endocrine target cells in the pars distalis of the hypophysis or adenohypophysis. According to some authors, the aminergic compound, mentioned sub (3), is likewise depleted in the primary capillary plexus of the hypophysial portal system to reach also the endocrine cells in the adenohypophysis supposedly cooperating with the hypophysiotropic factors in regulating the release and possibly the synthesis of the hormones, produced by these cells. Other authors, however, hold that this compound is not depleted in any vascular pathway, but acts, in the median eminence, on the terminals containing the hypophysiotropic factors regulating the depletion of these factors into the primary capillary plexus. In the latter case this aminergic compound should not be called a neurohormone because it is not being depleted into the blood.

From the foregoing it appears that mammalian neurohormones reach their elements of destination first along a neural pathway, the axons of the neurosecretory cells in which they are produced, and then along a post-linked vascular pathway, both pathways together constituting a neuro-vascular pathway.

Some of the axons of peptidergic neurosecretory cells of the magnocellular hypothalamic nuclei do not terminate in the infundibular process of the neurohypophysis, but on pituicytes and on endocrine cells of the intermediate part of the hypophysis. Because, ontogenetically, this pars intermedia originates from the posterior wall of Rathke's pouch, it does not belong to the central nervous system. Therefore, the axons ending in close contact to the endocrine cells of the pars intermedia have to leave the brain. As the proteinaceous mediators stored in the axon endings are not depleted into capillaries but act directly on the pars intermedia cells, they do not qualify as neurohormones although they are produced by neurosecretory cells. Due to various reasons these special mediators are classed in a category in between neurohormones and neurohumors. Similarly, some fibres transporting biogenic amines do not terminate in the median eminence, but in close contact to cells of the pars intermedia. Both, the peptidergic and the aminergic fibres ending on endocrine cells of the pars intermedia, are sometimes termed "neurosecretomotor fibres".

In some non-mammalian vertebrates, a caudal neurosecretory system showing features comparable to that of the hypothalamic magnocellular neurosecretory system, is present in the caudal end of the spinal cord. The axons of its neurosecretory cells terminate in a storage organ, the urophysis, from which the neurohormone is depleted into a capillary vascular system. In the present volume, this caudal secretory system will also be dealt with.

As is quite evident and has also been demonstrated by many authors, the function of the primary hypothalamic centres involved in the regulation of endocrine systems not only depends on the feedback activity of hormones produced in endocrine organs, reaching these centres by afferent vascular pathways, but also on neural stimuli contacting the nerve cells which constitute these primary centres. These stimuli are either excitatory or inhibitory. The axon terminals being in synaptic contact with the dendrites or the soma of the neurosecretory cells contain either biogenic amines, such as noradrenaline or serotonin, or acetylcholine. It can only be indicated here that these axons originate from nerve cells which are situated in various and quite different parts of the brain, such as for instance telencephalic limbic centres and the brain stem reticular formation. These centres, again, receive many impulses from various sources, such as from the sense organs, mostly via relay centres, and from the ascending multisynaptic pathway in cord and brain stem. It should, therefore, be clear that the function of the cells constituting the primary hypothalamic centres from which the efferent pathways for the regulation of endocrine systems originate, are, themselves, modulated by impulses from a multitude of various sources. To use a term, coined by Ernst Scharrer, the neurosecretory cells form a final common pathway for all stimuli reaching them.

The same holds for the centres in the spinal cord regulating the function of endocrine organs. Light stimuli entering the eye are, for instance, conveyed via a multisynaptic neural pathway, the links of which are now known, to that part of the intermediate lateral nucleus in the cord from which the preganglionic fibres originate to innervate the mammalian pineal gland via the superior cervical ganglia and their postganglionic noradrenergic fibres. In this way, the function of this gland depends, *i.a.*, on photic stimuli.

We will end this introduction to the central topic, primarily written from the standpoint of a neuro-anatomist, by pointing out that not only the blood, but also the cerebrospinal fluid probably serves as a vehiculum for the transport of hormones

6

which, by means of special ependymal elements or after stimulating special liquor-contacting neurones, may modulate the function of hypothalamic and other centres involved in neuro-endocrinological regulation. This relatively new and fascinating subject will also be mentioned in the present volume.

The proceedings of the Summer School testify to the industrious efforts of the participants to unravel, by various methods and techniques, the many structural and functional neuroendocrinological problems. I am most grateful to all participants cooperating by contributing so many important papers and taking such a lively and fruitful part in the discussions. The editors being responsible for the final script of the discussions, our apologies are offered in advance to anyone who would not be entirely satisfied with what has been published from his remarks and comments.

My sincere thanks are also due to the staff members of the Netherlands Central Institute for Brain Research, and more especially to Dr. Schadé. Without their assiduous help and experience the organization of the Summer School and the editing of its proceedings would scarcely have been possible.

The fact that, once again, the governing board of the Royal Netherlands Academy of Sciences and Letters has placed the mansion of the Academy at the disposal of the conference is much appreciated.

J. ARIËNS KAPPERS

Neuroendocrine Communication
(Neurohormonal, Neurohumoral, and Intermediate)

BERTA SCHARRER

Department of Anatomy, Albert Einstein College of Medicine, Bronx, N.Y. (U.S.A.)

Reports on current advances in neurobiology reflect a growing interest in control mechanisms involving close collaboration between the nervous and the endocrine systems. This trend reaches its culmination in the present program which addresses itself exclusively to Neuroendocrinology. In essence, this topic concerns two channels of communication, one conveying neural directives to the endocrine apparatus, the other providing the nervous system with information on hormonal events. Therefore, the central theme of a progress report on neuroendocrine phenomena will have to be an examination of the nature and mode of operation of these avenues of interaction. But the major share of our attention will be directed to the efferent link, *i.e.*, the varied means of communication between the neural and the endocrine systems, since it is even more important and considerably more complex than the afferent link. An introduction to this topic in general conceptual terms as provided in this first chapter can be concise, since several recent surveys along similar lines are available (see B. Scharrer, 1967–72; E. Scharrer, 1965, 1966).

Efficient operation of the endocrine system requires precise programming of rates of production and release of individual hormones in concert with others; it may be accomplished by active stimulation or inhibition, or by withdrawal of either kind of signal. There also seems to be an interplay among such varied directives. Since the effectors are subject to control by pluralistic and at times conflicting information, there is the possibility of confusion. Therefore, at any given time, instructions for action must be well integrated, *i.e.*, non-contradictory. They should reach endocrine effector cells of the same kind simultaneously, and their effects should be more or less sustained. Amplification of signals seems to be advantageous in cyclic control systems, and there is also an apparent requirement for trophic influences in the maintenance of endocrine organs.

The need for the conversion of a variety of simultaneous conditioning factors into uniform commands is met by the nervous system through which most of the afferent signals are channeled. In turn, the effectiveness of the "final common path" to the first way station in the endocrine system is assured by a multiplicity of means for the transfer of information. Their existence has become apparent as a result of correlative studies in which electron microscopy provided invaluable leads. A broad comparative approach has revealed the general validity of the conclusions to be discussed for all of the neuroendocrine systems thus far investigated.

References p. 14

TABLE I

MODES OF COMMUNICATION BETWEEN NEURONS AND NON-NEURAL EFFECTORS

		Endocrine effectors	*Nonendocrine effectors*
Conventional neuroeffector junctions	Contiguous	Neurohumoral	Pars intermedia Endopancreas Adrenal cortex { Ultimobranchial body Parafollicular cells Leydig cells, testis Interstitial cells, ovary Corpus allatum	Neuromuscular junctions Secretomotor junctions (exocrine cells)
Nonconventional mechanisms	Noncontiguous	Neurohormonal	Anterior pituitary (higher vertebrates) Prothoracic gland (insects)	Kidney tubule cells Uterine muscle Myoepithelial cells
		Nonhormonal (stromal pathway)	Some fish pituitaries Insect endocrines	Smooth muscle Some striated muscle Regeneration blastema (NTS) Muscle, *etc.* (insects)
	Contiguous (nonconventional)		Pars intermedia Corpus allatum	

The various modes of operation differ with respect to the type and amount of the neurochemical mediator in use, the manner in which it reaches its destination, and the duration of the signal. These parameters are related to the nature of the extracellular pathway. In addition, there are diagnostically useful ultrastructural and histochemical differences among the respective intracellular storage sites of the active principles.

The existing possibilities for neuroendocrine communication are listed in Table I which, for the sake of comparison, also includes non-neuronal effectors other than endocrine. Special adaptations to the needs of the endocrine system take precedence over control by conventional innervation, but it is difficult to decide which factors determine the choice of "language" used in different situations, and whether or not there are sharp lines of demarcation.

I. Conventional control mechanism

The presence of synaptic or synapse-like (synaptoid) configurations in electron micrographs of a variety of endocrine organs leads to the conclusion that at least some of the neurochemical signals in operation are the same as those in regular neuron-to-neuron communication. Quite often these junctional complexes resemble adrenergic elements, with the exception that some of the characteristics of conventional chemically transmitting synapses tend to be absent. Aside from those in the adrenal medulla and the pineal gland, putative secretomotor junctions also occur in a number of endocrine structures of non-neural derivation. Examples are the pars intermedia of the pituitary (Bargmann *et al.*, 1967; Follenius, 1968, 1970; Meurling and Björklund, 1970, and others); various components of the pancreatic islets (Legg, 1967; Esterhuizen *et al.*, 1968; Watari, 1968; Shorr and Bloom, 1970; Kern *et al.*, 1971), the adrenal cortex (Unsicker, 1969; Alvarez, 1970), various calcitonin producing cells (Robertson, 1967; Stoeckel and Porte, 1967; Young and Harrison, 1969), and interstitial elements in both male and female gonads (Baumgarten and Holstein, 1968; Unsicker, 1970; Dahl, 1970). Analogous observations obtain for invertebrates, *e.g.*, those reported for the corpus allatum of insects (for further details see Scharrer, 1970; Weitzman, 1964–71).

This kind of morphological information is substantiated by physiological data, for example in the case of the beta cells of the endocrine pancreas. The adrenergic nature of the transmitter operating at neuron terminals that are in contact with some of these glandular elements is suggested by their ultrastructure. The specific fluorescence for catecholamine displayed at these sites increases after the administration of monoamine oxidase inhibitors, and the measurable rise in catecholamine content is accompanied by a stimulation of insulin secretion (Gagliardino *et al.*, 1970; see also Tjälve, 1971; Tjälve and Slanina, 1971). Furthermore, alloxan-treated animals show fine structural alterations in the terminals that are indicative of neuronal hyperactivity in conjunction with stimulation of insulin secretion (Shorr and Bloom, 1970).

Another example is seen in the pars intermedia. The adrenergic nature of one class of fibers among those supplying this part of the adenohypophysis has been conclusively established by their uptake of adrenaline-^{3}H, as demonstrated by ultraautoradiography, and by their selective destruction with 6-hydroxydopamine (Doerr–Schott and Follenius, 1969; Hopkins, 1971).

The question may be raised as to how much control over endocrine systems can be accomplished by neurohumoral signals at such secretomotor junctions. It need hardly be stressed that the special features of synaptic transmission (strict localization of signal, high speed, rapid turnoff) which are so crucial in regular interneuronal communication, represent a disadvantage in the case of endocrine receptors. The efficiency of their operation requires types of signals that cannot be provided by the activity of neurotransmitters alone. As will become evident in the next section, the special requirements of endocrine receptors are in fact largely met by other than synaptic types of neurochemical input.

II. Nonconventional control mechanisms

(a) Neurohormonal mediation. Among the special means of neurochemical instruction available to endocrine cells, those conveyed by either a general or a limited (portal) circulatory pathway predominate. They seem to be made to order for maximum efficiency of the neuroendocrine axis. Here the mediator is not classified as a neurotransmitter but as a neurohormone. It is derived not from a conventional neuronal element but from a special "neurosecretory" neuron. The main distinction of the latter is that its capacity for the synthesis of specific secretory products is so highly developed as to overshadow all other neuronal functions (for more detailed information on the phenomenon of neurosecretion see Bargmann and Scharrer, 1970; Gabe, 1966; B. Scharrer, 1967, 1969a, c; 1970; B. Scharrer and Weitzman, 1970; E. Scharrer, 1965, 1966; E. Scharrer and B. Scharrer, 1963).

The material released from classical (A type) neurosecretory neurons is proteinaceous, but aside from these "peptidergic" elements there are aminergic (B type) fibers which also seem to manufacture enough active material to reach threshold concentrations sufficient for hormonal interaction. But here the mode of operation may be somewhat different from that of peptidergic mediators. This specialization in synthetic activity expresses itself morphologically by the presence of distinctive types of glandular products in considerable quantity.

The prolonged signals generated by blood-borne neurochemical messengers are in sharp contrast to those characteristic of synaptic function. A further advantage of neurohormones is their simultaneous availability to multiple effector cells. An A type neurohormone released into the general circulation by neurosecretory cell groups in the insect brain reaches the prothoracic gland, a receptor organ controlling postembryonic development. An analogous group of neurohormones in vertebrates is represented by the well known hypophysiotropic (releasing or regulating) factors of the hypothalamus that control adenohypophysial function via the portal circulation. As has been shown in several mammalian species, these neurohormonal factors originate in hypothalamic centers such as the arcuate nucleus and enter their restricted vascular route at the level of the median eminence. The thyrotropin releasing factor

(TRF) which may serve as a prototype has been identified as a tripeptide (see Meites, 1970a). LH release and synthesis, as well as FSH release, are stimulated by another hypothalamic hormone which seems to be an octapeptide (Schally *et al.*, 1971; Redding *et al.*, 1971). In addition to small peptides, aminergic elements may participate in the control of hypophysial cells that furnish adenotropic hormones. Cytological and cytochemical data indicate the presence of both peptidergic and aminergic fibers in the median eminence (see, for example, Konstantinova, 1970; Oksche *et al.*, 1970; Sharp and Follett, 1970). The possibility that the two types of neurochemical mediators act synergistically has been discussed (see Scott and Knigge, 1970). Experimental data from *in vivo* and *in vitro* tests suggest aminergic (especially dopaminergic) synaptic control over neurosecretory neurons that furnish various hypophysiotropic factors (Barry, 1970; Fuxe and Hökfelt, 1970; Müller, 1970; Schneider and McCann, 1970), but there is some disagreement as to which type of synapse is responsible for stimulatory and which for inhibitory signals.

In view of the known relationship between photoperiod and gonadotropic function, it is of interest that the activation of the hypothalamic-hypophysial system in frogs maintained on a long-day regime involves only the neurosecretory material released from the median eminence, and not that destined for the posterior lobe (Vullings, 1971). Comparable effects of relevant exteroceptive and interoceptive factors on the synthesis and release of hypophysiotropic factors have been demonstrated in mammals (Meites, 1970b).

(b) Intermediate mechanisms. Several types of nonconventional mediation operate without the intervention of neurohormones. It appears that in the dissemination of neurosecretory messengers vascular channels can be circumvented altogether. An interesting variant of such "directed delivery" occurs, for example in the adenohypophysis of some teleost fishes where axon terminals carrying neurosecretory material abut on areas of intercellular stroma that separate the release sites from the receptor cells (Vollrath, 1967).

Invertebrates in which no capillary system exists depend much more on extracellular channels, and are therefore particularly well suited for the exploration of their physiological features. For one, the relative closeness of the effector sites restricts the sphere of dissemination without pinpointing the signal to a single cell. But beyond this merely spatial issue, it is the physico-chemical nature of the pathway which deserves attention in that it may allow for temporary sequestration of the neurochemical mediator and thus determine the time course in this type of information transfer (see also Barer, 1967).

Another mode of action for which physiological correlates are still missing, is suggested by ultrastructural evidence indicating that "peptidergic" neurosecretory terminals can make direct contact with endocrine receptor cells. Examples of such "neurosecretomotor junctions" occur in the pars intermedia of the cat (Bargmann *et al.*, 1967), and the corpus allatum of insects (B. Scharrer, 1964). Although here the spatial relationships are the same as in standard types of synapses, the different nature of the chemical messenger involved sets these junctional configurations apart.

References p. 14

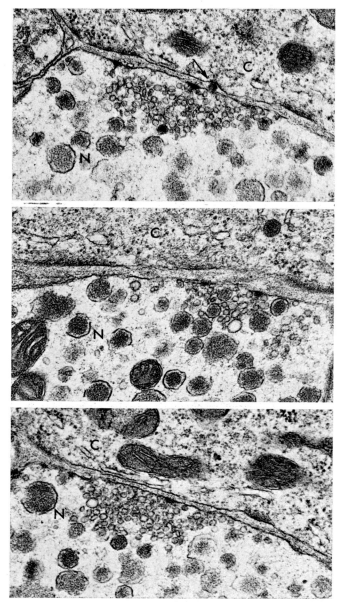

Fig.1. Three examples of neurosecretory fibers with synaptoid configurations in close proximity to endocrine cells (C) in corpus allatum of adult male of insect, *Periplaneta americana*. Note clusters of heterogeneous vesicles and small accumulations of electron dense (neurosecretory?) material close to axolemma or within narrow intercellular space (arrow). N, neurosecretory granules. Prior to fixation in Karnovsky's (1965) solution, the gland had been incubated for 30 min in insect Ringer's with excess of K^+ (*cf.* Sachs and Haller, 1968). Epon, uranyl acetate and lead citrate. $\times$ 40,000.

Fig. 1 shows three synaptoid elements in a corpus allatum that had been exposed to a stimulus effecting neurohormone release. The extracellular distances between the neurosecretory fibers and the putative endocrine effector cells are reduced almost to those observed in regular synaptic gaps. But the variability in the size and content of the synaptoid vesicles clustered near the axolemma, and several extravesicular accumulations of electron dense material, suggest that these configurations serve for the release of peptidergic neurosecretory material.

Nothing is known about the mechanism of inactivation for neurosecretory substances that do not reach the circulation and thus do not function in the capacity of neurohormones. It may be assumed that this process differs from those operating in the case of either acetylcholine or noradrenaline, and that the duration of the signals also belongs to a different range.

In sum, neural control of adenohypophysial functions can be accomplished by means other than those involving neurohormones and portal vascular channels. Therefore, the well established terms hypophysiotropic (releasing, or regulating) factors rather than hormones are preferable and should be retained.

CONCLUDING REMARKS

Further work may well provide us with additional examples of nonconventional situations. The multiplicity of possibilities already known to exist poses the question of whether specific types of neuroendocrine commands have to be carried out by specific mechanisms. Synaptic input, for example, is thought to be responsible for the control of hormone release rather than its synthesis (see Oshima and Gorbman, 1969; Unsicker, 1969). However, a more general answer to this question is not yet possible.

Since the present state of diversity must be the result of gradual specialization in the course of phylogeny, the possibility that a certain type of endocrine response can be elicited in more than one way must exist. Such alternative modes of operation with presumably similar results are illustrated by existing variations in the neural control over adenohypophysial function, where the extracellular route ranges from the smallest distance between contiguous cells, to the portal circulation. However, the fact remains that the greater the distance between the site of release and site of action of the messenger substance, the less pinpointed ("private") the signal becomes. Also the time course varies widely but, as has been indicated before, it is not determined by distance alone. Significant factors are the functional properties of the vehicle (blood, stromal matrix, possibly cerebrospinal fluid) and the mechanisms for inactivation of the neurochemical mediator (enzymatic action, recycling, *etc.*).

In conclusion, multiple avenues have been acquired in the course of specialization which allow for considerable versatility in neuroendocrine mediation. Our increasing familiarity with the dynamics of cellular interaction now directs our attention to the exploration of biochemical events at the receptor site, the results of which will transcend the scope of neuroendocrinology.

References p. 14

ACKNOWLEDGEMENT

This study was aided by U.S. Public Health Service Grants NB-00840, NB-05219, and 5P01-NS-07512.

REFERENCES

ALVAREZ, F. G. (1970) Estudio ultraestructural sobre la inervación de la corteza suprarenal. *An. Anat.*, **19**, 267–279.

BARER, R. (1967) Speculations on the storage and release of hormones and transmitter substances. Symp. electr. Activ. Innerv. Blood Vessels, Cambridge, 1966. *Bibl. anat. (Basel)*, **8**, 72–75.

BARGMANN, W., LINDNER, E. UND ANDRES, K. H. (1967) Über Synapsen an endokrinen Epithelzellen und die Definition sekretorischer Neurone. Untersuchungen am Zwischenlappen der Katzenhypophyse. *Z. Zellforsch.*, **77**, 282–298.

BARGMANN, W. AND SCHARRER, B. (Eds.) (1970) *Aspects of Neuroendocrinology*, Proc. Vth int. Symp. Neurosecretion. Springer, Berlin, 377 pp.

BARRY, J. (1970) Recherches sur le rôle des monoamines infundibulaires dans le contrôle de la sécrétion gonadotrope chez le cobaye et la souris. In *Aspects of Neuroendocrinology*, W. BARGMANN AND B. SCHARRER (Eds.), Springer, Berlin, pp. 245–252.

BAUMGARTEN, H. G. UND HOLSTEIN, A. F. (1968) Adrenerge Innervation im Hoden und Nebenhoden vom Schwan *(Cygnus olor)*. *Z. Zellforsch.*, **91**, 402–410.

DAHL, E. (1970) Studies of the fine structure of ovarian interstitial tissue. 3. The innervation of the thecal gland of the domestic fowl. *Z. Zellforsch.*, **109**, 212–226.

DOERR-SCHOTT, J. ET FOLLENIUS, E. (1969) Localisation des fibres aminergiques dans l'hypophyse de *Rana esculenta*. Etude autoradiographique au microscope électronique. *C. R. Acad. Sci. (Paris)*, **269**, Série D, 737–740

ESTERHUIZEN, A. C., SPRIGGS, T. L. B. AND LEVER, J. D. (1968) Nature of islet-cell innervation in the cat pancreas. *Diabetes*, **17**, 33–36.

FOLLENIUS, E. (1968) Innervation adrénergique de la méta-adénohypophyse de l'Epinoche *(Gasterosteus aculeatus* L.). Mise en évidence par autoradiographie au microscope électronique. *C. R. Acad. Sci. (Paris)*, **267**, Série D, 1208–1211.

FOLLENIUS, E. (1970) Mise en évidence, au microscope électronique, de l'innervation de l'hypophyse de *Gasterosteus aculeatus* L. par la technique de Maillet Champy. *C. R. Acad. Sci. (Paris)*, **271**, Série D, 1034–1037.

FUXE, K. and HÖKFELT, T. (1970) Participation of central monoamine neurons in the regulation of anterior pituitary function with special regard to the neuro-endocrine role of tubero-infundibular dopamine neurons. In *Aspects of Neuroendocrinology*, W. BARGMANN AND B. SCHARRER (Eds.), Springer, Berlin, pp. 192–205.

GABE, M. (1966) *Neurosecretion*. Pergamon Press, Oxford, London, New York.

GAGLIARDINO, J. J., ITURRIZA, F. C., HERNANDEZ, R. E. AND ZIEHER, L. M. (1970) Effect of catecholamine precursors on insulin secretion. *Endocrinology*, **87**, 823–825.

HOPKINS, C. R. (1971) Localization of adrenergic fibers in the amphibian pars intermedia by electron microscope autoradiography and their selective removal by 6-hydroxydopamine. *Gen. Comp. Endocr.*, **16**, 112–120.

KARNOVSKY, M. J. (1965) A formaldehyde–glutaraldehyde fixative of high osmolality for use in electron microscopy. *J. Cell Biol.*, **27**, 137A–138A.

KERN, H. F., HOFMANN, H. V. UND KERN, D. (1971) Licht- und elektronenmikroskopische Untersuchung der Langerhansschen Inseln vom Nutria *(Myocastor coypus)*, mit besonderer Berücksichtigung der neuroinsulären Komplexe. *Z. Zellforsch.*, **113**, 216–229.

KONSTANTINOVA, M. S. (1970) Adrenergic structures within the hypothalamo-hypophysial neurosecretory system in animals of different phylogenetic levels. *Proc. Leningrad Soc. Anat., Histol., Embryol.*, Issue 2, 109–113 (In Russian).

LEGG, P. G. (1967) The fine structure and innervation of the beta and delta cells in the islet of Langerhans of the cat. *Z. Zellforsch.*, **80**, 307–321.

MEITES, J. (Ed.) (1970a) *Hypophysiotropic Hormones of the Hypothalamus: Assay and Chemistry.*

Workshop conference on bioassay and chemistry of the hypophysiotropic hormones. Tucson, Arizona, January 1969. Williams and Wilkins, Baltimore, 338 pp.

MEITES, J. (1970b) Modification of synthesis and release of hypothalamic releasing factors induced by exogenous stimuli. In *Neurochemical Aspects of Hypothalamic Function*, Academic Press, New York and London, pp. 1–43.

MEURLING, P. AND BJÖRKLUND, A. (1970) The arrangement of neurosecretory and catecholamine fibres in relation to the pituitary intermedia cells of the skate, *Raja radiata*. *Z. Zellforsch.*, **108**, 81–92.

MÜLLER, E. E. (1970) Brain catecholamines and growth hormone release. In *Aspects of Neuroendocrinology*, W. BARGMANN AND B. SCHARRER (Eds.), Springer, Berlin, pp. 206–219.

OKSCHE, A., OEHMKE, H. J. UND FARNER, D. S. (1970) Weitere Befunde zur Struktur und Funktion des Zwischenhirn-Hypophysensystems der Vögel. In *Aspects of Neuroendocrinology*, W. BARGMANN AND B. SCHARRER (Eds.), Springer, Berlin, pp. 261–273.

OSHIMA, K. AND GORBMAN, A. (1969) Pars intermedia: Unitary electrical activity regulated by light. *Science*, **163**, 195–197.

REDDING, T. W., SCHALLY, A. V. and LOCKE, W. (1971) Stimulation of luteinizing hormone (LH) synthesis by porcine LH-releasing hormone. Proc. 53rd Meeting. Endocrine Soc. *Endocrinology*, **88**, Suppl., A-75.

ROBERTSTON, D. R. (1967) The ultimobranchial body in *Rana pipiens*. III. Sympathetic innervation of the secretory parenchyma. *Z. Zellforsch.*, **78**, 328–340.

SACHS, H. AND HALLER, E. W. (1968) Further studies on the capacity of the neurohypophysis to release vasopressin. *Endocrinology*, **83**, 251–262.

SCHALLY, A. V., ARIMURA, A., BABA, Y., NAIR, R. M. G., MATSUO, H., REDDING, T. W., DEBELJUK, L. AND WHITE, W. F. (1971) Purification and properties of the LH and FSH-releasing hormone from porcine hypothalami. Proc. 53rd meeting Endocrine Soc., *Endocrinology*, **88**, Suppl., A-70.

SCHARRER, B. (1964) Histophysiological studies on the corpus allatum of *Leucophaea maderae*. IV. Ultrastructure during normal activity cycle. *Z. Zellforsch.*, **62**, 125–148.

SCHARRER, B. (1967) The neurosecretory neuron in neuroendocrine regulatory mechanisms. *Amer. Zool.*, **7**, 161–169.

SCHARRER, B. (1969a) Neurohumors and Neurohormones: Definitions and Terminology. *J. neurovisc. Rel.*, Suppl. IX, 1–20.

SCHARRER, B. (1969b) Current concepts in the field of neurochemical mediation. *Med. Coll. Virginia Quart.*, **5**, 27–31.

SCHARRER, B. (1969c) Comparative aspects of neurosecretory phenomena. In *Progress in Endocrinology*, Proc., III int. Congr. Endocrinol., Mexico, 1968. pp. 365–367.

SCHARRER, B. (1970) General principles of neuroendocrine communication. In *The Neurosciences: Second Study Program*, F. O. SCHMITT (Ed.), The Rockefeller Univ. Press, New York, pp. 519–529.

SCHARRER, B. (1971a) Concepts of neurochemical mediation. *Neurocirurgía*, **29**, 257–262.

SCHARRER, B., (1971b) Comparative aspects of neuroendocrine communication. *Gen. comp. Endocr.*, Suppl., in press.

SCHARRER, B. (1972) Principles of neuroendocrine communication. In *The Median Eminence*, K. M. KNIGGE, D. E. SCOTT AND A. WEINDL (Eds.), Intern. Proc. Sympos. Brain-Endocrine Interaction, S. Karger, Basel, pp. 3–6.

SCHARRER, B. AND WEITZMAN, M. (1970) Current problems in invertebrate neurosecretion. In W. BARGMANN AND B. SCHARRER (Eds.), *Aspects of Neuroendocrinology*. Springer, Berlin, pp. 1–23.

SCHARRER, E. (1965) The final common path in neuroendocrine integration. *Arch. Anat. micr. Morph. exp.*, **54** 359–370.

SCHARRER, E. (1966) Principles of neuroendocrine integration. In *Endocrines and the Central Nervous System*, *Res. Publ. Ass. nerv. ment. Dis.*, **43**, 1–35.

SCHARRER, E. AND SCHARRER, B. (1963) *Neuroendocrinology*, Columbia Univ. Press, New York.

SCHNEIDER, H. P. G. AND McCANN, S. M. (1970) Dopaminergic pathways and gonadotropin releasing factors. In *Aspects of Neuroendocrinology*, W. BARGMANN AND B. SCHARRER (Eds.), Springer, Berlin, pp. 177–191.

SCOTT, D. E. AND KNIGGE, K. M. (1970) Ultrastructural changes in the median eminence of the rat following deafferentation of the basal hypothalamus. *Z. Zellforsch.*, **105**, 1–32.

SHARP, P. J. AND FOLLETT, B. K. (1970) The adrenergic supply within the avian hypothalamus. In *Aspects of Neuroendocrinology*, W. BARGMANN AND B. SCHARRER (Eds.), Springer, Berlin, pp. 95–103.

SHORR, S. S. AND BLOOM, F. E. (1970) Fine structure of islet-cell innervation in the pancreas of normal and alloxan-treated rats. *Z. Zellforsch.*, **103**, 12–25.

STOECKEL, M. E. ET PORTE, A. (1967) Sur l'ultrastructure des corps ultimobranchiaux du Poussin. *C.R. Acad. Sci. (Paris)*, Série D, **265**, 2051–2053.

TJÄLVE, H. (1971) Catechol- and indolamines in some endocrine cell systems. An autoradiographical, histochemical and radioimmunological study. *Acta physiol. scand.*, Suppl., **360**, p. 1–22.

TJÄLVE, H. AND SLANINA, P. (1971) Uptake of DOPA and 5-HTP in pancreatic islets and parafollicular cells studied by combined autoradiographic and fluorescence microscopic techniques. *Z. Zellforsch.*, **113**, 83–93.

UNSICKER, K. (1969) Zur Innervation der Nebennierenrinde vom Goldhamster. Eine fluoreszenz- und elektronenmikroskopische Studie. *Z. Zellforsch.*, **95**, 608–619.

UNSICKER, K. (1970) Zur Innervation der interstitiellen Drüse im Ovar der Maus (*Mus musculus* L.). Eine fluoreszenz- und elektronenmikroskopische Studie. *Z. Zellforsch.*, **109**, 46–54.

VOLLRATH, L. (1967) Über die neurosekretorische Innervation der Adenohypophyse von Teleostiern, insbesondere von *Hippocampus cuda* und *Tinca tinca*. *Z. Zellforsch.*, **78**, 234–260.

VULLINGS, H. G. B. (1971) Influence of light and darkness on the hypothalamo-hypophysial system of *Rana temporia* L. *Z. Zellforsch.*, **113**, 174–187.

WATARI, N. (1968) Fine structure of nervous elements in the pancreas of some vertebrates. *Z. Zellforsch.*, **85**, 291–314.

WEITZMAN, M. (Ed.) (1964–72) *Bibliographia Neuroendocrinologica, Vols. 1–9*. Albert Einstein College of Medicine, New York.

YOUNG, B. A. AND HARRISON, R. J. (1969) Ultrastructure of light cells in the dolphin thyroid. *Z. Zellforsch.*, **96**, 222–228.

DISCUSSION

SMELIK. I want to raise a puzzling question about the content of the nerve endings in the hypothalamus. I think that it is very difficult to say whether a neuron can possibly produce a peptide and a biogenic amine at the same time. We know that there are different types of granules in the nerve endings, big ones and small ones. This has been much discussed in the literature. I was very much impressed by your slides from insects, because I think that it appeared clearly that the small vesicles originate by fragmentation from big ones. I would like to ask whether you also observed this type of arrangement of vesicles in the posterior lobe of the mammalian pituitary. Do you think that it may be possible that various types of vesicles originate from the same source?

SCHARRER: I would in principle agree, at least on those grounds on which we can base our ideas at the moment. I think it is clear that a small vesicle of a certain size, let us say 500Å or so, having in an electronmicrograph a lucent content, is not necessarily the same as another vesicle which looks exactly alike. We do not know anything about the content except for the fact that our methods of preparation do not show any electron density when we fix it. It could be a vesicle which at some time has had a dense content which is probably true for aminergic terminals into which some of the released neurotransmitter is returned after the completion of the synaptic stimulus. I would think that in mammals there is some evidence that some of these small vesicles are derived from larger neurosecretory ones, in the same manner as they seem to be derived in this insect. In his extensive study on rodents Streefkerk showed similar results as the one I have shown. There are other cases in which we are not sure because the vesicles are seen to be very uniform, they look clustered in the way as they are in regular synaptic areas. We cannot be quite sure, but in principle I think this kind of fractionation cannot occur in higher vertebrates as it can in lower invertebrates.

KNOWLES: May I draw your attention to a problem which arises from the last question and also to the problem which you already mentioned, that is the origin of the releasing factors. Guillemin has advanced the theory that the main source would be the arcuate nucleus. Now some of us have just come from a conference in Munich where we have been considering the median eminence. The question of the localization of the releasing factors was one that we paid great attention to. However, this question still remained very much a problem at the end of the meeting. Certainly dopamine seemed to be present in the arcuate nucleus in considerable quantities. At one point the question whether dopamine could be present with the peptides in the same neuron was discussed. Dr. Fuxe believed that releasing factors were not present in the system; he thought that the endings were almost exactly the same as normal aminergic endings and also that the distribution of the releasing factors was not the same as the distribution of dopamine. A number of speakers considered the possibility that there is some intermediate cell between these dopaminergic fibres and the pituitary portal vessels. Porter showed that injection of dopamine itself into the portal vessels had no effect on the pituitary. But intraventricular injection of dopamine had an effect and this was yet another point in favour of some intermediate cell. It still remained an open question whether this intermediate cell lies in the ependyma or could be some other liquor-contacting neuron or an ependymal cell or yet some other neuron.

KAPPERS: Thank you very much Prof. Knowles for this recent information about a very difficult question. May I ask perhaps Prof. Halász to say a few words about this problem.

HALÁSZ: I just would like to comment briefly on terminology. Prof. Scharrer has pointed out that the substances produced by the neurosecretory cells and released into the portal system are neurohormones, but at the same time she favoured as terminology the term "factors". I think that in this case we should call these substances hormones.

SCHARRER: I hope I did not introduce an element of confusion, but what I meant was, considering mammals, that if it is true that neurosecretory neurones release mediators into the portal system which we call factors, then these products qualify as hormones and I want to call them hypophyseotropic hormones. However, if we go down in the phylogenetic scale, fishes and amphibians have the same hypophyseotropic mediators but they happen not to go into the blood stream. Then the term "factor" becomes a more generally applicable one. First of all I have no authority to determine the use of this term, but I think the term "factor" has been used for a very long time and in the sense that it allows for nonportal-system systems it is perhaps at the moment a more desirable one. We can still say that in the mammals these mediators have the nature of hormones.

GANONG: About the question of the secretion of the vesicles in peptidergic neurones Dr. Douglas has published interesting and rather good evidence that the peptidergic neurones in mammals can be secreted by exocytosis. He raised the possibility that these clear vesicles were simply the remains of the excess membrane which must be involved if exocytosis takes place. I would like to hear the comments on this question from Prof. Scharrer.

SCHARRER: I fully agree with this, Dr. Ganong. Excess membranous components of such granules in preterminal areas which have something to do with the production, sequestration and release of the mediators we are talking about have to be somehow either reincorporated or reused or in some way got rid of. This could apply to exocytocis systems and could happen in two ways. An exocytotic kind of release mechanism leaves an opening between a vesicle and the cell membrane and thus there will be some excess membrane. So this could be vesiculated and could then appear in little clusters. I have in my material evidence of a neurosecretory granule, a wide extra-granular space halo and a set of vesicles intracellularly, which indicates that perhaps in some systems this fractionation or rearrangement of membranous material occurs not at the cell surface but already intracellularly. I also think that a number of recent studies including those of Norman in Kopenhagen on insects indicate that exocytocis may occur on stimulation and that gradual release may already be in the beginning intracellularly and maybe more of a seeping out. There is no need for making the one or the other system exclusive. In either case the extra membrane, the surface membrane, might make its appearance as a group of small vesicles that simply come to pass by as membranes have a tendency to do.

KAPPERS: May I ask you one question. Does this membrane disappear later on?

SCHARRER: Yes, you have to look at the stages.

KAPPERS: This looks very familiar to me because in the pineal organ the same happens.

SCHARRER: Right.

SMITH: In the formal classical definition of a hormone this is a compound that must circulate in the blood stream. There is ample evidence that in fetal endocrinology this may not be so. There is experimental evidence very definitely showing this, and I think there is a danger in adhering too closely to the classical definition of the hormone following which this is an active agent that must circulate in the bloodstream in order to be effective. I have also a semantic question to you and to the neurophysiologists. Is it entirely justified to use the term target organ for the effector organ of a hormone? This term has been used so long that I don't think we could get away from it. But early in the science of endocrinology there has been some discussion whether there are target organs for hormones. Most hormones affect every cell in the body. But there are special receptors with which hormones act in a special way. Those receptor cells have to be called the target organs. May I ask your opinion on that?

SCHARRER: I did not call them target organs but effector cells. I fully agree with you, but I would like to draw a simple analogy. When a particular person is called in a public address system everybody hears it, but only one person goes to the telephone and answers it. In other words, the specificity is in the receptor. I am not using the term target, but rather effector cell or effector organ. In fetal endocrinology there may be a problem; is the pathway by which the hormones reach the effector cells comparable to that in insects in which there is no circulation system, but a hemolymph-blood space? In your fetal material what would you consider as the pathway for the hormone?

SMITH: In our experiments we are using organcultures, thus the situation is completely different from the one in the normal rat.

BERN: Can I make a comment on both things that just have been discussed? The first is that we have the term diffusion of a hormone still with us. Obviously this is only an elementary biological problem. How much diffusion do you believe to allow before we eliminate the word hormone? This again is a matter of distance between the source of the factor and the effector itself. So this is a terminological problem. It does not worry me and it does not worry you.

Then I want to make a point about small vesicles. A year ago I understood that Douglas also pointed out the probability that many of these lucent vesicles could arise as a result of endocrine activity after the secretory process had occurred. Since there is an awful lot of stuff that is going to be released at the axon ending as a result of whatever process release occurs by, the possibility of these vesicles being taken off very promptly by these nerve endings should not be overlooked.

Basic Electrophysiological Mechanisms in Neuroendocrinology

J. P. SCHADÉ AND H. VAN WILGENBURG

Central Institute for Brain Research, Amsterdam (The Netherlands)

INTRODUCTION

Progress in neurophysiology has resulted, in the past decade, in the development of a model which explains the functional characteristics of neurons at the cellular level. A generally accepted hypothesis holds that at the input site both excitatory and inhibitory neurotransmitters influence the polarization state of the membrane, and that, at the output site, a release of a neurotransmitter takes place after depolarization of the neuron. The communication between the input and output part of the neuron is accomplished by trains of action potentials.

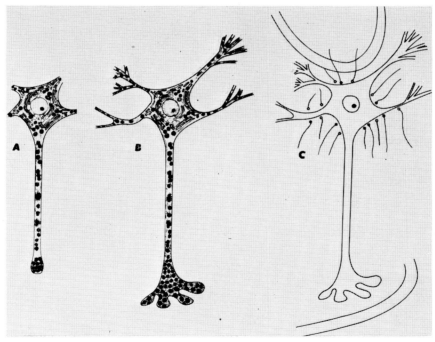

Fig. 1. A, Original diagram of E. Scharrer (1967), depicting the neuroendocrine integration unit. B, The diagram is extended with a large receptive surface, and a number of branches of the transmitting part. C, At the receptive surface information is transferred from excitatory and inhibitory synapses and from blood-borne substances. At the transmitting part the information is transferred to the blood stream.

References p. 28

From a system-analytical point of view, a generalized neuron possesses three parts that are involved in the transfer of information: a receptive part transducing signals from presynaptic endings, a conductive part transmitting action potentials, and a transmitting part releasing neurotransmitters. In order to establish a complete picture of a neuron as an information processing system one has to know the transfer functions of all these parts. This whole process may be called *transinformation*. Of the many topics dominating the current interest in the relationship between the nervous system and endocrine glands, one deals with the electrical properties of neuro-endocrine cells.

As a starting point for our discussion we will pursue a remark made by E. Scharrer in 1967: "Having established as a prerequisite the occurrence of hormone-sensitive and hormone-secreting nerve cells, we may now proceed with the formulation of some general principles governing the relationship between the endocrine and nervous system." (Fig. 1.)

It is not our intention to discuss all the literature on the electrical characteristics of neuroendocrine elements in both vertebrates and invertebrates. We will provide, however, some background information for the papers by Findlay and Hayward (see pages 163–189 and 145–161). In doing so we will draw up a model of a generalized neuroendocrine cell which may serve as a basis for further discussion.

Abundant evidence indicates that neuroendocrine cells in the central nervous system of vertebrates can be influenced both by neurotransmitters released from presynaptic terminals and by blood-borne substances. Effects from substances in the cerebrospinal fluid will here not be taken into account. The input signals resemble the input of a neuron in that they respond to excitatory and inhibitory neurotransmitters. The output of a generalized neuroendocrine cell is similar to the output of a true endocrine cell, in that it emits coded chemical messages that are delivered to all cells in the body, but provide information to only a relatively small population of receptor cells. The neuroendocrine cell is a part of a communication system that utilizes the circulation to transmit signals. By way of the circulation these cells are also influenced by substances like hormones. In order to function properly in a neuroendocrine communication system, these elements should be able to convert neuronal and hormonal signals into electrical potential changes—a process being accomplished by the receptive pole of the neuroendocrine element. At the output site a reverse action should take place: the electrical potentials must act as an intermediary link in the release of a hormone.

For didactic purposes the sequence of the discussion is as follows: *conductive part*, *transmitting part* and *receptive pole*.

Conductive part of a generalized neuroendocrine cell

A major step forward in elucidating the characteristics of axons of neuroendocrine cells has been made by Kandel (1964). Using intracellular recordings this author investigated the electrical properties of neurons in the goldfish hypothalamus. The magnocellular portion of the preoptic nucleus is made up exclusively of neuro-

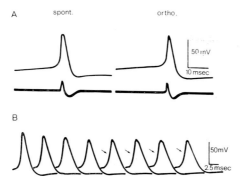

Fig. 2. Diagrams of Kandel (1964) depicting the various aspects of spike potentials in goldfish hypothalamic neuroendocrine cells. AB spikes with orthodromic, spontaneous, and direct stimulation. Part A, Spontaneous and orthodromic action potentials and their simultaneously recorded first derivatives (time constant of differentiating circuit 1 μsec). Note absence of AB inflection even in differentiated responses. Part B, Train of directly initiated spikes. Latency to the first spike: 10 msec. Interspike intervals, which have been omitted, are 52, 62, 105, 82, 89, 95, and 89 msec, respectively. Note the accentuation of the AB inflection in later members of the burst (indicated by arrows).

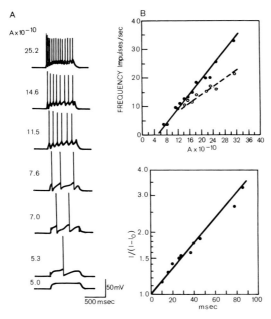

Fig. 3. Illustration of Kandel (1964) showing various aspects of the goldfish neuroendocrine cell upon direct stimulation. Part A, Patterns of response to progressively increasing direct current stimulation. The intensity of the current used is indicated to the left of the figures. Part B, The upper graph, is a plot of the reciprocal interval for the first two spikes (closed circles) and for steady-state firing (open circles) as a function of current intensity. The lower graph is a strength latency curve on a semilog scale. Both graphs are based on the experiment indicated in part A.

References p. 28

endocrine cells. An electrophysiological method of identification was afforded by antidromic activation of the impaled cell following stimulation of the pituitary gland. This method also permitted a measurement of the conduction velocity of the axons of the neuroendocrine elements.

An average conduction velocity of 0.46 m/sec was found which indicates that these axons belong to the class of C-fibres. These data are similar to the values of 0.5 m/sec obtained by Potter and Loewenstein (1955) for axons in the pituitary stalk of another teleost, *Lophius* (Figs. 2 and 3).

More than 60% of the cells in the preoptic nucleus could be activated antidromically. It seems reasonable to assume that a failure of preoptic cells to be activated by pituitary stimulation may be due to the impossibility of reaching sufficient depolarization levels of the axonal membranes or to the fact that not all preoptic cells send axons to the pituitary. Due to lack of sufficient histological data the latter assumption cannot be proved.

Recently, similar experiments were performed on the dog brain (Yamashita and Koizumi, 1971). These investigators recorded antidromic and orthodromic potentials from neurosecretory cells in the supraoptic nucleus. The neurons were identified by antidromic stimulation of the posterior pituitary. Of particular significance is the observation that both IS and SD spikes could be recorded, indicating that the mechanism of spike generation in these cells is identical to other neurons in the central nervous system.

The next point concerns the firing rate of neuroendocrine cells. Cells in the supraoptic and paraventricular nuclei and other hypothalamic areas in mammals tend to discharge rather slowly. The data in the literature reveal that the majority of neurons recorded have mean firing rates of under 10/sec. When the cells are excited by electrical or other stimuli the rate rarely exceeds 50/sec. In Table I a number of data are listed, but it is not justifiable to draw conclusions from the results of different investigators in firing rates, since in particular anesthetics have a significant effect on the firing pattern of neuroendocrine cells.

TABLE I

DATA ASSEMBLED BY CROSS AND SILVER (1966) ON THE
ELECTRICAL PROPERTIES OF CAT HYPOTHALAMIC UNITS

Anesthetic	Hypothalamic recording site	Frequency (spikes/sec)
urethane	anterior area	3.7– 27
pentobarbitone	supraoptic area	1 – 16
urethane	anterior and preoptic areas	<0.1–<50
chloralose	supraoptic area	0.1– 5
ether	ventromedial area	2 – 7
ether	lateral area	8 – 20

Spontaneous activity of the cells is usually first observed, but a full description of the activity of a neuron or neuroendocrine cell involves more than simply its mean firing rate. The interspike interval is one of the methods which may be used to characterize the details of the firing pattern. Few reports published provide information on the statistical analysis of firing patterns, so one is left in the dark as far as the information capacity of these cells is concerned. Oomura *et al.* (1969) fit their interspike interval data for cells in the ventromedial and lateral hypothalamus of the cat to Poisson and Gaussian distributions. On the basis of their results these authors suggest that hypothalamic neurons process very precise information. Our own data point to the same conclusion. During the course of an investigation on the electrophysiological concomitants of experimental atherosclerosis in rabbits, recordings were made of spontaneously firing neurons in various brain areas (van Emde Boas *et al.*, 1971; Schadé *et al.*, 1971). In general, the mean firing rate of hypothalamic neurons was rather low and the interspike interval distribution could be characterized by a high gamma-parameter. These results indicate that the spike trains transmit a rather simplified pattern of signals. These patterns may serve to transfer a specific relationship between input and output of the system.

The transmitting part

The transmitting part of the neuroendocrine cell has been subject to various kinds of electrical investigations. Most of the studies reported in the literature deal with the analysis of the relationship between the electrical activity in supraoptic and paraventricular neurons and the release of vasopressin and oxytocin. The so-called stimulus–secretion coupling hypothesis proposes that hormone release is initiated by a depolarization of the membrane of the neuroendocrine cell. In addition there should be a relationship between the number of action potentials conducted by the axons in a certain time span and the amount of hormone released. Dyball and Dyer (1971) compared the firing rate of identified rat paraventricular neurons and the plasma oxytocin concentration. Their results are consistent with the abovementioned hypothesis that an increase in firing rate is associated with oxytocin release from the posterior pituitary. In addition it was found that the hormone had no direct effect upon the electrical properties of the paraventricular neurons.

Characteristics of the receptive pole of neuroendocrine cells

Since it is obvious from the analysis of the conducting part of the neuroendocrine cells that these neurons exhibit regular electrical properties, a main question arises regarding the transducing features of the receptive pole. In general, neurons in the central nervous system of vertebrates are sensitive to at least two types of neurotransmitters, but are rather insensitive to blood-borne substances. Only major shifts in the concentration of electrolytes, *e.g.*, potassium, or amino acids, *e.g.*, glutamate, effect the polarization state of the neuronal membrane. The issue to discuss then concerns the mechanisms by which the receptive pole transduces the synaptic inputs and the blood-borne hormones. The questions are: do we have to account for an interaction of the two classes of substances; are the receptor mechanisms the same or different; should hormones, as far as the postsynaptic neuronal surface is concerned, be regarded as neurotransmitters?

Apparently, the receptive pole is able to respond to widely different substances which, after influencing the postsynaptic receptors, produce significant changes in the ionic permeability. These latter changes then generate synaptic potentials as a second step in the initiation of spike trains.

It is still unknown how blood-borne hormones affect the brain at the cellular level. Our knowledge in this field has recently been advanced by Ruf and Steiner (1967a, b), Steiner and coworkers (1968, 1969) and by York *et al.* (1971) who iontophoretically applied hormonal substances, *e.g.*, dexamethasone and ACTH, to the surface of cerebral neurons in the rat. They showed very elegantly the existence of steroid-sensitive neurons in the hypothalamus and midbrain reticular formation. Of 337 individual hypothalamic and mesencephalic neurons, only 57 showed a decrease or an increase in firing rate upon application of minute amounts of dexamethasone to the neuronal membrane. On the basis of these and other data, we suggest the presence of aggregates of neurons in the hypothalamus constituting a so-called steroidstat (Schadé, 1970). From a system-analytical point of view it seems likely to assume that the elements of the steroidstat can be divided into steroid-minus and steroid-plus sensors. The steroid-minus sensors show a decrease in firing rate upon application of dexamethasone, while the steroid-plus sensors exhibit an opposite effect.

In the rat brain the steroid-minus sensors exceed in number the plus sensors by far. The steroid sensitive neurons are scattered over a wide area in the hypothalamus. As far as other localizations of steroid sensors are concerned, no neurons in the cerebral cortex, dorsal hippocampus, or thalamus were found to respond to dexamethasone. Steroid-sensitive neurons were also exposed to the action of neurotransmitters in order to mimic the activity of excitatory and inhibitory presynaptic terminals upon the membrane of the steroid sensors. In general, acetylcholine increased the firing rate, while noradrenaline and dopamine decreased the basic activity of the neurons (Steiner *et al.*, 1968). Thus a dual sensitivity was observed, both to blood-borne substances and to regular neurotransmitters acting via presynaptic endings.

Backer *et al.* (1971) succeeded in recording the responsiveness of individual supra-optic neurons (decerebrate cat preparations) to direct iontophoretic application of catecholamines and acetylcholine. A stimulating electrode was placed in the posterior lobe of the pituitary for the purpose of antidromically identifying the supraoptic neurons. These authors confirmed the responsiveness to noradrenaline and acetyl-choline, as reported by other workers (*cf.* Steiner, 1971). Noradrenaline depressed the firing rate of 90% of the cells studied, while all others were unresponsive. Acetyl-choline did not show such a uniform response pattern. Both excitation and depression were observed. About 30% of the neurons showed no response at all to acetylcholine. The dual nature of the cholinergic response suggests the presence of two types of receptors. By using cholinergic agonists and antagonists, a differentiation could be made into muscarinic and nicotinic receptors.

The data of Steiner *et al.* (1969) and Backer *et al.* (1971) support the notion of the presence of two functionally distinct classes of receptors. In this respect the neuro-endocrine cells behave like ordinary neurons. In addition, the receptive pole shows a specific responsiveness to at least one blood-borne substance of high molecular weight.

Since no data are available on the interaction between the two classes of substances,

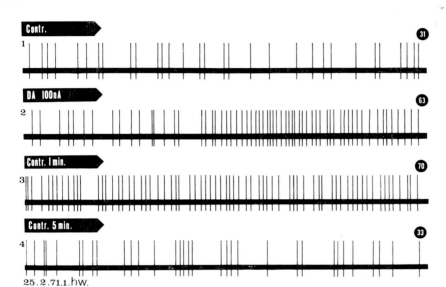

Fig. 4. Recording with a multibarrelled microelectrode from a neuron in the parietal ganglion of *Helix pomatia*. Iontophoretic application of dopamine (DA). nA, nanoamperes. The length of each record is equivalent to 1 min.

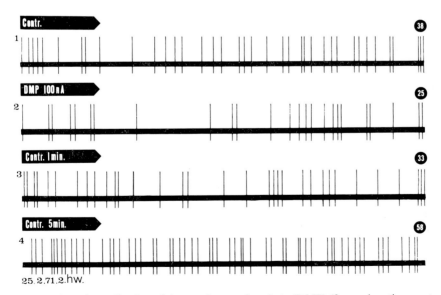

Fig. 5. Iontophoretic application of dexamethasonephosphate (DMP) (for explanation see text).

References p. 28

a search was made for a simplified model which would allow us to study these mechanisms simultaneously. The snail *(Helix pomatia)* provides a useful model, because neurons and neurosecretory cells have been shown to respond to iontophoretically applied neurotransmitters (van Wilgenburg, 1970).

Some preliminary results on the interaction of neurotransmitters and a steroid will be reported.

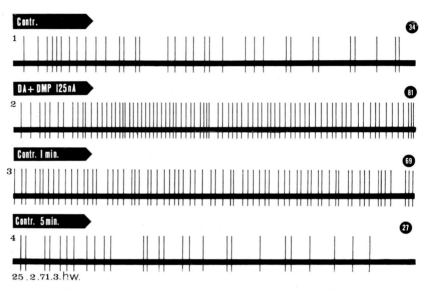

Fig. 6. Response of a neuron to the simultaneous application of dopamine (DA) and dexamethasone-phosphate (DMP).

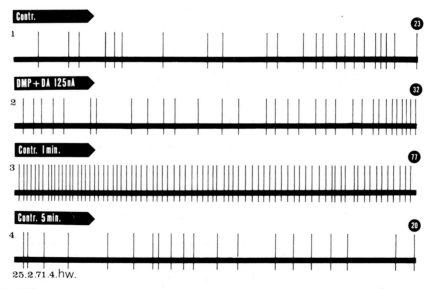

Fig. 7. Different response to the iontophoretic application of dopamine (DA) and dexamethasone-phosphate (DMP) (for explanation see text).

Figs. 4 and 6 show the difference between dopamine and dexamethasone on the firing rate of a snail neuron in the parietal ganglion. After 20 to 30 sec, a marked increase in firing rate is observed upon iontophoretic application of dopamine (Fig. 4). The effect may still be seen 1–2 min after cessation of the dopamine application, but 5 min after the onset of the experiment, a normal firing pattern is observed. In Fig. 5 a different response pattern is shown. Upon application of dexamethasone, initially a slight increase in firing rate is observed. A considerable time after the initial application an excitatory effect upon the firing rate is noted. Apparently, the substance has first to penetrate the neuronal membrane before an effect upon the membrane polarization state is accomplished. An additive effect is seen in Fig. 6, where the two substances have been applied simultaneously. The influence of dexamethasone apparently depends on the background level of synaptic inputs. In Fig. 7, the background level is considerably lower than in Fig. 6, resulting in a delayed increase in the firing rate.

DISCUSSION

These and other experiments lend support to the postulate that steroids do not act like neurotransmitters as far as a specific action on receptors is concerned. Probably one of the ionic pump mechanisms, such as ATP-ase activity, is effected, and thus, indirectly, the polarization state of the membrane will be affected.

Perhaps the most characteristic difference between the transmission of signals by neurotransmitters and by hormones lies in the specific molecular properties of the mechanisms which regulate the membrane potential. Among other things, the neurotransmitters alter the permeability for either sodium or potassium ions while the hormones seem to alter the regulatory mechanism of the membrane pump, probably by increasing or decreasing the speed of one of the systems involved in the synthesis of cyclic AMP or ATP-ase. In this way, a slow alteration in the polarization state of the neuronal membrane is achieved. This alteration in itself will not cause the generation of action potentials along the membrane, but if sufficient background synaptic activity is present, a considerable decrease or increase of the firing rate will occur. Neurotransmitters act via specific receptors of the postsynaptic surface of the neuroendocrine transducers, but the circulating hormones act in a more dynamic way. Any major alteration of the concentration of a circulating hormone will, depending on the product released by the neuroendocrine transducer, activate or slow down the pump mechanism of the membrane. Thus, either a great many more impinging sub-threshold stimuli will reach threshold value, or the resting value of the membrane is raised in such a way that considerably fewer action potentials are being generated. This mechanism seems to act as a modulator of membrane activity. In the absence of synaptic background activity the effect of a membrane modulator is nil, but with sufficient excitatory synaptic potentials a major influence is exerted on the generation of action potentials, and thus on the output of the system.

Oomura and coworkers (1971) have investigated a similar system in the rat hypothalamus. They arrived at an almost identical conclusion. Glucoreceptor neurons in the ventromedial and lateral hypothalamic areas respond to changes in blood glucose. A series of experiments was conducted to determine whether actual penetration of glucose through the receptor membrane or specific binding of glucose to the receptor membrane is essential to influence the polarization state of the neuron. For this purpose the authors mentioned studied the combined effects of glucose, glucose and insulin, and several glucose analogues. The firing rate of glucoreceptive neurons increased significantly when glucose and insulin were applied simultaneously, but no change was found upon application of insulin alone. Several glucose analogues had no effect at all. When a glucose analogue and insulin were applied simultaneously, the firing rate decreased. They concluded that glucose had to be incorporated into the cell through the receptor membrane in order to effect the polarization state of the membrane and so the firing level. No mention is made of the intraneuronal mechanism responsible for this effect.

The postulate of an involvement of cyclic AMP in the transducing properties of the neuronal membrane is also supported by studies of Siggins *et al.* (1971) on the response pattern of cerebellar Purkinje cells. Iontophoretic application of noradrenaline and cyclic AMP decreased the firing rate of rat Purkinje cells. Noradrenaline inhibition was brought about by hyperpolarization of the neuronal membrane and this effect is postsynaptically mediated by cyclic AMP. An enhanced formation of cyclic AMP was shown to occur in cerebellar slices treated with noradrenaline. These results imply operation of a metabolically dependent postsynaptic response in the cerebellum.

These results and our own data indicate that neurotransmitters and blood-borne substances probably interact at the receptive pole of neuroendocrine cells. The elucidation of this intriguing mechanism needs further investigation.

REFERENCES

BACKER, J. L., CRAYTON, J. W. AND NICOLL, R. A. (1971) Supraoptic neurosecretory cells: adrenergic and cholinergic sensitivity. *Science*, **171**, 208–210.

CROSS, B. A. AND SILVER, I. A. (1966) Electrophysiological studies on hypothalamus. *Brit. med. Bull.*, **22**, 254–260.

DYBALL, R. E. J. AND DYER, R. G. (1971) Plasma oxytocin concentration and paraventricular neurone activity in rats with diencephalic islands and intact brains. *J. Physiol. (Lond.)*, **216**, 227–235.

EMDE BOAS, W. VAN, SCHADÉ, J. P., CRANENBURGH, B. VAN AND SMITH, J. (1971) Neuronal spike trains in experimental atherosclerosis. *Proc. int. Congr. physiol. Sci.*, Munich, 578.

KANDEL, E. R. (1964) Electrical properties of hypothalamic neuroendocrine cells. *J. gen. Physiol.*, **47**, 691–717.

OOMURA, Y., ONO, T., SUGIMORI, M., NAKAMURA, T., GAWRONSKI, D. AND OOYAMA, H. (1971) Characteristics of the chemoreceptor neuron in the rat hypothalamus. *Proc. int. Congr. physiol. Sci.*, Munich, 432.

OOMURA, Y., OOYAMA, H., NAKA, F., YAMAMOTA, T., ONO, T. AND KOBAYASHI, T. (1969) Some stochastical patterns of single unit discharges in the cat hypothalamus under chronic conditions. *Ann. N. Y. Acad. Sci.*, **157**, 666–689.

POTTER, D. D. AND LOEWENSTEIN, W. R. (1955) Electrical activity of neurosecretory cells. *Amer. J. Physiol.*, **183**, 652–655.

RUF, K. AND STEINER, F. A. (1967a) Steroid-sensitive single neurons in rat hypothalamus and midbrain: identification by microelectrophoresis. *Science*, **156**, 667–669.

RUF, K. AND STEINER, F. A. (1967b) Feedback regulation of ACTH secretion: suppression of single neurons in rat brain by dexamethasone microelectrophoresis. *Acta endocr. (Kbh.)*, Suppl. 199, 38.

SCHADÉ, J. P. (1970) A system analysis of some hypothalamic functions. In *The Hypothalamus*, L. MARTINI, M. MOTTA AND F. FRASCHINI (Eds.), Academic Press, New York, pp. 69–82.

SCHADÉ, J. P., CRANENBURGH, B. VAN, EMDE BOAS, W. VAN AND SMITH, J. (1971) Neuronal firing patterns in various brain areas. *Proc. int. Congr. physiol. Sci.*, Munich, 495.

SCHARRER, E. (1967) Principles of neuroendocrine integration. *Res. Publ. Ass. nerv. ment. Dis.*, **43**, 1–35.

SIGGINS, G. R., OLIVER, A. P., HOFFER, B. J. AND BLOOM, F. E. (1971) Cyclic adenosine monophosphate and norepinephrine: effects on transmembrane properties of cerebellar Purkinje cells. *Science*, **171**, 192–194.

STEINER, F. A. (1971) *Neurotransmitter und Neuromodulatoren*. Thieme, Stuttgart.

STEINER, F. A., PIERI, L. AND KAUFMANN, L. (1968) Effects of dopamine and ACTH on steroid sensitive single neurones in the basal hypothalamus. *Experientia (Basel)*, **24**, 1133.

STEINER, F. A., RUF, K. AND AKERT, K. (1969) Steroid-sensitive neurones in rat brain: anatomical localization and responses to neurohumours and ACTH. *Brain Research*, **12**, 74–85.

YAMASHITA, H. and KOIZUMI, K. (1971) Study of neurosecretory neurons in supraoptic nuclei of dogs by intracellular recording. *Proc. int. Congr. physiol. Sci.*, 612.

YORK, D. H., BAKER, F. L. AND KRAICER, J. (1971) Transmembrane potentials of adenohypophyseal cells *in vivo*, after injection of hypothalamic releasing factors. *Proc. int. Congr. physiol. Sci.*, Munich, 614.

WILGENBURG, H. VAN (1970) *An Electrophysiological Analysis of Neurons in the Visceral and Parietal Ganglia of Helix pomatia*. Thesis, Free University, Amsterdam.

DISCUSSION

BERN: I believe that you have a nice model for testing steroid sensitivity, since the hormonal characteristics of invertebrate neurons are far easier to investigate than the central neurons of vertebrates. I would like to ask three questions.

1. Does it make any difference in applying steroid to neurosecretory cells or to neurons?
2. Does dexamethasonephosphate or cortisone circulate in the snail?
3. Is there any difference as far as spike duration is concerned in steroid sensitive neurons in invertebrates and vertebrates?

SCHADÉ: We applied iontophoretically dexamethasonephosphate to all kinds of cellular elements in the nervous system of snails. Neurosecretory cells can be recognized electrically by the long duration of the action potentials and by a slow firing rate. Steroid sensitivity occurs mainly in neurosecretory cells. As far as your second question is concerned; there are no data in the literature on the content of dexamethasonephosphate or cortisone in snails, however, the presence of corticosteroids has been demonstrated in the slug *Ariolimax*.

A significant difference exists between neurosecretory cells in vertebrates and invertebrates as fas as the electrical properties are concerned; the average spike duration of hypothalamic neuroendocrine cells in the goldfish amounts to about 3.5 msec, while the spike duration for neurosecretory cells in the snail is about 10–20 msec.

HAYWARD: In your generalized schema you restrict the receptive field to the cell body and its dendrites; does that mean that you exclude axo-axonal contacts?

SCHADÉ: Generally the receptive pole of an integrating neuron is comprised of the cell body and its dendrites. The transinformation properties of such a system are determined by the receptive, the conductive and the transmitting part of the integrating neuron. In order to draw up a transfer function of a generalized integrating neuron one has to deal with the neuronal and hormonal influences upon the three parts. Although we realize that axo-axonal contacts have been shown to be present in some vertebrates, the evidence for the snail nervous system is still circumstantial. Therefore we felt justified to leave out the axo-axonal contacts.

SLOPER: I would like to ask a question related to the possibility of recurrent collaterals. If I remember correctly Kandel showed the presence of inhibitory responses which he interpreted as antidromically conducted. The anatomical evidence was derived from silver-impregnation studies. Do you believe that the recurrent collateral hypothesis holds good for all types of neuroendocrine cells?

SCHADÉ: Kandel produced IPSP's by volleys which were subthreshold for the production of the antidromic action potential of the impaled neurons. The antidromic invasion of neuroendocrine cells in the hypothalamus of goldfish could only be obtained if the exposed tips of the microstimulating electrodes were in the sella turcica. The finding that the IPSP could be produced with stimuli which were below threshold for some of the neurohypophysial tract fibres makes the alternative of an intra-hypothalamic pathway unlikely. The results are therefore consistent with a recurrent collateral system. The situation in the snail nervous system is quite different. Up till now we have no firm evidence of a similar system in the visceral and parietal ganglion of the snail nervous system.

KNOWLES: Would it be possible that the neurohypophysial tract contains two types of fibres?

SCHADÉ: I think about 60% of the cells encountered in the preoptic nucleus could be activated anti-dromically. However, all cells in the nucleus, even those which could not be activated antidromically, showed otherwise identical properties which differed significantly from elements in the surrounding structures. Failure of certain preoptic cells to be activated by pituitary stimuli may perhaps be attributable to two factors: (a) the goldfish pituitary is quite large and the stimulating electrode may not always have been optimally placed for the activation of all axons; (b) not all preoptic cells send axons to the pituitary.

These findings leave open the possibility that the neurohypophysial tract is made up of two fiber systems.

KNOWLES: I have a comment about the axo-axonal contact. Certainly in the mammalian median eminence there are no normal axo-axonal contacts, that means with normal pre- and postsynaptic membrane specialisations.

STOECKART: Petersen described axo-axonal contacts in the supraoptic nucleus in the rat. In his pictures one can clearly distinguish axo-axonal contacts around the axon hillock.

SCHADÉ: Axo-axonal contacts in the nucleus itself can easily be included in the model of the generalized integrating neuron. The only problem we have regards the axo-axonal contact at the terminals of the axon of the integrating neuron, since the terminals are not involved in synaptic transmission, but in the release of a hormonal product.

BERN: I would like to make a comment about what I thought was Dr. Sloper's statement on different populations of fibres in a physiological sense, which might comprise the neurohypophysial tract. If one records single unit activity from the elements of the caudal neurosecretory system, one finds often long duration action potentials. The majority of the fibres show short duration action potentials, which may indicate the presence of two fibre systems.

SCHARRER: The results of Barker and co-workers indicate that the receptive pole of the neurosecretory cells may be influenced by various types of neurotransmitters, as has been put forward by Dr. Schadé for his model. I find it hard to believe that the axons are doing something else than conducting action potentials which may lead to the release of a hormone. So I would like to go along with the model.

BERN: Certainly, the nervous system contains many secrets.

The Isolated Neurohypophysis, a Model for Studies on Neuroendocrine Release Mechanisms

J. J. DREIFUSS, J. D. GRAU, J. J. LEGROS AND J. J. NORDMANN

Département de Physiologie de l'Université, Ecole de Médicine, 1211 Genève 4 (Suisse), and Laboratoire de Radioimmunologie, Institut de Médecine de l'Université, Liège (Belgique)

INTRODUCTION

It is now well established that neuroendocrine cells generate propagated action potentials as do conventional neurones. Thus the cell bodies in the hypothalamic

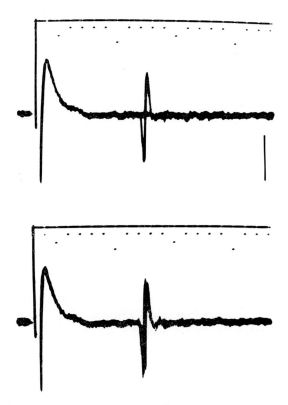

Fig. 1. Superimposed oscilloscope traces of extracellular records from a supraoptic neurone in response to stimulation of the pituitary stalk at threshold (upper traces) and at 1.1 times threshold intensity (lower traces). Note the "all-or-none" character of the response. Horizontal calibrations: msec; vertical calibration: 0.5 mV.

References p. 37

supraoptic and paraventricular nuclei, which give rise to the hypothalamo-neuro-hypophysial tract, are antidromically invaded by "all-or-none" action potentials elicited by electrical stimulation of the pituitary stalk (Fig. 1). Moreover, changes in the frequency of discharge of supraoptic and paraventricular neurones have been described in conditions associated with increased hormone release from the neurohypophysis (Brooks *et al.*, 1966; Dyball, 1971).

Much progress in the understanding of neuroendocrine release mechanisms has been made after Douglas' (1963) demonstration that the release of hormones from the nerve endings of the hypothalamo-neurohypophysial tract in the neurohypophysis can be readily studied *in vitro* in a preparation devoid of the parent cell bodies of the axons. It was shown that such isolated neurohypophyses liberate vasopressin on electrical stimulation of the cut end of the pituitary stalk or on exposure of the neural lobe to solutions containing excess potassium. The secretory process is dependent on the presence of external calcium and is inhibited by magnesium (Douglas and Poisner, 1964a). The release is accompanied by calcium uptake by the neurosecretory terminals (Douglas and Poisner, 1964b). Thus, as happens at presynaptic nerve endings, the entry of calcium which results from a decrease of the resting potential of the axon terminals appears to be the key event leading to hormone secretion. Although it is required for the generation and propagation of action potentials, extracellular sodium is not essential for the release process *in vitro*, since hormone secretion can be evoked in sodium-free solutions; rather, secretion evoked by an increase in external potassium seems to become more effective as the concentration of sodium is lowered (Douglas and Poisner, 1964a). We have reinvestigated whether the increase in hormone release evoked by electrical stimulation of the pituitary stalk *in vitro* is actually mediated by propagated action potentials, and have also studied the effect of changes in the sodium and calcium concentration of the incubation medium on secretion from isolated neurohypophyses.

METHODS

Rat neurohypophyses were dissected as described by Douglas and Poisner (1964a), and the neural lobe incised along the sagittal plane. A thread was tied around the cut end of the pituitary stalk, and the preparation was then tied by this thread to a platinum wire, and immersed in a test tube containing 1–2 ml of "Locke solution". The test tube rested in a water bath maintained at 37 °C and the Locke's solution it contained was continuously gassed with 5% CO_2/95% O_2. To stimulate, bipolar electrical pulses generated by a "constant-current" stimulator were applied between the platinum wire carrying the neurohypophysis and a platinum wire coil dipping into the incubation medium. During stimulation, the electrode holding the gland was raised so that only the inferior pole of the neurohypophysis remained in contact with the incubation medium by surface tension (Fig. 2). In other experiments, secretion was evoked by a ten-fold increase in external KCl concentration from 5.6 to 56 mM.

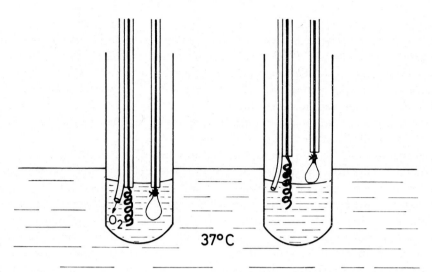

Fig. 2. Schematic drawing of the experimental arrangement used for chemical or electrical stimulation of the isolated neurohypophysis. Stimulation was evoked either by an increase in the KCl concentration in the bathing solution, or by short trains of current pulses applied as shown on the right hand drawing. The supply of gas was interrupted during such electrical stimulation in order to obtain stable conditions, but was restored once the neurohypophysis had been again lowered into the solution for the remainder of the incubation period (10 min).

A milk-ejection assay (Bisset *et al.*, 1967) was used to estimate the hormone content of the incubation media after successive incubation periods of 10 min each. Standards and unknowns were injected through a cannulated jugular vein to lactating rats, and the intra-mammary pressure changes recorded through a transducer. Since oxytocin was approximately four times more potent than equimolar amounts of lysine–vaso-pressin, results are expressed in international units of oxytocin.

Action potentials and hormone release in vitro

Resting hormone release during consecutive incubation periods was $\leqslant 1.5$ mU/neuro-hypophysis/10 min over a period of several hours. In normal Locke solution, electrical stimulation of the pituitary stalk with 1 min trains at 20–100 Hz, of 0.5–1.0 mA intensity, consistently increased hormone output approximately 5-fold (Dreifuss *et al.*, 1971). This increase in secretion was abolished if the incubation medium contained tetrodotoxin at a concentration of 10^{-7} g/ml, which completely suppressed the compound action potential recorded from the neurohypophysis following electrical stimulation of the stalk. Resting release continued however as in controls. As tetrodotoxin interferes selectively with the increase in sodium conductance responsible for the generation of propagated action potentials, the experiment indicates that action potentials may also initiate the release process in isolated neurohypophyses kept *in vitro*.

At presynaptic terminals, tetrodotoxin abolishes all action potentials, but does not reduce the spontaneous release of neurotransmitter, nor the increase in the rate of miniature synaptic potentials observed in response to presynaptic membrane depolarization (Katz and Miledi, 1967). Evidence that the release mechanism remains similarly operational in tetrodotoxin-poisoned neurohypophyses derives from their response to excess potassium. Exposure of the glands to solutions containing 56 mM KCl more than doubled hormone output above resting level, and a further increase in secretion occurred in incubation media containing 20 times the normal KCl concentration, *i.e.*, 112 mM (Dreifuss *et al.*, 1971).

The experimental uncoupling of the release process from the action potential generating mechanism by the use of tetrodotoxin represents yet another parallel between the mechanisms for the release of neurohypophysial hormones on one hand and those for the secretion of neurotransmitters from chemical synapses on the other.

In the above described experiments, the "high-KCl" solutions were hypertonic with respect to normal Locke solution, and no attempt was made to reduce the external NaCl concentration to keep them isotonic, since isolated neurohypophyses incubated in hypertonic media respond to stimulation in a way no different from that observed in mildly isotonic solutions. Actually, hormone release evoked by a standard membrane depolarization was *lower* in the medium kept hypertonic as compared to that observed in solutions in which the external NaCl was reduced for the sake of isotonicity.

Competition between calcium and sodium at neurohypophysial nerve terminals

These results, as well as Douglas and Poisner's (1964a) finding that potassium induced depolarization of neurohypophyses in sodium-free Locke solution leads to enhanced hormone output, raised the possibility that extracellular sodium might compete with extracellular calcium at the level of some cellular sites that trigger secretion, and may thereby partially inactivate the release process, just as has been described for neurotransmitter release at presynaptic nerve endings (Kelly, 1965).

We have therefore studied the hormone output in response to an increase in external potassium from isolated neurohypophyses incubated in sodium deficient solutions in which iso-osmolarity and ionic strength were maintained by the addition of equimolar amounts of choline chloride. Fig. 3 illustrates an experiment in which secretion was evoked by an external KCl concentration of 56 mM at three different NaCl concentrations, the $CaCl_2$ concentration in the incubation media being kept constant at 2.2 mM throughout. It may be readily seen that the standard stimulus is most effective at the lowest NaCl concentration tested (50 mM), and is still more effective at an intermediate (100 mM) than at the normal concentration (150 mM). This graded response was obtained with all possible permutations of the experimental design and qualitatively similar results were observed when NaCl in the medium was partially replaced by LiCl.

These observations could be explained by assuming that both calcium and sodium show an affinity for some common cellular binding sites, but that only the complexes formed with calcium are able to promote release; in media containing a high NaCl concentration, sodium ions might combine with numerous binding sites so as to form

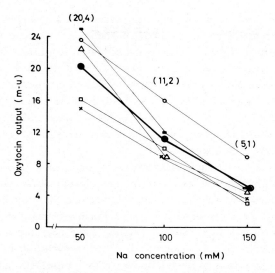

Fig. 3. Hormone output in response to excess KCl (56 mM) in relation to the NaCl concentration in the bathing solution. A total of 5 isolated neurohypophyses were studied each during three 10 min incubation periods in the "high-KCl"-solution at 50, 100 and 150 mM NaCl respectively, according to a random design. Isotonicity was maintained with appropriate amounts of choline chloride. The black dots represent the mean hormone output (value in parenthesis) at each NaCl concentration tested.

inactive complexes. If such an antagonism did exist, hormone release would be expected to depend on the $[Ca^{++}]/[Na^+]^2$ ratio in the incubation solution. In order to test this possibility, experiments were done in which this ratio was either kept constant or deliberately varied in the bathing solution. We found the release of

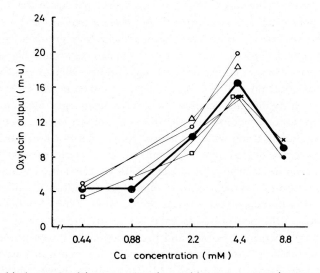

Fig. 4. Relationship between calcium concentration and hormone output in response to excess KCl (56 mM).

hormones increases approximately linearly with the $[Ca^{++}]/[Na^+]^2$ ratio. The fact that the release process depends *indirectly* on the square of the external sodium concentration, whereas the height of the action potential is a direct function of external NaCl, represents further experimental evidence that hormone secretion and the generation of propagated action potentials depend on different ionic conductance changes of the axon membrane. Moreover, since a major part of the currents flowing across the axon terminals in the neurohypophysis are, under normal conditions, carried in all probability by sodium ions, the release mechanism is not fully operational *in vivo* or in standard saline solutions.

Whereas hormone secretion is determined by the $[Ca^{++}]/[Na^+]^2$ ratio over an approximately ten fold range of external calcium concentration (Dreifuss *et al.*, 1971), the relationship does not hold for calcium concentrations much above normal, in keeping with the observation of Douglas and Poisner (1964a) that hormone output decreases in this range (Fig. 4). Similar findings have been reported for neurotransmitter release at presynaptic axon terminals. Thus, Brown and Feldberg (1936) have described that the secretion of acetylcholine from sympathetic ganglia evoked by a rise in external KCl is depressed in the presence of high $CaCl_2$, and Gage and Quastel (1966) have shown that the frequency of miniature endplate potentials in rat diaphragm increases steadily with calcium concentration in the range of 0.3 to 2.0 mM, but diminishes with a further rise in $CaCl_2$.

Release of neurophysins

The nature of the cellular mechanisms involved in hormone secretion from the neurohypophysis following the influx of calcium into the nerve endings has not yet been fully clarified. For a review of recent theories the reader is referred to an article by Thorn (1970). While some authors have suggested that secretion occurs from an extragranular pool, others have proposed that release may occur by exocytosis, *i.e.*, the extrusion of the whole content of the neurosecretory granules (Douglas, 1968). Recently, electron micrographs from neurohypophyses of rats and hamsters have been published that show images consistent with secretion by exocytosis (Nagasawa *et al.*, 1970). If release does indeed occur as a result of collision between neurosecretory granules and axon membrane, leading thereby to temporary membrane fusion and discharge of the granular contents into the pericapillary space, one would expect neurophysins to escape along with the neurohypophysial hormones during secretion.

Neurophysins represent as much as half of the soluble proteins found in the neurosecretory granules (Ginsburg and Ireland, 1966). On density gradient centrifugation, the distribution of oxytocin follows that of neurophysin I, while vasopressin is mainly associated with neurophysin II (Dean and Hope, 1968). Studies on the binding of the hormones to the neurophysins have led to the suggestion that the latter are involved in the intraneuronal storage and transport of the hormones. However, after the introduction of a sensitive radioimmunoassay for neurophysins (Legros *et al.*, 1969; Cheng and Friesen, 1971; Legros, 1971), it has been shown that their level in the blood is elevated in conditions associated with increased neurohypophysial activity in man (Legros *et al.*, 1969) and in experimental animals (Cheng and Friesen, 1970). We have employed the isolated rat neurohypophysis in order to examine the release of hormones and of neurophysins following electrical stimulation *in vitro*. The milk-ejection activity of the incubation media was determined in a rat bioassay (Bisset *et al.*, 1967), and its neurophysin content was estimated by radioimmunoassay.

Preliminary findings indicate that neurophysins and hormones are released in a fixed ratio (Nordmann *et al.*, 1971).

This finding represents necessary—but not yet sufficient—evidence for the contention that polypeptide hormone release may occur by exocytosis. Even more convincing evidence of this type suggests that release of catecholamines from the adrenal medulla occurs in multimolecular packets.

At the level of presynaptic axon terminals there is ample electrophysiological evidence to indicate that neurotransmitter is released in multimolecular "quanta". The axon terminals in the neurohypophysis are not presynaptic terminals in the usual sense, as they form neurovascular junctions and as their secretion product diffuses from the depolarized endings into capillaries and from there reaches distant target organs. However, the isolated neurohypophysis represents a remarkably homogeneous collection of some 10^4–10^5 unmyelinated, small diameter nerve fibres and terminals which share many characteristics with presynaptic nerve endings. We feel that the clustered axons that form the bulk of the neurohypophysis may further contribute to a better understanding of neurosecretion at prejunctional axon endings, as well as represent a useful model for the study of neuroendocrine release processes. Some functional differences must however be kept in mind. Thus, while neural transmitter substances can be synthetized in the axon terminals, synthesis of polypeptide hormones in the hypothalamo-neurohypophysial system takes place apparently in the perikarya only. Moreover, reuptake of the secretion product or of one of its metabolites by the axon terminal through a transport mechanism in the membrane is unlikely to play a major role in replenishing hypothalamic neuroendocrine cells.

ACKNOWLEDGEMENTS

This work was supported by grants from the Swiss National Science Foundation (Nr 5340.3) and the F. Hoffmann-La Roche Foundation. J. J. Legros is a fellow of the Belgian FNRS.

REFERENCES

BISSET, G. W., CLARK, B. J., HALDAR, J., HARRIS, M. C., LEWIS, G. P. AND ROCHA E SILVA, M. (1967) The assay of milk-ejecting activity in the lactating rat. *Brit. J. Pharmacol.*, **31**, 537–549.

BROOKS, C. McC., ISHIKAWA, T., KOIZUMI, K. AND LU, H. H. (1966) Activity of neurones in the paraventricular nucleus of the hypothalamus and its control. *J. Physiol. (Lond.)*, **182**, 217–231.

BROWN, G. L. AND FELDBERG, W. (1936) The action of potassium on the cervical superior ganglion of the cat. *J. Physiol. (Lond.)*, **86**, 290–305.

CHENG, K. W. AND FRIESEN, H. G. (1970) Physiological factors regulating secretion of neurophysin. *Metabolism*, **19**, 876–890.

CHENG, K. W. AND FRIESEN, H. G. (1971) A radioimmunoassay for vasopressin-binding proteins—neurophysin. *Endocrinology*, **88**, 608–619.

DEAN, C. R. AND HOPE, D. B. (1968) The isolation of neurophysin-I and -II from bovine pituitary neurosecretory granules separated on a large scale from other subcellular organelles. *Biochem. J.*, **106**, 565–573.

DOUGLAS, W. W. (1963) A possible mechanism of neurosecretion: release of vasopressin by depolarization and its dependance on calcium. *Nature (Lond.)*, **197**, 81–82.

DOUGLAS, W. W. (1968) Stimulus–secretion coupling: the concept and clues from chromaffin and other cells. *Brit. J. Pharmacol.*, **34**, 451–474.

DOUGLAS, W. W. AND POISNER, A. M. (1964a) Stimulus–secretion coupling in a neurosecretory organ: the role of calcium in the release of vasopressin from the neurohypophysis. *J. Physiol. (Lond.)*, **172**, 1–18.

DOUGLAS, W. W. AND POISNER, A. M. (1964b) Calcium movement in the neurohypophysis of the rat and its relation to the release of vasopressin. *J. Physiol. (Lond.)*, **172**, 19–30.

DREIFUSS, J. J., GRAU, J. D. AND BIANCHI, R. E. (1971) Antagonism between Ca and Na ions at neurohypophysial nerve terminals. *Experientia (Basel)*, **27**, 1295–1296.

DREIFUSS, J. J., KALNINS, I., KELLY, J. S. AND RUF, K. B. (1971) Action potentials and release of neurohypophysial hormones *in vitro*. *J. Physiol. (Lond.)*, **215**, 805–817.

DYBALL, R. E. J. (1971) Oxytocin and ADH secretion in relation to electrical activity in antidromically identified supraoptic and paraventricular units. *J. Physiol. (Lond.)*, **214**, 245–256.

GAGE, P. W. AND QUASTEL, D. M. J. (1966) Competition between sodium and calcium ions in transmitter release at mammalian neuromuscular junctions. *J. Physiol. (Lond.)*, **185**, 95–123.

GINSBURG, M. AND IRELAND, M. (1966) The role of neurophysin in the transport and release of neurohypophysial hormones. *J. Endocr.*, **35**, 289–298.

KATZ, B. AND MILEDI, R. (1967) Tetrodotoxin and neuromuscular transmission. *Proc. roy. Soc. B (Lond.)*, **167**, 8–22.

KELLY, J. S. (1965) Antagonism between Na^+ and Ca^{2+} at the neuromuscular junction. *Nature (Lond.)*, **205**, 296–297.

LEGROS, J. J. (1971) Discussion. In *Radioimmunoassay Methods*, K. E. KIRKHAM AND W. M. HUNTER (Eds.), Livingston, Edinburgh, p. 228.

LEGROS, J. J., FRANCHIMONT, P. ET HENDRICK, J. C. (1969) Dosage radioimmunologique de la neurophysine dans le sérum de femmes normales et de femmes enceintes. *C.R. Soc. Biol. (Paris)*, **163**, 2773.

NAGASAWA, J., DOUGLAS, W. W., AND SCHULZ, R. A. (1970) Ultrastructural evidence of secretion by exocytosis and of "synaptic vesicle" formation in posterior pituitary glands. *Nature (Lond.)*, **227**, 407–409.

NORDMANN, J. J., DREIFUSS, J. J. AND LEGROS, J. J. (1971) A correlation of release of polypeptide hormones and of immunoreactive neurophysin from isolated rat neurohypophyses. *Experientia (Basel)*. **27**, 1344–1345.

THORN, N. A. (1970) Mechanism of release of neurohypophysial hormones. In *Aspects of Neuroendocrinology*, W. BARGMANN AND B. SCHARRER (Eds.), Springer, Berlin, pp. 140–152.

DISCUSSION

HAYWARD: I wonder if you care to generalize about a few points. Where do oxytocin and vasopressin fit in the supraoptic-paraventricular-neurohypophysial system? There are two general theories neither of which are very much substantiated, but I wonder if you could tell us first a little bit about neurophysin and its role in the hormone production and release. And secondly I wonder what is the relationship of vasopressin and oxytocin in the supraoptic and paraventricular system.

DREIFUSS: It is now generally believed that the supraoptic nucleus is mainly concerned with the synthesis of antidiuretic hormone and probably a small part of it only with the synthesis of oxytocin, in contrast to the paraventricular nucleus which seems to be mainly the place where oxytocin is synthetized, and vasopressin either not, or to a much lesser extent. The question whether one has two completely different types of neurones, one producing oxytocin and the other vasopressin, is likely but far from being proven, so that one cannot exclude at present that neurones may produce the two, although this seems somewhat unlikely to neurophysiologists according to the principle of Sir Henry

Dale. Hope and others in Oxford have shown that, in fact, one can separate several neurophysins; they are proteins with a molecular weight of approximately 10.000.

Depending on the species one can isolate 2, 3, or more neurophysins but it seems to be accepted that there are essentially two types of neurophysins, neurophysin I and neurophysin II. I would not be able to tell you what the biochemical difference between the two is, but Hope and collaborators have postulated or shown that neurophysin I seems to bind oxytocin to a larger extent, although *in vitro* the two have some affinity and there is no specificity at this level. It seems that, *in vivo*, neurophysin I is mostly associated with oxytocin and vasopressin with neurophysin II.

The regular amino-assay which we have used seems to be most sensitive to neurophysin II and to a lesser extent to neurophysin I. The bio-assay we have been using is more sensitive to oxytocin and to a lesser extent to vasopressin. We measure about 100% of the oxytocin activity and 25% of the vasopressin activity, so at this stage we cannot do any stochiometry. Now that we know this we will look with our bio-assay for pressure changes and diuretic changes which are most specific for vasopressin. But at this time I am not too unhappy to see that a rather unspecific bio-assay is related to neurophysin levels. Of course this has some implication in tests, because the determination of neurophysin is related in a fixed ratio to vasopressin. This may be very useful because of the technical difficulties in measuring these small peptides.

HAYWARD: Dr. Bodian has shown a number of years ago the presence of a chemical substance that produced a passive release of material from the pituitary. The neurosecretory vesicles were dumped into the bloodstream. The question remains how physiological is the stimulus in terms of release of the contents of the vesicles in the bloodstream.

DREIFUSS: In respect to what Dr. Scharrer has said, strong stimulation may work by exocytosis and weak stimulation by some other means. This is absolutely possible of course. But at this stage I see no need to postulate two different mechanisms. In our experiments it is the same whether we stimulate with a weak or strong stimulus, the ratios remaining the same. This is no good evidence because we have the artifacts of electrical stimulation. It has now been shown that neurophysin levels are increased in humans, if they are prevented from drinking for a few hours. We would call this a weak and physiological stimulus. I am not saying there are not two mechanisms, but there is no need to postulate this.

SCHARRER: I would like to avoid some misunderstanding: Your use of the term exocytocis is primarily concerned with the release of, or maybe comparable with, the right kind of ratio of neurophysins. The ultrastructural term exocytocis is one in which the whole granule, as it were, is dumped. I have not tried to say or to indicate by the fact that some ultrastructural evidence of the kind of vesiculation inside the cytoplasma occurs prior to the release of the contact of these granules, would necessarily result in retaining of neurophysin or pouring out the active principle. I think the exocytocis concept is one of morphology and I would be perfectly willing to assume that, since there is evidence of intracellular vesiculation before release of neurophysin, these mechanisms may function along the same lines. So I do not want to make the impression that I make biochemical conclusions from morphological observations.

JONGKIND: I did some quick calculations about the amount of moles of neurophysin which were released together with the amount of oxytocin. I don't know if I am wrong but I made a calculation of about 30 to 1. I calculated that the released amount of neurophysin is related to the amount of oxytocin as follows. About 30 moles of oxytocin are released with one mole of neurophysin with a molecular weight of 20.000.

DREIFUSS: The ratio is 1 to 4 but both calculations are not too useful in this stage as can be deduced from the figure I showed, since the levels of neurophysin and oxytocin can not be compared in a direct way.

JONGKIND: With the extrapolation of a straight line you can get every kind of relationship you want, because if you are very high on the line then you will get a relationship of 30 to 1; when you are at the intersection with the x-axis, then you have a ratio of 0 to 20.

DREIFUSS: That is just what I want to avoid by keeping it exactly the same. Hope and others have shown that it should be one neurophysin molecule to two polypeptide molecules, but again I think it is too early to draw definite conclusions.

JAMIESON: Referring back to your graphs am I correct in assuming that when you are plotting the results of the bio-assays against the current strength you believe that the strong stimulus might give rise to oxytocin release? I just wonder what sort of stimulus you are using and whether you don't think a stimulus of 10 milliamp to the hypophysis might not in fact give you either heat or electrolytic injury or perhaps both.

DREIFUSS: Certainly not. The slope of the line is the same all along, so whenever we refer to weak and strong stimuli I was only referring to what Dr. Scharrer had said this morning. In fact, weak stimuli, of 5 or 1 milliamp give also proportional release of both. So I don't agree with the first part of your comment.

JAMIESON: I was just wondering whether a stimulus of 10 milliamp which I think is a powerful current for the tissue, may not give heat or electrolytic damage to the tissue. What kind of stimulus are you using?

DREIFUSS: We are using biphasic pulses, 2 millisecond biphasic pulses; in other words there are 2 milliseconds for each of the phases and we apply this pulse at 50 per second. The highest level is 10 milliamp, peak to peak. This is done again in sodium free media so we don't have the complication of action potentials. In order to get high amounts released we withdraw the calcium. In our preparations a lot of current flows extracellularly and we have to use high intensities of stimulation in order to really depolarize the axonal endings. So if we have heat and if we burn the preparation, this is in the worse case of no importance as we are only testing depolarization which occurs locally at the terminal level.

BATTA: We have some experience with birds, in which the temperature is lower. I think that the temperature of the pituitary in the rat is higher in the living animal than you mention. Would not this affect the stimulus itself and the sensitivity of the pituitary to the stimulus?

DREIFUSS: This is a very complicated matter because I think the preparation has a Q_{10}, which is negative at least for very low temperatures. Douglas has shown that if you cool the neurohypophysis at very low temperatures you get a big release of substances. I don't know if anybody has studied the Q_{10} at more physiological values, let's say 27° or 28 °C. Being a few degrees off represents no serious problem as long as we look at such a fundamental and such an unphysiological situation. This is not an experiment in which we look at a living animal. We take out the neurophysis, incubate it in a medium, which is of course poor in terms of what the animals need normally, then we withdraw the external sodium and, nevertheless, we still are able to make some inferences on what the release-mechanism itself is, when placed in the artificial conditions.

BATTA: What will be the effect of increasing or decreasing the calcium concentration?

DREIFUSS: I do not know.

BATTA: Do you know whether the hormone contains a di-sulphate bond?

DREIFUSS: The polypeptide does.

Pharmacological Aspects of Neuroendocrine Integration

WILLIAM F. GANONG

Department of Physiology, University of California, San Francisco, San Francisco, Calif. 94122 (U.S.A.)

In view of the close relationship between the nervous and endocrine systems, it is not surprising that drugs that act on the nervous system modify endocrine function. This is only one of the ways that drugs affect endocrine function (Table I; see also Gold

TABLE I

DRUGS AFFECTING ENDOCRINE FUNCTION*

I.	Hormone congeners that
	A. Act like naturally occurring hormones
	B. Block the effects of naturally occurring hormones
II.	Drugs that act directly on endocrine organs to stimulate or inhibit secretion.
III.	Drugs that inhibit the actions of hormones on their target organs.
IV.	Drugs that alter hormone secretion by acting on the nervous system (including drugs that act as stressful stimuli).

* From Gold and Ganong, 1967.

and Ganong, 1967), but it is an important one, since the endocrine system is in large part an effector arm of the nervous system. The effectors by which neural integration is brought about are summarized in Fig. 1. It now appears that the link between the

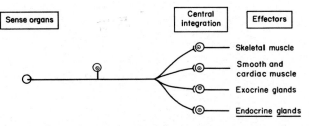

Fig. 1. Diagram of the reflex arc, showing the effectors by which the integrative action of the nervous system is brought about. From Ganong, 1966.

* Previously unpublished data included in this paper were obtained in experiments supported by U.S. Public Health Service Grant AM06704 and performed in collaboration with Drs. Jeffrey Caren, Umberto Scapagnini and Augusto Cuello, Miss Angela Borcyzka, Mr. Norman Kramer and Mr. Roy Shackelford.

References p. 52

nervous and endocrine systems is at least in part adrenergic, and it is this theme of adrenergic control which I would like to explore and develop in the present paper.

The catecholamines that mediate transmission at adrenergic synapses are dopamine and norepinephrine. The third physiologically important catecholamine, epinephrine, is formed in the adrenal medulla. Catecholamine biosynthesis is summarized in Fig. 2. The steps through the formation of norepinephrine are common to adrenal

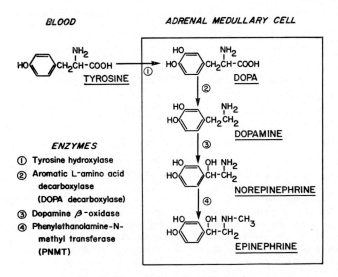

Fig. 2. Biosynthesis of catecholamines.

medullary cells and adrenergic nerve endings (Wurtman, 1966). The adrenal medullary cells contain in addition the enzyme phenylethanolamine-N-methyltransferase (PNMT) which catalyzes the conversion of norepinephrine to epinephrine. The catecholamines are metabolized to inactive products by O-methylation or by oxidative deamination.

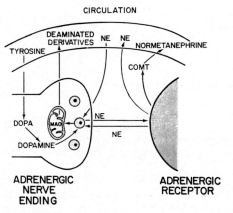

Fig. 3. Formation, uptake and metabolism of norepinephrine at adrenergic nerve endings. From Ganong, 1971a.

The former reaction is catalyzed by the enzyme catechol-O-methyltransferase (COMT), and the latter by monoamine oxidase (MAO). MAO is a mitochondrial enzyme, while COMT is primarily extracellular. Therefore, some of the intracellular catecholamines are metabolized to deaminated derivatives in the adrenergic nerve endings, while O-methylation occurs outside cells. The formation, uptake, and metabolism of norepinephrine are summarized in Fig. 3.

The receptors on which secreted catecholamines act are divided into two general categories: α-adrenergic receptors are those at which in the case of vascular smooth muscle norepinephrine acts to produce contraction, while β-adrenergic receptors are those at which epinephrine acts to produce relaxation. There is considerable evidence that the β-mediated effects are brought about via increased intracellular formation of cyclic AMP, and there is some evidence that α-mediated effects are exerted by way of inhibition of the formation of this intracellular 'second messenger' (see Robison and Sutherland, 1970).

There are a variety of drugs that affect catecholamine synthesis and metabolism. Alpha-methyl-para-tyrosine (α-MT) inhibits tyrosine hydroxylase, preventing the formation of L-dopa and therefore leading to depletion of catecholamine stores. Reserpine also produces a profound depletion of these amines and of serotonin by blocking cellular amine concentrating mechanisms. FLA-63 and a number of other compounds inhibit dopamine β-oxidase, preventing the conversion of dopamine to norepinephrine. Dihydroxyphenylserine (DOPS) is the amino acid that corresponds to norepinephrine, and it can be decarboxylated to form norepinephrine, bypassing dopamine β-oxidase. Drugs that inhibit monoamine oxidase increase intracellular stores of catecholamines because they prevent their intracellular oxidative deamination. There are in addition a variety of drugs that selectively block α- or β-adrenergic receptors. Phenoxybenzamine is a frequently used α-adrenergic blocking agent, while propranolol is an effective β-adrenergic blocking agent.

Cholinergic mechanisms are also involved in neuroendocrine control. The adrenal medulla, for example, is controlled by cholinergic neurons. However, it is really a special case, since the adrenal medullary cells are in effect postganglionic sympathetic neurons that have lost their axons and become specialized for the secretion of norepinephrine and epinephrine directly into the bloodstream.

Another endocrine organ that appears to be in part under the control of the sympathetic nervous system is the renin-secreting organ, the juxtaglomerular cells in the kidneys. Other factors in addition to sympathetic activity play important roles in the regulation of renin secretion. These probably include the degree to which the juxtaglomerular cells themselves are stretched, and the amount of sodium crossing the cells of the macula densa, the receptor-like region in the distal tubule. However, there are many adrenergic nerve fibers among the juxtaglomerular cells, and synapse-like structures between the nerves and the hormone-secreting cells have been described (Barajas, 1964). In addition, sympathetic stimuli are known to increase renin secretion. For instance, hypoglycemia leads to increased renin secretion (Otsuka et al., 1970). So does stimulation of the pressor region of the medulla oblongata (Passo et al., 1971a, b) and stimulation of the renal nerves (Vander, 1965; Lee, Loeffler, Stockigt and Ganong, unpublished observations). The response to hypoglycemia is blocked by adrenal denervation, while that to stimulation of the pressor region of the medulla oblongata is blocked by section of the renal nerves, indicating that circulating catecholamines and catecholamines liberated at adrenergic endings both can stimulate renin secretion (Fig. 4). The close association of adrenergic nerves and the secretory

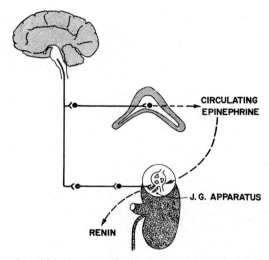

Fig. 4. Pathways by which the sympathetic nervous system stimulates renin secretion.

cells plus the observation by Michelakis *et al.* (1969) that norepinephrine, epinephrine, and cyclic AMP increase the release of renin *in vitro*, support the view that the action of the sympathetic nervous system on the juxtaglomerular cells is a direct one.

The increase in renin secretion produced by sympathetic stimulation appears to be mediated by way of a β-adrenergic receptor. The responses to hypoglycemia, stimulation of the medulla oblongata and stimulation of the renal nerves are all unaffected or potentiated by α-adrenergic blockade with phenoxybenzamine but blocked by the β-adrenergic blocking agent, propanolol (Assaykeen *et al.*, 1970; Passo *et al.*, 1971a; Loeffler, Stockigt and Ganong, unpublished observation). Additional support for the concept of β-mediation of the sympathetic effects on renin secretion is provided by the observation that theophylline, which increases intracellular cyclic AMP, causes an increase in renin secretion that is unaffected by propranolol (Reid and Ganong, 1971).

Adrenergic stimuli also affect the secretion of insulin by the β cells of the pancreatic islets. The major controls of insulin secretion are, of course, the level of glucose in the blood perfusing the pancreatic islets, the blood level of certain amino acids, and 'gut factors' secreted by the mucosa of the gastrointestinal tract. However, it is clear from the work of Porte and associates that catecholamines can inhibit insulin secretion through an α-adrenergic action and stimulate it through a β-mediated action (see Williams, 1968). A cholinergic mechanism also affects insulin secretion; stimulation of the right vagus nerve causes an increase in the secretion of this hormone although the physiological significance of this fact remains uncertain (see Williams, 1968).

The adrenergic effects on renin and insulin secretion are mediated via the sympathetic nervous system. The hypothalamus contains dopamine and norepinephrine, and the question arises whether adrenergic mechanisms in this part of the brain affect the secretion of the pituitary gland. Evidence that they do is accumulating at an accelerating rate; indeed, there is now at least some evidence that adrenergic mechanisms affect the secretion of every one of the hormones known to be secreted by the pituitary gland.

O'Connor and Verney (1945) reported that epinephrine inhibited vasopressin secretion, but their epinephrine injections were administered systemically and this amine does not penetrate the blood–brain barrier. On the other hand, Mills and Wang observed that stimulation of the ulnar nerve led to increased vasopressin secretion, and that this stimulatory effect was blocked by administration of α-adrenergic blocking drugs (see Sawyer and Mills, 1966). Many adrenergic nerve fibers end on the cell bodies of the supraoptic and paraventricular neurons (see Fuxe and Hökfelt, 1969), and these pathways are presumably excitatory. Reserpine and chlorpromazine have also been reported to reduce vasopressin secretion. Cholinergic mechanisms are also involved in the regulation of vasopressin secretion, although their role is debated. Much less is known about the secretion of oxytocin, but it is interesting that Grosvenor and Turner (1957) found that α-adrenergic blocking agents as well as cholinergic blocking agents inhibited milk excretion. This suggests that oxytocin may be under stimulatory control by adrenergic pathways.

The intermediate lobe of the pituitary is believed to be innervated by nerve fibers which tonically inhibit its secretion, and there may be MSH-releasing and inhibiting factors as well. Very little is known about the synaptic mediators involved in the control systems, but it has been demonstrated that phenothiazines increase MSH secretion in frogs (Scott and Nading, 1961). Since phenothiazines have antiadrenergic activity, this raises the possibility that adrenergic mechanisms normally inhibit the secretion of MSH.

The hypothalamic pathways that regulate the secretion of TSH by the anterior pituitary have not been mapped in detail, but it has been reported that injection of epinephrine into the hypothalamus increases TSH secretion. This claim has been disputed, but it has also been reported that the antiadrenergic drugs reserpine and chlorpromazine inhibit TSH secretion in the rat (for references, see Gold and Ganong, 1967). Tentatively, therefore, one may assign TSH to the group of hormones whose secretion is stimulated by adrenergic mechanisms.

In the case of growth hormone, adrenergic mechanisms also appear to affect secretion. In man, growth hormone secretion increases at the onset of sleep. This increase is unaffected by chlorpromazine, but in two of four subjects studied, it was abolished by imipramine (Takahashi et al., 1968). This antidepressant is believed to increase available free catecholamines by inhibiting their re-uptake. On the other hand Blackard and Heidingsfelder (1968) have shown that α-adrenergic blockade inhibits the increase in growth hormone secretion produced by insulin-induced hypoglycemia, while β-adrenergic blockade potentiated the response in their patients. In addition, L-dopa has been shown to stimulate growth hormone secretion (Boyd et al.,

References p. 52

1970) and chlorpromazine to inhibit growth hormone secretion in the fasting state and following the administration of insulin (Sherman et al., 1971). More recently, chlorpromazine has been reported to reduce growth hormone secretion in patients with acromegaly (Kolodny et al., 1971). In rats, Mueller and his associates (1970) reported that injection of dopamine or norepinephrine into the ventricles of the brain increased the amount of growth hormone-releasing factor in the plasma and decreased its content in the hypothalamus. On the other hand, Takahashi et al. (1971) found that epinephrine decreased plasma growth hormone levels in the rat, and that this decrease was unaffected by α- or β-adrenergic blocking agents. It should be noted, however, that Mueller et al. measured growth hormone by the tibia test bioassay, while Takahashi and his associates used a radioimmunoassay, and it is well known that results with these two assays do not agree. In addition, the regulation of the secretion of radioimmunoassayable growth hormone in the rat seems to be fundamentally different from that in the primates and man, since the level of growth hormone falls rather than rises with hypoglycemia and other stresses. It seems fair, therefore, to tentatively assign growth hormone to the list of hormones whose secretion is affected by adrenergic mechanisms, and to speculate that the effect of adrenergic discharge is stimulatory.

The secretion of FSH and LH is clearly affected by catecholamines. It is simplest to treat these hormones together, since it is known that there is a peak in the secretion of both at the time of ovulation and since the secretion of both may be controlled by a single hypothalamic releasing factor (Schally et al., 1971).

The classical studies of Sawyer, Markee and Everett indicate that there are adrenergic and cholinergic links involved in the burst of hormone secretion responsible for ovulation in the rat and the rabbit (see Sawyer, 1963). The antiadrenergic compounds they used to block ovulation were α-adrenergic blocking agents. Reserpine and chlorpromazine have also been shown to block ovulation (see Gold and Ganong, 1967).

Subsequently, Schneider and McCann (1969) demonstrated that addition of dopamine to hypothalamic and pituitary tissue incubated together would produce release of LH. They then demonstrated that injection of dopamine in the third ventricle produced increased secretion of LH in male and female rats. Norepinephrine was less effective (Schneider and McCann, 1970a). In addition, they observed that dopamine caused an increase in the circulating levels of LRF in hypophysectomized rats (1970b). Kamberi et al. (1970) also found that injection of dopamine in the ventricles increased LH in the circulation, and they showed that infusion of dopamine directly into a portal vessel or into an artery supplying the primary plexus of the portal system had no effect on LH secretion. They obtained similar results with FSH (Kamberi et al., 1971a). Epinephrine and norepinephrine also released LH and FSH, but larger doses were required. Thus, it appears that discharge of dopaminergic neurons stimulates the secretion of LRF and the factor that stimulates FSH secretion, with a resultant increase in the secretion of these two pituitary gonadotropins. Schneider and McCann (1970a) have reported that the effects of dopamine on LH secretion are inhibited by α-adrenergic blocking agents but unaffected by β-blocking drugs. Dopamine is known to act on α-adrenergic receptors in other parts of the body (see Goodman and Gilman, 1970).

There are two slightly discordant notes in this otherwise apparently clearcut story. Rubinstein and Sawyer (1970) found epinephrine more effective than dopamine in producing ovulation upon injection into the third ventricle in rats. However, they agree that adrenergic mechanisms are involved, finding that reserpine blocks ovulation and that monoamine oxidase inhibitors block the inhibitory effect of reserpine. Kalra (1971) has presented evidence that in one particular circumstance, norepinephrine rather than dopamine is the mediator that produces increased LH secretion. She studied the burst of LH secretion that is produced in ovariectomized rats given an injection of estrogen followed in 24 h by an injection of progesterone. This burst was abolished by drugs which deplete brain catecholamines, but it was also abolished by compounds which block dopamine β-oxidase, presumably producing norepinephrine depletion while leaving dopamine intact. Conversely, it was present in animals treated with α-MT and DOPS, in which brain dopamine would be expected to be low but brain norepinephrine normal.

In their experiments on intraventricularly injected catecholamines, Kamberi et al. (1971b) found that prolactin secretion appeared to vary inversely with that of FSH and LH. Thus, intraventricular injections of dopamine and, less effectively, norepinephrine and epinephrine lowered plasma prolactin. Injections into a portal vessel or into an artery supplying the primary plexus of the portal system had no effect. A role of brain catecholamines in inhibiting prolactin secretion has been postulated by others as well. Lu et al. (1970) showed that reserpine, chlorpromazine, α-MT and α-methyl-meta-tyrosine all increase circulating prolactin. Several of these anti-adrenergic drugs had previously been reported to produce lactation (see Gold and Ganong, 1967), and chlorpromazine has recently been shown to increase circulating prolactin in humans (Kleinberg et al., 1971). Lu et al. (1970) noted that there was no effect of systemically injected dopamine, norepinephrine, epinephrine, or serotonin on plasma prolactin, presumably because these amines failed to cross the blood–brain barrier to reach the part of the central nervous system where the adrenergic effect is exerted. More recently, it has been demonstrated that L-dopa inhibits prolactin secretion (Donosa et al., 1971). Catecholamines do exert a direct effect on the release of prolactin from the pituitary in vitro (Koch et al., 1970), but it seems unlikely that direct effects play any role in the normal regulation of the secretion of this hormone. The inhibition of prolactin secretion produced by the ergot alkaloid, ergocornine, appears to be unique (Wuttke et al., 1971). This compound is a relatively potent α-adrenergic blocking agent, but there is evidence that it inhibits prolactin secretion by a direct effect on the pituitary gland. Thus, it appears that in rats and humans, a central adrenergic system inhibits prolactin secretion. The mediator involved is probably dopamine and inhibition is probably brought about by stimulation of the secretion of the PIF, but this has not been definitely proved.

Adrenergic mechanisms affecting the secretion of ACTH have been under study in my laboratory for some years (see Ganong, 1965, 1970, 1971b, 1972). The experiments indicate that both in the dog (Van Loon et al., 1971a, 1971b) and in the rat (Scapagnini *et al.*, 1970a, 1970b), there is a central adrenergic system which inhibits stress-induced ACTH secretion. We have found that the dopamine β-oxidase inhibitor, FLA-63, which lowers hypothalamic norepinephrine without affecting dopamine, increases ACTH secretion (Scapagnini *et al.*, 1970b). We have also found that DOPS counteracts the increase in ACTH secretion produced by α-MT, and that the magnitude of this inhibition of the response to α-MT is proportional to the degree to which hypothalamic norepinephrine is repleted (Cuello, Scapagnini and Ganong, unpublished observations). The effects of α-MT and of α-MT plus DOPS are summarized in Fig. 5.

We have also undertaken a series of experiments in dogs to determine the type of receptor involved in the ACTH response to adrenergic stimulation. The adrenocortical

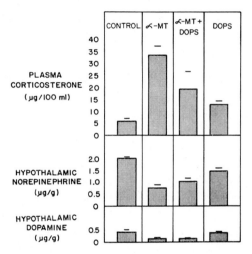

Fig. 5. Effect of α-MT and DOPS on plasma corticosterone and hypothalamic norepinephrine and dopamine concentrations. From Ganong, 1972.

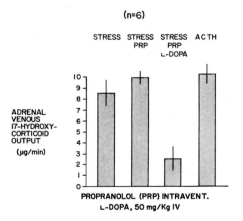

Fig. 6. Effect of injecting propranolol into the third ventricle on the adrenocortical response to stress and L-dopa in the dog. From Ganong, 1971b.

response to surgical stress is first determined. A drug is next injected directly into the third ventricle and the response to stress is tested again. L-Dopa is then injected systemically and the effect of this blocking agent on the inhibition of ACTH secretion normally produced by L-dopa is determined. In these experiments we found that intraventricular propranolol had no effect on the stress response (Fig. 6) and no effect on the inhibition produced by L-dopa (Kramer, Boryczka, Shackelford and Ganong, unpublished observations). Phenoxybenzamine also had no effect on the response to stress, but it abolished the inhibition produced by L-dopa (Fig. 7). One disturbing

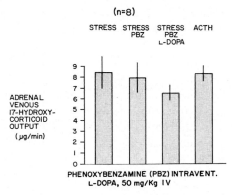

Fig. 7. Effect of injecting phenoxybenzamine into the third ventricle on the adrenocortical response to surgical stress and L-dopa in the dog. From Ganong, 1971b.

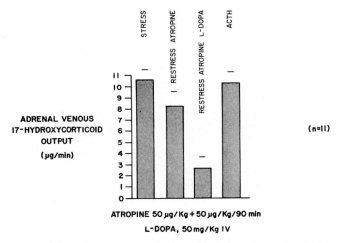

Fig. 8. Effect of injecting atropine into the third ventricle on the adrenocortical response to stress and L-dopa in the dog.

note is the fact that phentolamine, another type of α-adrenergic blocking agent, fails to alter the inhibition of ACTH secretion produced by L-dopa. However, there is precedent for blockade of a neuroendocrine response by phenoxybenzamine and not by phentolamine; Sawyer and his associates observed a similar selective effect of phenoxybenzamine on ovulation (see Sawyer, 1963). The data therefore support the conclusion that the adrenergic inhibition of ACTH secretion is due to activation of an α-adrenergic receptor.

Since atropine has been reported to inhibit stress-induced ACTH secretion in the rat (Hedge and Smelik, 1968; Hedge and De Wied, 1971), and since phenoxybenzamine has anticholinergic activity (Goodman and Gilman, 1970), we tested the effect of atropine in the third ventricle on the response to stress and L-dopa. Results are summarized in Fig. 8. Atropine had no inhibitory effect on the response to stress and did not modify the inhibitory effect of L-dopa. The explanation of the discrepancy between these data and the results in the rat is not apparent. It may be significant, however, that atropine was implanted in the rat experiments, and high concentrations of atropine exert a local anesthetic effect (Goodman and Gilman, 1970).

Thus, it seems clear that there is a central adrenergic system that inhibits ACTH secretion. The mediator in this system appears to be norepinephrine rather than dopamine, and an α-adrenergic receptor is probably the type of receptor involved.

The picture that emerges from the data presented above is one of extensive involvement of adrenergic neural pathways in the regulation of hormone secretion. The hormones affected are listed in Table II. It should be emphasized that this list is

TABLE II

EFFECTS OF ADRENERGIC DISCHARGE (NORADRENERGIC OR DOPAMINERGIC)
ON ENDOCRINE FUNCTIONS

Tentative List

Secretion stimulated	Secretion inhibited
FSH, LH	prolactin
GH	ACTH
TSH	
vasopressin	MSH
oxytocin	
renin	
insulin	insulin

highly tentative, that it is based in some instances on very tenuous data, and that it may be modified as additional data become available. However, it does appear that the secretion of FSH and LH is stimulated by a neural circuit in which dopamine is a key synaptic mediator. The same system or a similar system inhibits the secretion of prolactin. The receptor involved, at least in the case of FSH and LH, is blocked by α-adrenergic blocking drugs. In the case of growth hormone, an adrenergic neural circuit appears to stimulate secretion, and the evidence leans toward norepinephrine rather than dopamine being the mediator involved. Contrariwise, a noradrenergic circuit inhibits the secretion of ACTH. In both cases, a receptor that is blocked by α-adrenergic blocking agents appears to be involved. TSH secretion may also be stimulated by adrenergic mechanisms in the hypothalamus. There is some evidence for an adrenergic pathway which stimulates the secretion of vasopressin and oxytocin, and in the case of vasopressin, an α-adrenergic receptor appears to be involved. The secretion of MSH may be inhibited by an adrenergic system, but the receptor involved is unknown.

The secretion of renin is stimulated by circulating catecholamines or by catecholamines liberated at the endings of the renal sympathetic nerves. A β- rather than an α-adrenergic receptor is involved in this case, and the action of catecholamines may well be directly on the secretory cells. Insulin secretion is unique in that it is inhibited by α-adrenergic stimulation and stimulated by β-adrenergic stimulation.

The significance of the adrenergic components in the regulation of the secretion of each hormone remains to be determined. It should be emphasized that catecholamines are not the only regulators. In the case of renin, for instance, secretion also appears to be regulated by the sodium concentration at the macula densa and the degree to which the juxtaglomerular cells are stretched. In the case of insulin, secretion varies in response to the plasma levels of glucose, amino acids, and 'gut factors'. The same consideration applies to the pituitary hormones; there are, for instance, feedback effects of steroids and thyroid hormones directly on the pituitary gland. Thus, catecholamines affect the secretion of many different hormones, and they are one, but only one of the many regulatory factors involved in adjusting the secretion of individual hormones to the demands of the environment.

SUMMARY

Changes in endocrine function can be produced by drugs that act on the nervous system because a large segment of the endocrine system is under neural control. The link between the nervous and endocrine systems appears in many instances to be adrenergic, or at least to have an adrenergic component in it. Circulating catecholamines and the catecholamines secreted at the endings of the renal nerves increase renin secretion by a mechanism involving a β-adrenergic receptor. Catecholamines inhibit insulin secretion by an α-adrenergic mechanism and stimulate it by a β-adrenergic mechanism. Hypothalamic catecholamines affect the secretion of most if not all pituitary hormones, generally via receptors that are blocked by α-adrenergic blocking agents. Dopaminergic pathways apparently stimulate FSH and LH secretion and inhibit prolactin secretion. Noradrenergic pathways stimulate growth hormone secretion and inhibit ACTH secretion. There is evidence that the secretion of TSH, MSH, oxytocin and vasopressin are also regulated by catecholamine-containing neurons in the hypothalamus. The interactions between adrenergic mechanisms and the other unique factors that affect the secretion of renin, insulin and the pituitary hormones merit further study.

References p. 52

REFERENCES

ASSAYKEEN, T. A., CLAYTON, P. L., GOLDFIEN, A. AND GANONG, W. F. (1970) The effect of alpha- and beta-adrenergic blocking agents on the renin response to hypoglycemia and epinephrine in dogs. *Endocrinology*, **87**, 1318–1322.

BARAJAS, L. (1964) The innervation of the juxtaglomerular apparatus. *Lab. Invest.*, **13**, 916–929.

BLACKARD, W. F. AND HEIDINGSFELDER, S. A. (1968) Adrenergic receptor control mechanisms for growth hormone secretion. *J. clin. Invest.*, **47**, 1407–1414.

BOYD, A. E., III, LEBOVITZ, H. E. AND PFEIFFER, J. B. (1970) Stimulation of human-growth-hormone secretion by L-dopa. *New Engl. J. Med.*, **283**, 1425–1429.

DONOSO, A. O., BISHOP, W., McCANN, S. M. AND ORIAS, R. (1971) Effects of alternations in brain monoamine concentrations on plasma prolactin. *Abstracts, 53rd Meeting of the Endocrine Society*, San Francisco, p. A–127.

FUXE, K. AND HÖKFELT, T. (1969) Catecholamines in the hypothalamus and the pituitary gland. In *Frontiers in Neuroendocrinology*, W. F. GANONG AND L. MARTINI (Eds.), Oxford Univ. Press, New York, pp. 47–96.

GANONG, W. F. (1965) The effect of chlorpromazine and related drugs on ACTH release. *Proc. 2nd int. Congr. Endocrinol., Excerpta med. int. Congr. Ser.*, No. 83, Part 1, pp. 624–628.

GANONG, W. F. (1966) Neuroendocrine integrating mechanisms. In *Neuroendocrinology, Vol. 1*, L. MARTINI AND W. F. GANONG (Eds.), Academic Press, New York, pp. 1–13.

GANONG, W. F. (1970) Control of ACTH and MSH secretion. In *The Hypothalamus*, L. MARTINI, M. MOTTA AND F. FRASCHINI (Eds.), Academic Press, New York, pp. 313–333.

GANONG, W. F. (1971a) *Review of Medical Physiology*, 5th ed., Lange Medical Publications, Los Altos, Calif.

GANONG, W. F. (1971b) Brain amines and ACTH secretion. *Proc. Third int. Congr. Hormonal Steroids, Excerpta med. int. Congr. Ser.*, No. 219, Excerpta Medica, Amsterdam, 814–821.

GANONG, W. F. (1972) Evidence for a central noradrenergic system that inhibits ACTH secretion. In *Brain-Endocrine Interaction*, K. KNIGGE, D. E. SCOTT AND A. WEINDL (Eds.), Karger, Basel, pp. 254–266.

GOLD, E. M. AND GANONG, W. F. (1967) Effects of drugs on neuroendocrine processes. In *Neuro-endocrinology, Vol. 2*, L. MARTINI AND W. F. GANONG (Eds.), Academic Press, New York, pp. 377–437.

GOODMAN, L. AND GILMAN, A. (1970) *The Pharmacological Basis of Therapeutics*, 4th ed., MacMillan, New York.

GROSVENOR, C. C. AND TURNER, C. S. (1957) Evidence for adrenergic and cholinergic components in milk let-down reflex in lactating rat. *Proc. Soc. exp. Biol. (N.Y.)*, **95**, 719–722.

HEDGE, G. A. and DE WIED, D. (1971) Corticotropin and vasopressin secretion after hypothalamic implantation of atropine. *Endocrinology*, **188**, 1257–1259.

HEDGE, G. A. AND SMELIK, P. G. (1968) Corticotropin release: inhibition by intrahypothalamic implantation of atropine. *Science*, **159**, 891–892.

KALRA, P. S. (1971) Involvement of norepinephrine in transmission of the stimulatory influence of progesterone on gonadotropin release. *Abstracts, 53rd Meeting of the Endocrine Society*, San Francisco, p. A–78.

KAMBERI, I. A., MICAL, R. S. AND PORTER, J. C. (1970) Effect of anterior pituitary perfusion and intraventricular injection of catecholamines and indolamines on LH release. *Endocrinology*, **87**, 1–12.

KAMBERI, I. A., MICAL, R. S. AND PORTER, J. C. (1971a) Effect of anterior pituitary perfusion and intraventricular injection of catecholamines on FSH release. *Endocrinology*, **88**, 1003–1011.

KAMBERI, I. A., MICAL, R. S. AND PORTER, J. C. (1971b) Effect of anterior pituitary perfusion and intraventricular injection of catecholamines on prolactin release. *Endocrinology*, **88**, 1012–1020.

KLEINBERG, D. L., WHARTON, R. N. AND FRANTZ, A. G. (1971) Rapid release of prolactin in normal adults following chlorpromazine stimulation. *Abstracts, 53rd Meeting of the Endocrine Society*, San Francisco, p. A–126.

KOCH, Y., LU, K. H. AND MEITES, J. (1970) Biphasic effect of catecholamines on pituitary prolactin release *in vitro*. *Endocrinology*, **87**, 673–675.

KOLODNY, H. D., SHERMAN, L., SINGH, A., BENJAMIN, F. AND KIM, S. (1971) Chlorpromazine treatment of human acromegaly, *Abstracts, 53rd Meeting of the Endocrine Society*, San Francisco, p. A–213.

Lu, K.-H., Amenomori, Y., Chen, C. L., and Meites, J. (1970) Effects of central acting drugs on serum and pituitary prolactin levels in rats. *Endocrinology*, **87**, 667–672.

Michelakis, A. M., Caudle, J. and Liddle, G. W. (1969) *In vitro* stimulation of renin production by epinephrine, norepinephrine and cyclic AMP, *Proc. Soc. exp. Biol. (N.Y.)*, **130**, 748–753.

Mueller, E. E., Pecile, A., Felici, M. and Cocchi, D. (1970) Norepinephrine and dopamine injections into lateral brain ventricle of the rat and growth hormone-releasing activity in the hypothalamus and plasma. *Endocrinology*, **86**, 1376–1382.

O'Connor, W. J. and Verney, E. B. (1945) The effect of increased activity of the sympathetic system in the inhibition of water-diuresis by emotional stress. *Quart. J. exp. Physiol.*, **33**, 77–90.

Otsuka, K., Assaykeen, T. A., Goldfien, A. and Ganong, W. F. (1970) The effect of hypoglycemia on plasma renin activity in dogs. *Endocrinology*, **87**, 1306–1317.

Passo, S. S., Assaykeen, T. A., Goldfien, A. and Ganong, W. F. (1971a) Effect of α- and β-adrenergic blocking agents on the increase in renin secretion produced by stimulation of the medulla oblongata in dogs. *Neuroendocrinology*, **7**, 97–104.

Passo, S. S., Assaykeen, T. A., Otsuka, K., Wise, B. L., Goldfien, A. and Ganong, W. F. (1971b) Effect of stimulation of the medulla oblongata on renin secretion in dogs. *Neuroendocrinology*, **7**, 1–10.

Reid, I. A. and Ganong, W. F. (1971) Effect of theophylline on renin secretion. *Fed. Proc.*, **30**, 449 (Abstract).

Robison, G. A. and Sutherland, E. W. (1970) Sympathin e, sympathin i and the intracellular level of cyclic AMP. *Circulation Res.*, Suppl. I, **26**, **27**, 147–161.

Rubinstein, L. and Sawyer, C. H. (1970) Role of catecholamines in stimulating the release of pituitary ovulating hormone(s) in rats. *Endocrinology*, **86**, 988–995.

Sawyer, C. H. (1963) Discussion. In *Advances in Neuroendocrinology*, A. V. Nalbandov (Ed.), Univ. of Illinois Press, Urbana, pp. 445–457.

Sawyer, W. H. and Mills, E. (1966) Control of vasopressin secretion. In *Neuroendocrinology*, Vol. 1, L. Martini and W. F. Ganong (Eds.), Academic Press, New York, pp. 187–216.

Scapagnini, U., Van Loon, G. R., Moberg, G. P. and Ganong, W. F. (1970a) Effect of α-methyl-*p*-tyrosine on the circadian variation of plasma corticosterone in rats. *Europ. J. Pharmacol.*, **11** 266–268.

Scapagnini, U., Van Loon, G. R., Moberg, G. P., Preziosi, G. P. and Ganong, W. F. (1970b) Evidence for central adrenergic inhibition of ACTH secretion in the rat. *Communications Joint Meeting Italian-German Soc. Pharmacol.*, Heidelberg (Abstract).

Schally, A. V., Arimura, A. R., Baba, Y., Nair, R. M. G., Matsuo, H., Redding, T. W., Debeljuk, L. and White, W. (1971) Purification and properties of the LH- and FSH-releasing hormone from porcine hypothalami. *Abstracts, 53rd Meeting of the Endocrine Society*, San Francisco, p. A–70.

Schneider, H. P. G. and McCann, S. M. (1969) Possible role of dopamine as transmitter to promote discharge of LH-releasing factor. *Endocrinology*, **85**, 121–132.

Schneider, H. P. G. and McCann, S. M. (1970a) Mono- and indolamines and control of LH secretion. *Endocrinology*, **86**, 1127–1133.

Schneider, H. P. G. and McCann, S. M. (1970b) Release of LH-releasing factor (LRF) into the peripheral circulation of hypophysectomized rats by dopamine and its blockage by estradiol. *Endocrinology*, **87**, 249–253.

Scott, G. T. and Nading, L. K. (1961) Relative effectiveness of phenothiazine tranquilizing drugs causing release of MSH. *Proc. Soc. exp. Biol. (N.Y.)*, **106**, 88–90.

Sherman, L., Kim, S., Benjamin, F. and Kolodny, H. D. (1971) Effect of chlorpromazine on serum growth hormone concentration in man. *New Engl. J. Med.*, **284**, 72–74.

Takahashi, K., Daughaday, W. H. and Kipnis, D. M. (1971) Regulation of immunoreactive growth hormone secretion in male rats. *Endocrinology*, **88**, 909–917.

Takahashi, Y., Kipnis, D. M. and Daughaday, W. H. (1968) Growth hormone secretion during sleep. *J. clin. Invest.*, **47**, 2079–2090.

Vander, A. J. (1965) Effect of catecholamines and the renal nerves on renin secretion in anesthetized dog. *Amer. J. Physiol.*, **209**, 659–662.

Van Loon, G. R., Hilger, L., King, A. B., Boryczka, A. T. and Ganong, W. F. (1971a) Inhibitory effect of L-dihydroxyphenylalanine on the adrenal venous 17-hydroxycorticosteroid response to surgical stress in dogs. *Endocrinology*, **88**, 1404–1414.

Van Loon, G. R., Scapagnini, U., Cohen, R. and Ganong, W. F. (1971b) Effect of the intraventricular administration of adrenergic drugs on the adrenal venous 17-hydroxycorticosteroid response to surgical stress in the dog. *Neuroendocrinology*, **8**, 257–272.

WILLIAMS, R. H. (1968) The pancreas. In *Textbook of Endocrinology*, R. H. WILLIAMS (Ed.), 4th ed., Saunders, Philadelphia, pp. 613–802.

WURTMAN, R. J. (1966) *Catecholamines*, Little, Brown and Co., Boston.

WUTTKE, W., CASSELL, E. AND MEITES, J. (1971) Effect of ergocornine on serum prolactin and LH, and on hypothalamic content of PIF and LRF, *Endocrinology*. **88**, 737–741.

DISCUSSION

SMELIK: I have a couple of questions to Dr. Ganong about this very intriguing lecture. First of all I would suppose, otherwise you should correct me, that the action of the catecholamines occurs at the hypothalamic level presumably. If this is so then there is one interesting feature: in your last slide you showed that the secretion of some pituitary hormones was stimulated, while in some others it was inhibited. The latter group includes ACTH, prolactin and MSH. If you take it for granted that there is a central inhibition of MSH and prolactin that means, and the evidence in the literature is very clear, in respect to prolactin that in fact there is an adrenergic stimulation of all the releasing or inhibiting factors we know of, except for CRF. This would put ACTH or control of ACTH in a very peculiar situation. I think it would be more correct to "translate" the hormones into their releasing factors. I do not know why you did not do this, but I suppose since you injected the substances into the third ventricle that this is at the level of the hypothalamic neurosecretory cells. This is just a remark I wanted to make because it was somewhat unexpected to me that CRF would be in such a separate place. The other question is: do you know anything about the more precise site of action of the adrenergic drugs, be it noradrenergic or dopaminergic. You injected these compounds into the third ventricle in dogs. I have always had the feeling that perhaps with implantation of crystalline substances you might come to know something about the precise site of action. Did you do any experiments suggesting whether this is really within the hypothalamus, or some part of it?

Coming to the point of atropine, I may disappoint you in so far that when I did my implantation studies with adrenergic substances I could never see any effect. You could not see any effect either with atropine and the difference between both studies is that you put it into the third ventricle and I did crystalline implantation. As far as atropine is concerned it is a very specific site where you have to implant it. Could you speculate, when you put the substances in the third ventricle, where the substances can be picked up or to where they are transported? Would that give you any lead to the site of action? As far as I recall, the implants were not very close to the wall of the ventricle and it might be that, when you inject into the third ventricle, the compound does not reach that particular site which is apparently very small.

GANONG: The point about the releasing factors is well taken since the secretion of prolactin is usually held to be inhibited by a prolactin inhibitory factor. I may remind you, however, that there is now pretty good evidence that there is also a releasing factor and as far as I know there is no conclusive evidence either way whether this adrenergic effect is mediated by the releasing factor or by the inhibiting factor. If one believes that there is a growth hormone inhibiting factor I suppose the same thing can be said for growth hormone. It was largely for this reason that I chose to put them in terms of the hormones themselves rather than in terms of the releasing factors. However, the point is still correct and a growth hormone releasing factor is involved. Our situation with CRF is a rather unique one.

The question of the site of action of these compounds is an interesting one. It will probably interest the rest of the audience to hear what conclusions can be drawn about possible sites of action of the aminergic substances.

Point 1 is that I can make a broad general statement and say that there is no good evidence for either norepinephrine or dopamine, injected into the portal vessels in physiological amounts, leading to changes in pituitary secretion, at least as far as the anterior pituitary hormones are concerned. If you give large doses of dopamine and incubate dopamine with the anterior pituitary, it will activate ACTH or activate FSH and LH but this is a chemical reaction which appears to be totally out of the range of anything physiologically significant. I think it is unlikely that the catecholamines are liberated into the portal vessels. They could be acting at the endings of releasing factors secreting neurons, if neurons could secrete releasing factors. The possibility of ionic mechanisms acting like presynaptic inhibition such as at the spinal cord level, is an attractive one because we know that the dopaminergic endings are very abundant in the median eminence. If dopamine is not acting directly on the pituitary then one would more or less expect it is acting somewhere at the endings of the neurons which are liberating the releasing factors. But there are some problems here too.

We know that the median eminence itself, its ventral portion, is outside of the blood–brain barrier. Why then do not systemically administered substances have an inhibitory effect? I think that this point has not received as much attention as it deserves. This suggests that the site of action of nor-epinephrine and probably also of dopamine is well up from the ventral median eminence region, some-what higher in the hypothalamus. Now you are correctly implying that on the basis of our intraven-tricular injection experiments we have no evidence to say that this site of action is hypothalamic. It could be anywhere along the wall of the third ventricle. Presumably the material sweeps into the fourth ventricle and from there to the foramen of Luschka. However, we also did experiments in which we stimulated points in the brain stem and administered a sympathomimetic agent studying the effect of stimulation on ACTH secretion before and after administration of the drugs. The only place we found where stimulation would overcome the inhibition was in the hypothalamus. So this suggests, although it does not prove, that the site of action of this aminergic compound and catecholamine releasing substance is probably at the level of the hypothalamus.

Now it is possible that the adrenergic inhibition is diffuse and is acting somewhere in the midbrain, but another point is that, in addition to stimulating ascending pathways in our brain stem stimulation studies, we also carried out stimulation studies in the limbic system. We showed that amygdala stimulation would increase ACTH secretion and that the response to stimulation of the amygdala was also blocked by sympathomimetic agents. It is entirely possible of course that there are many sites of aminergic inhibition on all of these incoming pathways but I think it would be better if there were single sites. Where I am leading up to is that all the data presently available are consistent with, but far from proving, the theory that there are adrenergic synapses directly on the neurons which liberate the releasing factors.

Your last point about atropine I cannot directly answer at the moment, but it is entirely possible that our atropine did not reach the particular point where your crystalline implants had this effect on CRF secretion. I think the atropine was acting in the third ventricle because the needle was put down just over the median eminence where the compound was injected. At least in this area there should be a high concentration. Evidence was presented showing that very little of various substances was taken up by the median eminence; instead the material acted laterally in the region around the median eminence.

HAYWARD: The problem of intraventricular injection is probably as difficult as placing substances within the brain itself. In terms of my own area of interest concerning the neurohypophysis and osmo-reception, the intraventricular routes have been used to study in a convenient way the nervous system. Experiments that have been done to test the physiological routes are twofold. Thinking about the hypothalamus one route would be by way of the vascular system. The second would be by way of the ventricular system. At the Munich meeting two papers were presented, one by Sawyer and his group where they injected LRF, the releasing factor for LH, into the ventricle and into the vascular system. And as I recall the doses for the vascular route were considerably lower to get a release of LH than in the ventricular route. So from this system at least it seemed as if the vascular route reaches the effective sites in the pituitary system more easily. The second paper was by Feldberg and his group who studied the intraventricular route extensively in thermoregulation. They now use a substance that is released from leucocytes and produces fever in mammals. This substance circulates to the hypothalamus and it causes fever. Feldberg and his group injected this substance into the ventricle and into the vascular system and again found that with vascular injection a lower amount of the substance was needed to produce the same amount of temperature rise. So these are some of the early experiments that begin to assess a ventricular approach physiologically versus a vascular route. The reason I discuss this is that the ventricular approach is a very convenient one to study the hypothalamus. I am sure Sir Francis Knowles and others will discuss this problem. To relate pharmacological data to physiological systems is not easy.

GANONG: Just to add to what you said: TRF has also been injected into the ventricle and has been found no more effective upon third ventricular injection than it is upon administration into the vas-cular system. Again fitting with the concept there is not any very rapid transport out of the ventricular system but I think we are going to hear more about this later.

DE WIED: I just want to ask you about the drug phenoxybenzamine. When did you study the effect of stress on the influence of this particular drug?

GANONG: This drug is given by a loading dose and a constant infusion. As I remember testing starts half an hour later.

DE WIED: You never tried to study, because it is quite a long duration of action, the effect, *e.g.*, 24 hours after the administration?
The entire cholinergic effect of this drug might disappear after about such a time.

GANONG: No, we did not perform such an experiment but it is an interesting idea.

DREIFUSS: I just want to come back to the supraoptic and paraventricular neurons; it has already been said that microiontophoretic application of norepinephrine seems to inhibit these neurons and although we have not done any studies of this type, there are two other papers that come to my mind that confirm this. Cross and some of his collaborators have published a short note presenting the data at one of the meetings of the Physiological Society in England. They found that the supraoptic and paraventricular neurons were again inhibited by norepinephrine. There is also an old paper by Pickford and collaborators in which epinephrine this time was injected prior to an injection of acetylcholine. The second injection was an excitant and the epinephrine inhibited the effect of acetylcholine. I just want to add that I also feel that vasopressin and oxytocin should belong to the other side of the table.

GANONG: I just wanted to stimulate the discussion. I am not an expert in the field, but I thought that there were some conflicting results about the effects of norepinephrine on supraoptic neurons.

DREIFUSS: There is some problem with acetylcholine. Some people have not found the inhibitory effect of acetylcholine. I think there is no dispute as far as norepinephrine is concerned.

VAN REES: Please would you give some comments on some inhibitory effects of serotonin, because it has been shown that inhibition of ovulation occurs by neon light due to increase of serotonin levels at the site of the hypothalamus. Do you know of any other evidence about the other pituitary hormones?

GANONG: There is a considerable piece of evidence indicating that serotonin and possibly other indole amines may exert effects on pituitary secretion, particularly on gonadotropins. According to Fuxe and associates, however, there are relatively few endings that contain serotonin in the ventral hypothalamus. Most of them seem to sweep forward in the dorsal hypothalamus and distribute to other areas in the brain but it is still possible that serotonin may play some role.

LEENEN: Dr. Ganong, you found a difference in the effects of phenoxybenzamine and pentolamine on ACTH secretion. I think you can find the same difference in effect on renin secretion because it has been shown by the group of Pesca in Vienna that pentolamine can cause an increased release of renin 5 times higher or something like that in rats, whereas you could not find any change after the phenoxybenzamine injection.

GANONG: Excuse me, I may not have phrased it correctly but phenoxybenzamine potentiates the response to hypoglycemia in data I did not show. If one gives a big dose of phenoxybenzamine to an anaesthetized animal one knocks out the peripheral receptors and the blood pressure of course falls. Now we have been able to show that blood pressure drops because rise in renin is totally blocked by the drug I mentioned.

BATTA: You have shown one table indicating that administration of catecholamines does effect the release of LH. Is there any difference in ovulation in rabbits.

GANONG: I don't know. Perhaps anybody else? This is not my work.

SMELIK: Perhaps I might come back to one aspect: You said that one of the problems was that the substances do not act when you give them systemically. So you concluded that perhaps this means that the site of action is outside the blood–brain barrier. If I go back to atropine again, of course if you give atropine systemically it also does not block. There are some indications because of the work of Krieger in the cat, that it might block or have some effect on the control of ACTH because it blocks the diurnal rhythm. This might mean that the circadian rhythm has a greater sensitivity to its blocking action than the stress inducing release of this substance. In other words I think that the fact that systemic injection works, does not need to mean that the site of action is outside the blood–brain barrier. When we either implant or bring the substance into the hypothalamus using a micro-injection we have a much higher local concentration than I think we ever can get systemically. Another point is, and I would like to hear your comment on this, that, if you look at pictures of the fluorescent–histochemical preparations, you see fluorescent fibres everywhere in the hypothalamus which are supposed to be adrenergic. I think this is not true for acetylcholine because as far as I can remember cholinesterase is concentrated in a few small areas of the hypothalamus one of them being the supra-optic nucleus, while another one is more dorsal to it. I do not know whether this is the region of the paraventricular nucleus or not. I am wondering whether, if there is any adrenergic inhibition, this could be due to a more diffuse effect on the whole hypothalamic area or on mechanisms which are much more diffuse than, for instance, in the case of the atropine effect which suggests to me that there might be a cholinergic synapse on the cell bodies of the CRF neurons. If this is true you would expect a localized effect and then implants of noradrenaline and of atropine would certainly have an effect. It could be that there is still a difference between the two. The only thing is that I do not know how to think about such a very diffuse effect without a special localized action and I do not know how you or anybody else thinks about all these noradrenergic fibres which you see everywhere in the hypothalamus and which do not seem to end specifically on certain cells.

GANONG: Two points: one about atropine not working systemically. This is interesting, particularly because I believe that atropine does get into the brain. I am surprised that it does not produce inhibition of ACTH secretion. There is considerable pharmacological evidence that atropine does act centrally but it may not act centrally as well as the others. The point that I made, however, concerns the amines which we know are crossing the blood–brain barrier poorly if at all. If we administer them directly into the arterial blood supply going to the median eminence, they do not produce the expected change in the secretion of the particular pituitary hormones.

This is a piece of evidence which makes me lean toward a more dorsal site of action. The point about the fluorescence in the hypothalamus is correct; I am not sure that I go as far as you saying that there is no localization. Some centres are more innervated than others, but Fuxe himself has made the point effectively that this is a diffuse system. I could comment better on this question of endings on the CRF secretory neurons if I knew where they were. But I would like to emphasize this point about systemical injection versus either intraventricular injection or implants. Perhaps I may get reaction from the audience because this bothers me as far as postulated dopaminergic systems are concerned. The dopamine in the hypothalamus is almost exclusively well-localized in those arcuate neurons that end around the portal vessels. This area should be penetrated by systemically administered compounds and yet I think uniformly in one laboratory and another these compounds were not found to be active. This makes me wonder whether dopamine in the experiments where it is given in the ventricles is acting higher up. If that is true then that leaves us with nothing for the dopaminergic neurons to do.

Neurophysin

JOHAN F. JONGKIND

Netherlands Central Institute for Brain Research, Amsterdam (The Netherlands)

INTRODUCTION

Morphological investigations into the presence and function of neurosecretory systems were greatly stimulated by the introduction of Gomori's chrome-alum haematoxylin technique by Bargmann (1949). A microscopical comparison of this rather aspecific staining technique with those selectively demonstrating protein-bound cystine suggested that both, aspecific and specific methods, stained identical substances present in the mammalian hypothalamo-neurohypophysial system (HNS) (Sloper, 1966; Gabe, 1966a).

As for the specific nature of the substance demonstrated by these staining techniques some controversy exists. Truly, the hormonal principles vasopressin and oxytocin are somewhat richer in cystine than the carrier protein. However, histochemical investigations (for a review see: Adams, 1965) and the consideration that the preservation of small peptides such as vasotocin, vasopressin and oxytocin is improbable due to the conditions of histological fixation (Gabe, 1966b) pointed to the carrier protein as responsible for the staining reactions in the HNS.

Not only has this carrier protein played a major role in morphological studies of neurosecretory phenomena, but in biochemical investigations of the HNS as well has this remarkable protein with its specific hormone-binding properties been used as an analytical tool.

In the present paper dealing especially with the analytical use of neurophysin no attempt will be made to cover all the literature on the chemistry of this carrier protein. For this subject and for the general biochemistry of the HNS, the reader is referred to the reviews by Sachs (1969, 1970) and Ginsburg (1968).

'ACHER'S' NEUROPHYSIN

Chemical studies on neurohypophysial proteins and hormones started with the isolation of a protein fraction from bovine posterior pituary glands with oxytocic, vasopressor and antidiuretic activities (Van Dyke *et al.*, 1941). Using electrodialysis, Acher *et al.* (1956) were able to dissociate the hormonal principles from the protein. They concluded that the 'Van Dyke' protein was a complex compound consisting of two active peptides and at least one inactive carrier protein for which they suggested the name 'neurophysin'. In the course of their studies, Acher and collaborators could demonstrate that the dissociation of the hormonal principles from the Van Dyke protein could also be accomplished easily by relatively mild procedures such as countercurrent distribution, and dialysis against dilute acids. On the other hand, the protein–hormone complex was resistant to simple dialysis with water, ultrafiltration or precipitation by strong solutions of sodium chloride. These techniques, together with ion exchange chromatography, were used in the purification of the active hormonal peptides and neurophysin from other peptides and proteins of the bovine neurohypophysis (Acher *et al.*, 1958). This isolation and purification scheme is schematically shown in Fig. 1a, b.

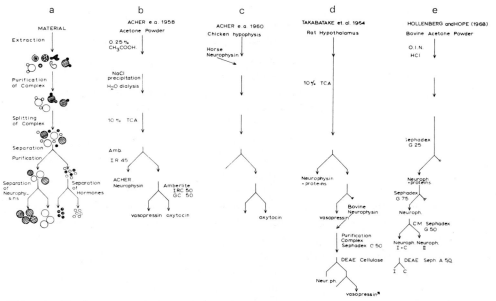

Fig. 1. Purification and application schemes for neurophysin. a, Schematical representation of the different purification steps. b, Isolation procedure of Acher, Light and de Vigneaud (1958). c, Application of horse neurophysin in the isolation procedure of chicken oxytocin (Acher, Chauvet and Lenci, 1960). d, Application of bovine neurophysin in the isolation of radioactive vasopressin (Takabatake and Sachs, 1964). e, Isolation procedure of Hollenberg and Hope (1968).

The first use of the specific binding properties of neurophysin was made by Acher and co-workers in order to isolate the neurohypophysial hormones of various mammals (Chauvet *et al.*, 1960a) and other classes of vertebrates (Acher *et al.*, 1960a; Acher *et al.*, 1960b; Acher *et al.*, 1965). The introduction of ovine neurophysin was necessary since the species-specific neurophysins did not precipitate in the original purification procedure (Fig. 1b, c). A drawback of the method is the introduction of foreign hormones by using impure neurophysin. An example of this phenomenon is given in the study of Chauvet *et al.* (1960b) which reported the isolation of two 'vasopressins' in the fowl extract to which horse neurophysin has been added to facilitate precipitation. Avian Vasopressin II contained the amino acids of arginine vasopressin, a conclusion which seemed, however, to be ruled out by the pharmaco-logical and chromatographic studies of Munsick et al. (1960).

Acher's neurophysin has been used extensively as an analytical tool in the radio-active tracer studies of Sachs and collaborators. Since the hypothalamic vasopressin content is very low (about 2 % of that present in the neurohypophysis), the introduc-tion of the carrier protein in the isolation procedure of radioactive vasopressin (Fig. 1d) was an ingenious tool to isolate submicrogram quantities of labeled hormone from the large hypothalamic pool of radioactive impurities (Takabatake and Sachs, 1964). In the hands of these authors, the purification method had a vasopressin recovery of 30%; the labeled hormone represented 10^{-4} of the counts originally present in the hypothalamus.

Many important conclusions were drawn from in vitro experiments with hypo-thalamic median eminence slices and intact hypothalamo-neurohypophysial tissue of the guinea pig (Takabatake and Sachs, 1964). The in vitro synthesis of vasopressin showed a lag phase of approximately $1-1\frac{1}{2}$ h, which could not be attributed to a general failure of synthetizing activity since the radioactivity was incorporated in the TCA-insoluble proteins during this lag phase. The failure of vasopressin synthesis during the first hour was explained by supposing that first, an inactive vasopressin precursor molecule is formed. In contrast with the isolated hypothalamus, it appeared that, in the isolated neurohypophysis, no vasopressin synthesis occurs.

The in vivo pretreatment of the animals was reflected in the in vitro hypothalamic vasopressin synthesis, as was also shown by Takabatake and Sachs (1964). A thirsting period of 4 days resulted in the incorporation of about a double amount of $[^{35}S]$-cysteine into vasopressin. Similar in vitro work with slices of canine hypothalami, however, failed to label vasopressin (Sachs and Takabatake, 1964), while no detectable increase in in vitro vasopressin biosynthesis occurred after in vivo stimulation by hemorrhage (Sachs et al., 1967).

Sachs and Haller (1968) also used Acher's neurophysin as an isolating tool to prove a compartmentation in neurohypophysial vasopressin. In their in vitro work on isolated dog posterior lobes they were able to show, that under basal conditions of incubation the secreted hormone, labelled by an elaborate in vivo scheme, had a specific activity which was somewhat less than that of the hormone remaining in the gland. After raising the potassium concentration in the medium, the $[^{35}S]$vasopressin secreted had a specific activity of 1.6–2.4 times that of the hormone remaining in the tissue.

'OXFORD' NEUROPHYSIN

The introduction of gel electrophoresis as a new analytical technique, introduced between 1960 and 1970, made it doubtful that Acher's bovine neurophysin was homogeneous. As many as 4 different fractions could be isolated, all of which bind oxytocin and vasopressin with almost equal affinity (Breslow and Abrash, 1966). Comparing the results of gel electrophoretic studies of Acher's protein with those obtained from the proteins of isolated bovine neurosecretory granules (Dean et al.,

1967) it was revealed that none of the proteins in Acher's 'protein' was identical with the two major protein components present in these organelles. Since the components, absent from the neurosecretory granules, could not be detected in any other subcellular fraction of the neurohypophysis, it was evident that the composition of neurophysin changes during the isolation procedure. Formation of artifacts during this procedure could be avoided by destroying the activity of protein-splitting enzymes by means of acid treatment (pH 1.6) of the acetone-desiccated glands. A raise in pH to 3.9 resulted in an increase in the number of electrophoretically distinct components (Dean et al., 1967).

This improved isolation procedure of Dean, Hollenberg and Hope (see Fig. 1e) must be considered an important milestone in the application of the neurophysins as a more specific analytical tool. The first experiments with these now purified substances were directed to the question of specific hormone-binding properties. Binding experiments with vasopressin and oxytocin, however, indicated that both hormones could equally well associate with either of the three bovine neurophysins (Hollenberg and Hope, 1968; Hope and Hollenberg, 1968; Rauch et al., 1969). Although, at that time, it was not possible to define the role of the different neurophysins, it was felt that they should have different roles; one might be responsible for the transport and storage of oxytocin, the other for that of vasopressin and the third (Neurophysin C), present in much smaller quantities, might be bound in vivo to another related peptide. The only study directed to the question of the binding properties of the neurophysins in vivo is rather conclusive about the specific roles of these proteins (Dean et al., 1968). Equilibrium-density centrifugation of neurosecretory granules showed evidence that neurophysin I and oxytocin are stored together in neurosecretory granules which are different from those which store neurophysin II and vasopressin. The difficulty of interpretation using this centrifugation technique is illustrated by comparing the results obtained by these authors with another study of this group (Dean and Hope, 1968), in which under identical circumstances completely different vasopressin and oxytocin distributions were obtained. Whether the third neurophysin, present in the bovine posterior lobe, is bound in vivo to a new oxytocic principle (Hope and Watkins, 1969) remains to be established.

Other studies with the now purified bovine neurophysins are relatively scarce. A significant contribution concerning the role of Ca^{++} in hormone–carrier dissociation was made by the optical rotary dispersion studies of Breslow (1970) utilizing bovine neurophysin II and oxytocin. Her data indicated, that, at pH 7.7, 10 mM Ca^{++} produced maximally only a twofold change in the affinity of bovine neurophysin II for oxytocin, a finding which sheds serious doubt on the suggestion that increase in Ca^{++} concentration in vivo plays a direct role in the release of oxytocin by dissociating the hormone–neurophysin complex. On the ground of the above-mentioned studies of Dean et al. (1968) it must, however, also be doubted whether neurophysin II and oxytocin are ever present together in the same neurosecretory vesicle. Therefore, the role of Ca^{++} as a dissociator of the carrier–hormone complex should be reinvestigated in the neurophysin I–oxytocin as well as in the neurophysin II–arginine vasopressin complex.

The latest contribution to the field of bovine neurophysins is the determination of the complete amino acid sequence of neurophysin II by Walter *et al.* (1971). The amino acid composition of this protein is close to that reported earlier by Hollenberg and Hope (1968).

One of the obvious difficulties in the application of purified bovine neurophysins seems to be that neither neurophysin I nor neurophysin II produce antibodies in the rabbit (Livett *et al.*, 1971).

PORCINE NEUROPHYSINS

In contrast with the neurophysins from bovine origin, the porcine carriers of hormones played a very important role in immunological applications. At this moment, three groups are working with antibodies against porcine neurophysins: Ginsburg and Jayasena (1968), Cheng and Friessen (1970, 1971), and Livett *et al.* (1971). The extraction procedures and purification schemes of the carrier proteins are, however, so varied that comparison of the results obtained by these three groups is not easy.

TABLE I

CROSS REACTIONS OF RABBIT ANTI-PORCINE NEUROPHYSIN SERA WITH PROTEINS

	Anti-porcine neurophysin (Ginsburg et al., 1968)	*Anti-porcine peptide II (Cheng and Friessen, 1970, 1971)*	*Anti-porcine peptide III (Cheng and Friessen, 1970, 1971)*	*Anti-porcine neurophysin II (Uttenthal et al., 1971)*
neurophysin I				−
peptide II		+	+	
neurophysin II				+
peptide III		+	+	
rat neurohypophysis	−	+	+	
bovine neurohypophysis	−	+	+	−
guinea pig neurohypophysis	−	+	+	
rabbit neurohypophysis		+	+	
canine neurohypophysis		+	+	
monkey neurohypophysis		+	+	
ovine neurohypophysis		+	+	
human neurohypophysis		+	+	
porcine liver	−	−	−	
porcine spleen	−	−	−	
porcine kidney	+	+	+	−
porcine uterus	+			
porcine mammary gland	+			
porcine brain	−			
porcine skeletal muscle	∼			
porcine serum	+	+	+	
porcine small intestine		−	−	
porcine colon		−	−	

Furthermore, no extensive investigations have been carried out concerning the question as to the optimal extraction procedure, as was done in the case of the neuro-physins of bovine origin. Thus, the significance of the results obtained must be considered with some caution.

The nonidentity of the rabbit anti-porcine neurophysin sera of the different groups is perhaps best indicated by comparing the cross reactions of these antisera with other proteins (Table I).

A comparison of the amino acid composition of the antigens, used by the above-mentioned authors, indicates that porcine neurophysin I (Uttenthal and Hope, 1970) is probably identical with peptide II used by Cheng and Friessen (Rudman et al., 1970). The identity of peptide III with porcine neurophysin II is not yet established.

By using the antibody against peptide III, which seemed to be a sensitive system for peptide II (neurophysin I), Cheng and Friessen (1970) estimated the normal neurophysin levels in pig and rat plasma to be around 5 ng/ml. Under a variety of experimental conditions leading to blood volume depletion or to an increase in serum osmolality, conditions which are known to increase the vasopressin release from the neurohypophysis, neurophysin concentration in the plasma was also shown to be raised considerably (Cheng and Friessen, 1970) indicating an increased concomitant release of vasopressin and neurophysin. This finding was supported by studies on the *in vitro* release of neurophysin in rat (Cheng and Friessen, 1970) and porcine (Utten-thal et al., 1971) neurohypophysis, which showed a steep increase during incubation in a high potassium Locke.

The radioimmunoassay was also used to determine the neurophysin content of the different compartments of the porcine HNS (Cheng and Friessen, 1971). The hypo-thalamic amount of neurophysin, which was very low (0.4 μg), proved to be 2% of the stalk neurohypophysial content, a distribution which is comparable with that of vasopressin.

The aspecific staining methods that started morphological research on the HNS have got a most specific immunological successor as demonstrated by the immuno-fluorescence studies of Livett et al. (1971). These authors showed that an antibody against porcine neurophysin II reacts nearly exclusively with proteins in the supra-optic nucleus, median eminence and neurohypophysis, a finding which is highly suggestive of the association of this neurophysin with lysine vasopressin in the supra-optic nucleus of the pig.

In the near future this immunohistochemical staining method will surely be used by electron microscopists. Techniques are now available to make antibodies sufficiently electron opaque without destroying their immunological reactivity. The study of synthesis, storage and secretion of neurophysins at the ultrastructural level will be a most fascinating subject in the coming years.

REFERENCES

ACHER, R., CHAUVET, J., CHAUVET, M. T. ET CREPY, D. (1965) Phylogénie des peptides neuro-hypophysaires: Isolement d'une nouvelle hormone, la glumitocine (Ser^4-Gln^8-oxytocine) présenté chez un poisson cartilagineux, la raie *(Raia clavata)*. Biochim. biophys. Acta *(Amst.)*, **107**, 393–396.

ACHER, R., CHAUVET, J. AND LENCI, M. T. (1960a) Isolement de l'oxytocine du poulet. *Biochim. biophys. Acta (Amst.)*, **38**, 344–345.

ACHER, R., CHAUVET, J., LENCI, M. T., MOREL, F. ET MAETZ, J. (1960b) Présence d'une vasotocine dans la neurohypophyse de la grenouille. *Biochim. biophys. Acta (Amst.)*, **42**, 379–380.

ACHER, R., CHAUVET, J. ET OLIVRY, G. (1956) Sur l'existence éventuelle d'un hormone unique neurohypophysaire. Relation entre l'ocytocine la vasopressine et la protéine de Van Dyke extraites de la neurohypophyse de boeuf. *Biochim. biophys. Acta (Amst.)*, **22**, 421–427.

ACHER, R., LIGHT, A. AND DU VIGNEAUD, V. (1958) Purification of oxytocin and vasopressin by way of a protein complex. *J. biol. Chem.*, **233**, 116–120.

ADAMS, C. W. M. (1965) *Neurohistochemistry*, Elsevier, Amsterdam, p. 310.

BARGMANN, W. (1949) Über die neurosekretorische Verknüpfung von Hypothalamus und Neurohypophyse. *Z. Zellforsch.*, **34**, 610–634.

BRESLOW, E. (1970) Optical activity of bovine neurophysins and their peptide complexes in the near ultraviolet. *Proc. nat. Acad. Sci. (Wash.)*, **67**, 493–500.

BRESLOW, E. AND ABRASH, L. (1966) The binding of oxytocin and oxytocin analogues by purified bovine neurophysins. *Proc. nat. Acad. Sci. (Wash.)*, **56**, 640–646.

CHAUVET, A., LENCI, M. T. ET ACHER, R. (1960a) L'oxytocine et la vasopressine du mouton: Reconstruction d'un complexe hormonal actif. *Biochim. biophys. Acta (Amst.)*, **38**, 266–272.

CHAUVET, A., LENCI, M. T. ET ACHER, R. (1960b) Présence de deux vasopressines dans la neurohypophyse du poulet. *Biochim. biophys. Acta (Amst.)*, **38**, 571–573.

CHENG, K. W. AND FRIESSEN, H. G. (1970) Physiological factors regulating secretion of neurophysin. *Metabolism*, **19**, 876–890.

CHENG, K. W. AND FRIESSEN, H. G. (1971) A radioimmunoassay for vasopressin binding proteins—Neurophysin. *Endocrinology*, **88**, 608–619.

DEAN, C. R., HOLLENBERG, M. D. AND HOPE, D. B. (1967) The relationship between neurophysin and the soluble proteins of pituitary neurosecretory granules. *Biochem. J.*, **104**, 8C–10C.

DEAN, C. R. AND HOPE, D. B. (1968) The isolation of Neurophysin-I and II from bovine pituitary neurosecretory granules separated on a large scale from other subcellular organelles. *Biochem. J.*, **106**, 565–573.

DEAN, C. R., HOPE, D. B. and KAŽIĆ, T. (1968) Evidence for the storage of oxytocin with neurophysin-I and of vasopressin with neurophysin-II in separate neurosecretory granules. *Brit. J. Pharmacol.*, **34**, 192P–193P.

GABE, M. (1966a) *Neurosecretion*, Pergamon Press, Oxford, p. 25.

GABE, M. (1966b) *Neurosecretion*, Pergamon Press, Oxford, p. 615.

GINSBURG, M. (1968) Production, release, transportation and elimination of the neurohypophyseal hormones. In *Neurohypophyseal Hormones and Similar Polypeptides, Handbook of Experimental Pharmacology, Vol. 23*, B. BERDE (Ed.), Springer, Berlin, p. 286.

GINSBURG, M. AND JAYASENA, K. (1968) The occurrence of antigen reacting with antibody to porcine neurophysin. *J. Physiol. (Lond.)*, **197**, 53–63.

HOLLENBERG, M. D. AND HOPE, D. B. (1968). The isolation of the native hormone-binding proteins from the bovine pituitary posterior lobes. Crystallization of Neurophysin-I and -II complexes with (8-arginine)-vasopressin. *Biochem. J.*, **106**, 557–564.

HOPE, D. B. AND HOLLENBERG, M. D. (1968) Crystallization of complexes of neurophysins with vasopressin and oxytocin. *Proc. roy. Soc. B.*, **170**, 37–47.

HOPE, D. B. AND WATKINS, W. B. (1969) Isolation of a new oxytocic peptide from bovine posterior pituitary lobes. *Brit. J. Pharmacol.*, **37**, 533P–535P.

LIVETT, B. G., UTTENTHAL, L. O. AND HOPE, D. B. (1971) Localization of neurophysin-II in the hypothalamo-neurohypophyseal system of the pig by immunofluorescence histochemistry. *Phil. Trans. B.*, **261**, 371–378.

MUNSICK, R. A., SAWYER, W. H. AND VAN DYKE, H. B. (1960) Avian neurohypophyseal hormones: pharmacological properties and tentative identification. *Endocrinology*, **66**, 860–871.

RAUCH, R., HOLLENBERG, M. D. AND HOPE, D. B. (1969) Isolation of a third bovine neurophysin. *Biochem. J.*, **115**, 473–479.

RUDMAN, D., DEL RIO, A. E., GARCIA, L. A., BARNETT, J., HOWARD, C. H., WALKER, W. AND MOORE, G. (1970) Isolation of two lipolytic pituitary peptides. *Biochemistry*, **9**, 99–107.

SACHS, H. (1969) Neurosecretion. *Advanc. Enzymol.*, **32**, 327–372.

SACHS, H. (1970) Neurosecretion. In *Handbook of Neurochemistry, Vol. IV*, A. LAJTHA (Ed.), Plenum Press, New York, 1970, p. 373.

Hormonal Regulation of Rat Brain Development
II. Biochemical Changes Induced by β-Estradiol

CARLO CAVALLOTTI AND LUIGI BISANTI

Department of Anatomy, Università Cattolica del S. Cuore, 00168 Rome (Italy)

INTRODUCTION

Various hormones may modify brain activity during the early stages of development as well as after complete maturation of the central nervous system (Harris, 1964; Dörner and Döcke, 1966; Arai and Kusuma, 1967; Chowers *et al.*, 1967; Martini, 1969).

The neonatal rat brain is a unique object for the study of neuronal maturation because it is comparatively immature at birth, maturing gradually in the course of postnatal life within a short well-defined period, when structural, biochemical, functional and behavioural changes are observed (Himwich, 1951, 1962; Jilek and Fischer, 1965; Patel and Balazs, 1968; Kollros, 1968). Estrogen treatment modifies the development, growth and maturation of neonatal rat brain (Heim and Timiras, 1963; Casper *et al.*, 1967; Dörner, 1970; McEwen and Pfaff, 1970; Dörner *et al.*, 1971).

The present report deals with changes induced by β-estradiol treatment during rat brain development in water and protein content as well as in lipid composition and in glycoproteins. Moreover, some specific and glycolytic enzymatic activities have been studied during rat brain development.

These investigations will provide a basis for further studies on some electrophysiological parameters and behavioural manifestations of rat brain activity.

MATERIALS AND METHODS

Treatment of animals

Ten litters of female Sprague–Dawley rats, 1–28 days of age, were used. Each litter consisted of 8 females kept with their lactating mothers until sacrificed. The experimental groups consisted of a normal control group, a β-estradiol-treated group, an ovariectomized group and a similar group receiving a replacement therapy with β-estradiol.

Normal control group. In each litter two animals served as controls. They were sham-operated and injected with the vehicle alone.

References p. 82

RESULTS

Effect of experimental treatment. All animals were autopsied after being sacrificed in order to demonstrate the efficiency of the experimental treatments. In estrogenized rats the ovaries were studied in 5 μm thick serial sections stained with hematoxylin and eosin. Controls were made in castrated rats to exclude an incomplete ovariectomy. Animals of both groups with unclear pictures were rejected from the experiment.

Body weight. Data obtained in all experimental groups are shown in Fig. 1. As can be seen, β-estradiol treatment results in a statistically significant increase of body weight, while in ovariectomized rats this was slightly reduced. At 21 days of age the gap between the treated groups and the control group is larger. Replacement therapy with β-estradiol in ovariectomized animals restores the normal level of body weight.

Brain weight. Fig. 2 shows statistically significant differences between the brain weights of normal and β-estradiol-treated animals. Ovariectomy, performed 14 days after birth, induces a slight decrease of brain weight. Replacement therapy with β-estradiol after ovariectomy restores brain weight to the normal level. It is evident

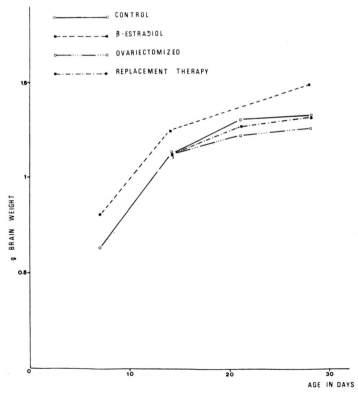

Fig. 2. Effect of β-estradiol on the brain weight of rat. Experimental conditions as in Fig. 1.

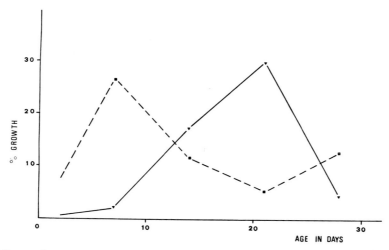

Fig. 3. Effect of β-estradiol on the growth of rat. The mean values are expressed as percentage of that in the normals. Triangles: body weight; squares: brain weight.

from Fig. 3 that there are no significant correlations between the increases of body and brain weight induced by β-estradiol treatment.

Dry weight and water content of brain. Values for dry weight were expressed as mg/g tissue. As can be seen in Fig. 4, estrogen treatment results in an increase of dry weight and in a decrease of brain water content. In contrast, ovariectomy induces a decrease in dry weight and an increase in water content. β-Estradiol treatment in ovariectomized animals restores normal values.

Protein. In Fig. 4 the protein contents of developing rat brain are shown in the 4 experimental groups. As can be seen in the normal control rats, one gram of brain tissue contains approximatively 50 mg protein during the first 7 days of age. Between the 14th and 21st day of age brain proteins amount to 105–135 mg/g tissue. At 28 days of age this value is about 150 mg/g wet tissue. In β-estradiol-treated animals the protein content of cerebral tissue was slightly but significantly increased, while in ovariectomized rats it was reduced. Replacement therapy with β-estradiol restores normal content of proteins in brain tissue.

The results of this series reveal the following facts: (i) body and brain weights were slightly higher in the estradiol-treated animals and slightly lower in the ovariectomized rats; (ii) dry weight of brain was higher after estradiol treatment and lower after ovariectomy; (iii) proteins were increased in β-estradiol-treated animals while they were reduced in ovariectomized rats.

Lipids. Data reported in Fig. 4 include total lipids minus gangliosides, which were removed during washing of the lipids' extract. Therefore, they were determined as NANA. In normal rats lipids increase during development from 60 mg/g tissue in the

References p. 82

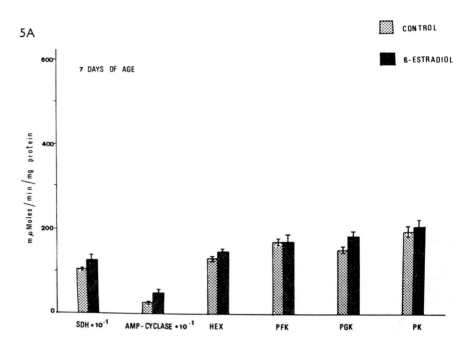

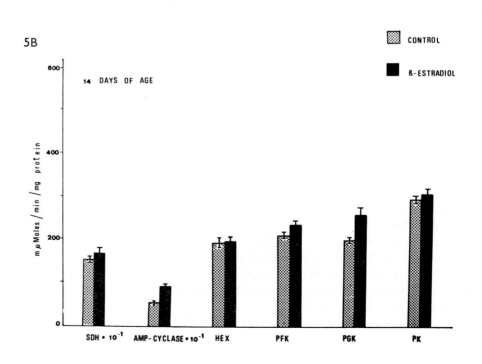

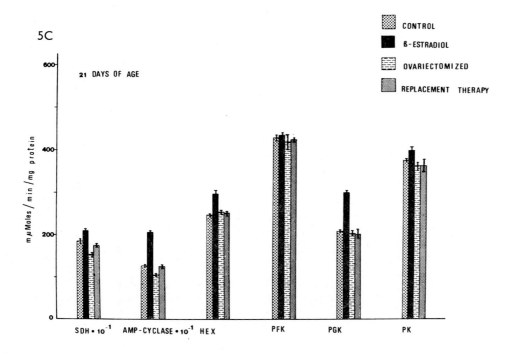

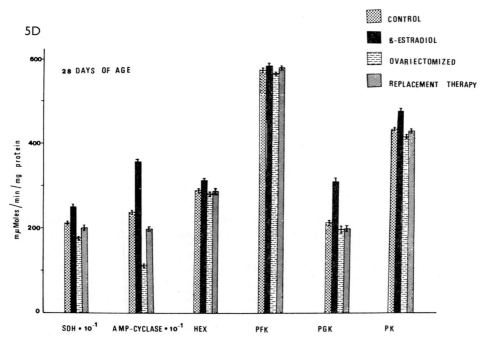

Fig. 5. Effect of β-estradiol on some enzymic activities of rat brain (mean $\pm$ S.E.M.; $P < 0.005$).

References p. 82

during rat brain development imply those of proteins, lipids, glycoproteins, glycolytic enzymes (kinases), and finally, enzymes involved in specific functions of nerve cells.

Proteins. β-Estradiol treatment induces an increased synthesis of proteins in the brain as well as in the uterus in order to produce specific estrogen-binding proteins required for β-estradiol action (Martini, 1969).

The biochemical study of the receptors that bind hormones to brain cells are, so far, unknown. It is expected that a correct knowledge of these hormonal receptors can clarify the hormone–brain relationship.

Lipids. The lipid concentration in the brain markedly increases during the period of early development parallel to myelination. In particular, cerebrosides and sulphatides are believed to be typical myelin lipids. The increase in lipids, cerebrosides and sulphatides after β-estradiol treatment suggests that the process of myelination is highly accelerated in these experimental conditions, while it is retarded after ovariectomy.

Enhanced myelination occurring at an early period of development after neonatal administration of β-estradiol may partly induce a precocious functional maturation of rat brain (Casper *et al.*, 1967).

Glycoproteins. The sensitivity to β-estradiol is not a special feature of the uterus. β-Estradiol treatment, for instance, induces in glycoproteins of brain the same modifications recently described by Iacobelli (1971) for cervical mucus of the uterus. Moreover, the ratio NANA/fucose was modified in β-estradiol-treated rats in the brain as well as in the uterus. On the basis of the evidence presently available it is difficult to explain the mechanism of action of β-estradiol on the brain. Nevertheless, the data obtained suggest that rat brain contains specific receptors for estrogens.

Glycolytic enzymes. Enzymes involved in glycolysis largely participate in metabolic energy production in nervous tissue. A detailed knowledge of phosphofructokinase in brain is particularly required since this enzyme, together with hexokinase, controls the energy-yielding reactions of the glycolytic pathway in rabbit brain (Miani *et al.*, 1969). 3-Phosphoglycerate kinase and pyruvate kinase participate in lipid metabolism and, therefore, their activity is stimulated after β-estradiol treatment. Both the enzymatic production of energy and lipid metabolism are an essential prerequisite for brain development; β-estradiol treatment and ovariectomy may modify these functions through a specific control on these enzymatic activities.

Enzymes involved in nervous functions. The enzymes investigated in the present study are distinctly related to morphological differentiation and functional adaptation of the brain. They exhibit an increased activity during the critical period of rat brain maturation under hormonal control. The levels of activity of all these enzymes are highly affected both by β-estradiol-treatment and by ovariectomy. Experimental treatment may control brain development by way of these specific changes.

AMP cyclase can be considered a receptor-enzyme system. Therefore, it plays an important role in the mechanism of action of several hormones. β-Estradiol treatment induces a greater increase in activity of this enzyme but it is not established whether estrogen hormones act on brain through AMP cyclase activity or by way of a specific receptor.

The above results indicate a clear relationship between β-estradiol levels and brain development which may be at the base of alterations observed in the electroencephalogram as well as in the patterns of behaviour and learning capacity of rat (Bisanti and Cavallotti, 1972).

Unfortunately it is difficult at the present time to bring all these biochemical data into a single comprehensive picture. Although differences have been observed both in β-estradiol-treated and in ovariectomized rats, the fundamental cortical developmental processes are essentially the same in all experimental groups. On the basis of the evidence presently available it is impossible to explain why β-estradiol treatment influences brain development. It is expected that further investigations will clarify the mechanism of action of hormones on rat brain development.

SUMMARY

The results of the experiments performed demonstrate that rat brain development is sensitive both to β-estradiol treatment and ovariectomy. Specific biochemical changes are induced by experimental treatment during the critical period of brain development.

The increase in body and brain weight induced by β-estradiol are not significantly correlated. Dry weight, proteins and lipids of developing brain vary interestingly under each hormonal condition. β-Estradiol treatment causes an increase of glycoproteins with inversion of the ratio NANA/fucose.

The values of cerebrosides and sulphatides are higher in the β-estradiol-treated rats than in controls, suggesting that hormones may influence the process of myelination which is very active at this period of age.

The activities of the following enzymes involved in the glycolytic pathway have been found modified under each hormonal condition: hexokinase, phosphofructokinase, 3-phosphoglycerate kinase and pyruvate kinase. Moreover succinate dehydrogenase, choline acetyltransferase, acetylcholinesterase and adenosine triphosphatase are enzymes directly involved in specific nerve cell functions and are highly affected both in β-estradiol-treated and in ovariectomized rats.

AMP cyclase plays an important role in hormone–brain relationships. The activity of this enzyme appears markedly stimulated by β-estradiol treatment, while it is unaffected by ovariectomy.

At present it is impossible to bring all biochemical data found into a single comprehensive picture. As yet, the specific mechanism by which the estrogen hormones exert their effects on brain development is unknown.

References p. 82

ACKNOWLEDGEMENTS

The authors are greatly indebted to Dr. N. Miani for his continuous encouragement and criticisms during this investigation.

REFERENCES

ARAI, I. AND KUSUMA, T. (1967) Effect of neonatal estrogen treatment on hypothalamic neurons and regulations of gonadotrophin secretion. *Anat. Record.*, **157**, 207–219.

BISANTI, L. AND CAVALLOTTI, C. (1972) Hormonal regulation of rat brain development. III. Effect of β-estradiol on electrical activity and behaviour. In *Progress in Brain Research, Vol. 38, Topics in Neuroendocrinology*, J. ARIËNS KAPPERS AND J. P. SCHADÉ (Eds.), Elsevier, Amsterdam, pp. 327–335.

BÜCHER, T. AND PFLEIDERER, G. (1955) In *Methods in Enzymology, Vol. I*, S. P. COLOWICK AND N. O. KAPLAN (Eds.), Academic Press, New York, p. 435.

BÜCHER, T. AND PFLEIDERER, G. (1955) *Methods in Enzymology*, S. P. COLOWICK AND N. O. KAPLAN (Eds.), *Vol. I*, Academic Press, New York, p. 435.

CASPER, R., VERNADAKIS, A. AND TIMIRAS, P. S. (1967) Influence of estradiol and cortisol on lipids and cerebrosides in the developing brain and spinal cord of the rat. *Brain Research*, **5**, 524–526.

CAVALLOTTI, C. (1968) Presenza di una attività ATPasi nella mielina purificata da nervo periferico. *Acta med. Romana*, **6**, 1–14.

CHOWERS, I., CONFORTI, N. AND FELDMAN, S. (1967) Effects of corticosteroids on hypothalamic corticotropin releasing factor and pituitary ACTH content. *Neuroendocrinology*, **2**, 193–199.

DÖRNER, G. (1970) The influence of sex hormones during the hypothalamic differentiation and maturation phases on gonadal function and sexual behaviour during the hypothalamic functional phase. *Endokrinologie*, **19**, 280–291.

DÖRNER, G. AND DÖCKE, F. (1966) The influence of intrahypothalamic and intrahypophysial implantation of estrogen or progesterone on gonadotrophin release. *Abstr. 2nd int. Congr. Hormonal Steroids*, Excerpta med. int. Congr. Ser., III, p. 194.

DÖRNER, G., DÖCKE, F. AND HINZ, G. (1971) Paradoxical effects of estrogen on brain differentiation. *Neuroendocrinology*, **7**, 146–155.

ELLMAN, G. L., COURTNEY, K. D., ANDRES, V. AND FEATHERSTONE, R. M. (1961) A new and rapid colorimetric determination of acetylcholinesterase activity. *Biochem. Pharmacol.*, **7**, 88–92.

FOLCH, J., LEES, M. AND SLOANE STANLEY, G. H. (1957) A simple method for the isolation and purification of total lipids from animal tissues. *J. biol. Chem.*, **226**, 497–509.

FONNUM, F. (1970) Surface charge of choline acetyltransferase from different species. *J. Neurochem.*, **17**, 1095–1100.

HARRIS, G. W. (1964) Sex hormones, brain development and brain function. *Endocrinology*, **75**, 627–648.

HAUSER, G. (1968) Cerebroside and sulphatide levels in developing rat brain. *J. Neurochem.*, **15**, 1237–1238.

HEIM, L. M. AND TIMIRAS, P. S. (1963) Gonad-brain relationship: Precocious brain maturation after estradiol in rats. *Endocrinology*, **72**, 598–606.

HEPP, K. D., EDEL, R. AND WIELAND, O. (1970) Hormone action on liver adenyl cyclase activity. *Europ. J. Biochem.*, **17**, 171–177.

HIMWICH, H. E. (1951) *Brain Metabolism and Cerebral Disorders*, Williams and Wilkins, Baltimore.

HIMWICH, W. A. (1962) Biochemical and neurophysiological development of the brain in the neonatal period. In *Int. Rev. Neurobiology, Vol. 4*, C. C. PFEIFFER AND J. R. SMYTHIES (Eds.), Academic Press, New York, London, pp. 117–158.

IACOBELLI, S. (1971) personal communication.

IACOBELLI, S. AND CAVALLOTTI, C. (1971) Hormonal regulation of rat brain development. I. Effect of thyroid hormones. *Biochem. J.*, in press.

JILEK, J. AND FISCHER, J. (1965) Development of LDH and SDH activities in various regions of the CNS in rats during ontogeny. *Acta Univ. Carol. Med. (Praha)*, Suppl. 21, 195–199.

KOLLROS, J. J. (1968) Endocrine influences in neural development. In *Growth of the Nervous System*, A Ciba Foundation Symposium, G. E. W. WOLSTENHOLME AND M. O'CONNOR (Eds.), Churchill, London, p. 179–199.

LOWRY, D. H., ROSENBROUGH, N. J., FARR, A. L. AND RANDALL, R. J. (1951) Protein measurement with the Folin-phenol reagent. *J. biol. Chem.*, **193**, 265–271.

MÅRTENSSON, E. (1963) Quantitative estimation of sulphates in lipid extracts. *Biochim. biophys. Acta (Amst.)*, **70**, 1–8.

MARTINI, L. (1969) Action of hormones on the central nervous system. *Gen. comp. Endocr.*, Suppl. 2, 214–226.

MCEWEN, B. S. AND PFAFF, D. W. (1970) Factors influencing sex hormone uptake by rat brain regions. I. Effect of neonatal treatment, hypophysectomy and competing steroid on estradiol uptake. *Brain Research*, **21**, 1–16.

MIANI, N., CAVALLOTTI, C. AND CANIGLIA, A. (1969) Synthesis of adenosine triphosphate by myelin of spinal nerves of rabbit. *J. Neurochem.* **16**, 249–260.

PATEL, A. J. AND BALAZS, R. (1968) Development of metabolic compartmentation in rat brain. *Biochem. J.*, **3**, 170.

RACKER, E. (1947) Enzymatic synthesis and breakdown of desoxyribose phosphate. *J. biol. Chem.*, **196**, 347–365.

SLATER, E. C. AND BONNER, W. D. (1952) The effect of fluoride on the succinic oxidase system. *Biochem. J.*, **52**, 185–197.

SPERRY, W. M. (1954) Method for determination of total lipids and water in brain tissue. *J. biol. Chem.*, **209**, 377–386.

SVENNERHOLM, L. (1956) The quantitative estimation of cerebrosides in nervous tissue. *J. Neurochem.*, **1**, 42–53.

SVENNERHOLM, L. (1957) Quantitative estimation of sialic acids. *Biochim. biophys. Acta (Amst.)*, **24**, 604–612.

Some Questions on the Nature and Function of Cranial and Caudal Neurosecretory Systems in Non-Mammalian Vertebrates

HOWARD A. BERN

Department of Zoology and its Cancer Research Genetics Laboratory,
University of California, Berkeley, Calif. 94720 (U.S.A.)

This brief overview of established neurosecretory systems in non-mammalian vertebrates will attempt to consider several questions (by no means all) that seem to deserve attention at the present time. The literature on these subjects is enormous, and only some of the most recent and most directly pertinent references will be cited.

1. How many distinct neurosecretory systems exist in non-mammalian vertebrates?

The answer to this question depends upon the clear recognition that the hypothalamic neurosecretory system is in fact a dual entity, even in piscine vertebrates (*cf.* Kobayashi and Matsui, 1969; Kobayashi *et al.*, 1970; Zambrano *et al.*, 1972). The well-recognized neurosecretory nuclei (paired preoptic in fishes and amphibians; paired supraoptic and paraventricular in amniotes) are apparently distinct from the less understood and often highly complex paired lateral tuberal nuclei in fishes and the largely undefined comparable nuclei in tetrapods (*cf.* Jørgensen, 1968). Neurosecretory tracts originating from the former nuclei terminate in the pars nervosa (neural lobe) of the hypophysis, and fibers from the latter terminate in the median eminence. Although the accepted terminology that refers to the anterior median eminence and the posterior pars nervosa as divisions of the neurohypophysis is anatomically useful, functionally it tends to detract from the concept of the separateness of the two hypothalamic systems. However, in non-teleostean bony fishes and amphibians (Rodríguez *et al.*, 1970) the preoptic fiber system may indeed contribute to median eminence function, judging from ultrastructural indications.

Thus, it is useful to recognize two distinct cranial neurosecretory systems. In addition, in some fish groups, notably teleosts and elasmobranchs, there is also a caudal neurosecretory system (Fridberg and Bern, 1968; Bern, 1969), located in the posterior spinal cord and projecting to a neurohemal zone at the base of the spinal cord, which is organized into a prominent urophysis in most teleost fishes.

There are other stainable neuronal groups and fiber tracts that have been described in various vertebrates, along with modified glandular ependymal areas. Whether any of these histologically defined areas is neurosecretory or ependymosecretory in a truly endocrine sense remains uncertain.

References p. 94

2. *Is control of adenohypophysial function by the median eminence a feature of all vertebrate brains?*

Until a short time ago, it was thought that a functional median eminence (*cf*. Knigge and Scott, 1970) controlling adenohypophysial secretion was characteristic of tetrapods and of only one piscine group, the lungfishes. Adenohypophysial control was considered to be accomplished primitively by 'neurosecretory innervation', with fibers from the hypothalamic nuclei projecting to various areas of the adenohypophysial complex. It now appears that a true median eminence may be absent only from the teleosts (*cf*. Perks, 1969), although functional division of the neurohypophysis may occur in the teleosts also, especially the more primitive ones (Henderson, 1969). Adenohypophysial control by nerve fibers, once considered 'primitive', seems more likely to be a specialization of the teleosts (*cf*. Zambrano *et al*., 1972). Evidence for the presence of a median eminence-like structure and of a hypophysial portal system connecting it with the adenohypophysis exists for the hagfish (Kobayashi and Uemura, 1972; but see Fernholm, 1972), elasmobranchs (albeit not for the important ventral lobe) (Meurling, 1967a), holocephalans (Jasinski and Gorbman, 1966; Meurling, 1967b) ganoids (Lagios, 1968, 1970; Hayashida and Lagios, 1969) and *Latimeria* (Lagios, 1972), as well as lungfishes and tetrapods (see also Jasinski).

From this last statement, one should not conclude that neurosecretory innervation is confined to teleosts, but only that it is likely that much of the adenohypophysis, pars distalis as well as pars intermedia, is so controlled in the advanced bony fishes.

3. *Is control of adenohypophysial function by neurosecretory innervation a feature of all vertebrate brains?*

As noted above, possible control of total adenohypophysial function by nerve fibers may occur in teleosts. The aminergic fibers (Knowles's type 'B', large granulated

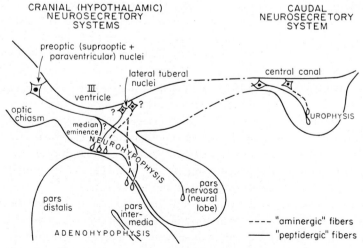

Fig. 1. Generalized diagram of vertebrate neurosecretory systems.

vesicle-, LGV-containing) from parts of the lateral tuberal nucleus and the peptidergic fibers (Knowles's type 'A', elementary neurosecretory granule-, ENG-containing) from the preoptic nucleus may both influence synthesis and release of all adenohypophysial hormones. Such fibers may end in direct contact with adenohypophysial cells, making non-synaptic or synaptoid 'junctions'; in intercellular spaces adjacent to the glandular cells; on basement membranes and even connective tissue 'capsules' separating them from the effector cells; on short blood vessels which may serve a portal role in transporting 'hypophysiotropins' to the adenohypophysis. In addition, at least the 'A'-type fibers may terminate on capillaries emptying into the venous drainage, thus forming a true neurohemal organ (the posterior part of the neurohypophysis) which would permit discharge of octapeptides (arginine vasotocin, isotocin) into the systemic circulation (*cf.* Henderson, 1969). Scharrer (1972, and this volume) has considered the variety of terminations open to fibers involved in regulation of effector cells.

Dual control of the fish pars intermedia, especially that of the elasmobranchs, has been well delineated, both type 'A' and type 'B' fibers appearing to participate. For the remainder of the adenohypophysial cell types (gonadotropes, thyrotropes, corticotropes, somatotropes and prolactin cells), type 'B' (presumably aminergic) inner-

TABLE I

OCCURRENCE OF 'NEUROSECRETORY INNERVATION' OF ADENOHYPOPHYSIS AND OF MEDIAN EMINENCE IN VERTEBRATES

Based on the recent studies of Kobayashi, Fernholm, Olsson, Knowles, Vollrath, Nishioka, Follenius, Jasinski, Meurling, Mellinger, Lagios, Zambrano, Henderson, Abraham, Kasuga, Urano, Iturriza, Rodríguez, Dierickx, Gorbman, Gabe, LaPointe, Pandalai, Bargmann, Anand Kumar, Belenky and others.

	Innervation of pars intermedia	Innervation of pars distalis	Median eminence and portal vessels
Cyclostomes			
Hagfishes	± ? occasional	−	+ ?
Lampreys	±	−	− ?
Ratfishes	+	−	+
Elasmobranchs	+	−	+*
Chondrosteans,			
Polypteriforms	+	−	+
Holosteans	+	±	+
Teleosts	+	± to +	−**
Lungfishes	+	+	+
Latimeria	+	?	+
Amphibians	+	− (some species +)	+
Reptiles	−†	−	+
Birds		−	+
Mammals	± (occasional)††	− (rare)	+

* Not to ventral lobe.
** Anterior neurohypophysis may serve as median eminence, especially in clupeiform.
† Control by portal transport from pars nervosa.
†† Especially in cat, ferret.

References p. 94

vation seems to be of major significance. Innervation of the pars intermedia, however, is not confined to fish groups, but extends to amphibians, where the innervation is similar to that seen in elasmobranchs and teleosts, and even to mammals (see Belenky *et al.*, 1970, for references). In the cat, synaptoid terminations of fibers upon pars intermedia cells are prominent. In reptiles, there are species where no nerve fibers enter the pars intermedia; however, the immediately adjacent pars nervosa could influence pars intermedia function by the diffusion, or even by the short vascular transport, of agents across the thin septum separating the two parts (Nayar and Pandalai, 1963; Rodríguez and LaPointe, 1970). This would still represent a kind of neurosecretory innervation such as seems to occur in the rostral pars distalis (corticotropes and prolactin cells) in some teleosts. In birds, no pars intermedia as such exists, and the neural lobe is totally separated from the pars distalis. Innervation of MSH-secreting cells, although unlikely, has neither been described nor denied.

Table I summarizes in a general fashion the information available on innervation of the adenohypophysis in the several vertebrate groups.

4. *Is the physiological nature of the hypothalamic control over adenohypophysial function the same in all vertebrates?*

This question is difficult to answer at present for two principal reasons. Firstly, although the mammalian adenohypophysial hormones are considered to be either under stimulatory control (gonadotropins, ACTH, STH, TSH) or under inhibitory control (prolactin, MSH), there is increasing evidence for dual control (especially in regard to prolactin and MSH). And some investigators feel that control over hormone synthesis and control over hormone release may be influenced by different factors. Secondly, the studies on non-mammalian vertebrates involving electrolytic lesions, ectopic transplantations, pharmacological treatments, etc., have been conducted on too few species to warrant the kind of generalization one would like to be able to make. For example, hypophysiotropic control over avian prolactin secretion is considered to be primarily stimulatory; however, in the duck, prolactin secretion seems to be regulated by an inhibitory factor (Tixier-Vidal and Gourdji, 1972), as in mammals. In teleosts and in amphibians, there may be varying degrees of autonomy of adenohypophysial function, depending upon the species investigated.

Some notable differences at the level of major taxa can be recorded, however. Thus, prolactin secretion in teleosts, amphibians and mammals does appear to be primarily under tonic inhibition from the hypothalamus; in reptiles and birds (except the duck) a stimulatory factor seems to be required. Thyrotropin secretion in teleosts seems also to be under tonic inhibition (Ball *et al.*, 1972), unlike the dependence on a stimulatory hypophysiotropin evident in most other vertebrates. Generalized differences in the control of the other hormones have not been noted, although autonomous secretion of various tropic hormones has been reported for species in several vertebrate groups (Jørgensen, 1968; Ball *et al.*, 1972). The primary control over MSH secretion seems to be consistently through tonic inhibition, whether this message be conveyed by nerve fibers or by portal vessels or by both (*cf.* Schally and Kastin, 1972;

Rodríguez and Gimenez, 1972). And evidence for a second, stimulatory influence, again be it by nervous or vascular connections or both, is available for most vertebrate groups.

5. What is the chemical nature of the hypophysiotropic factors operating in non-mammalian vertebrates?

The question of our knowledge of the chemistry of the factors regulating adenohypophysial function in non-mammalian vertebrates would be easy to answer (negatively), were the answer not complicated by two problems which also continue to obfuscate our understanding of the situation in mammals, albeit to a lesser degree. Succinctly, there is no knowledge of the nature of special chemical mediators involved in adeno-hypophysial regulation in vertebrates other than mammals. The peptidic nature of various hypophysiotropins (including TRH, GRH, LRH/FRH and MIH) is established for some mammalian species only (cf. Schally and Kastin, 1972).

However, the first problem concerns the neurohypophysial octapeptides (neural lobe hormones). If these hormones contribute to adenohypophysial regulation in teleosts, amphibians, etc., then obviously something is known about the chemistry of 'lower' vertebrate hypophysiotropins (arginine vasotocin, isotocin, glumitocin, mesotocin are all possible candidates). The second problem concerns the role of monoamines, an issue much debated by mammalian hypothalamists. The cells secreting the peptidic hypophysiotropins may be regulated—through axodendritic, axosomatic and axo-axonic contacts—by monoamine-secreting neurons. Presumably aminergic fibers extend directly to adenohypophysial cells of various types in anamniote vertebrates. If they release adrenalins, or dopamine, or other biogenic amines, to stimulate or inhibit the several cell types, then again we may know something of the chemistry of 'lower' vertebrate hypophysiotropins. If, as Zambrano (1972) suggests, the amines are concerned with regulating the release of peptides carried by the same type 'B' fibers—and it is these peptides which are the hypophysiotropins—then we are totally ignorant of their chemistry.

6. Is the caudal neurosecretory system present in all tailed vertebrates?

At present, this question can be answered in two ways by appropriate investigative techniques: cytological and pharmacological. Earliest studies indicated the presence of recognizable caudal secretory neurons in elasmobranchs, teleosts and holosteans. Similarly prominent cells occur in chondrosteans (Saenko, 1970) and Polypterus; however, they have also been sought but not found to date in representatives of other fish groups and of tailed amphibians. There is no a priori reason, of course, why such cells must be marked by large size or by distinctive inclusions. In view of the presence of characteristic elementary neurosecretory granules in at least many of the cells of the caudal system in all teleost and elasmobranch species examined, electron micro-scope study may prove rewarding in other vertebrates. Some of the cells of the system in teleosts are obviously monoaminergic and project into the urophysis (Baumgarten *et al.*, 1970). Their presence raises questions not unlike the questions posed by the presumed aminergic neurons of the nucleus lateralis tuberis in the hypothalamus of the same fishes. Do the caudal aminergic neurons secrete products into the capillary network (which drains ultimately into the renal portal system), or do they play a role, along with cholinergic neurons, in regulating the hormonogenic activity of the 'real' neurosecretory neurons?

By using one or more of the biological activities present in teleost urophysial extracts as a marker, one can survey the caudal spinal cords of a variety of vertebrates for the occurrence of this activity. Such a survey has been conducted for the trout bladder-contracting activity of Lederis, with the tentative results indicated in Table II.

TABLE II

OCCURRENCE OF TROUT BLADDER-CONTRACTING ACTIVITY IN THE CAUDAL SPINAL CORD
OF REPRESENTATIVES OF VARIOUS VERTEBRATE GROUPS

Group	Activity*	Cytological evidence
Cyclostomes	−	−
Elasmobranchs	+ +	+
Holocephalans	±	−
Polypterus	±	+
Chondrosteans	+	+
Holosteans	+ +	+
Teleosts	+ + +	+
Dipnoans	− ?	−
Urodeles	−	− ?
Larval anurans	−	− ?

* Bern, Gunther, Johnson and Nishioka, unpublished.

(In all cases, activity in the caudal spinal cord is compared with that present in the abdominal spinal cord of the same animal before deciding whether the specific activity may be present). Where the cells have been positively identified, activity is most prominent. However, activity in the holocephalans (ratfish) is strongly suggested, and no specific cells have yet been described in this group. Eel-hypertensive activity has also been found in elasmobranchs (as well as teleosts) but other fish groups have not yet been examined (Chan and Ho, 1969). Hydrosmotic activity has been examined in only three of eleven teleost species so far (Lacanilao and Bern, 1972).

7. In what ways does the caudal neurosecretory system resemble and differ from the hypothalamic neurosecretory systems?

a. What is the nature of the biologically active factors? At present, there seem to be at least three factors (urotensins, see Table III) present in extracts of the teleost caudal system (studies have been confined largely to the goby *Gillichthys mirabilis*, to the

TABLE III

PRINCIPAL BIOLOGICALLY ACTIVE PRINCIPLES IN THE TELEOST UROPHYSIS

Activity	Chemistry	References
Rat hypotensive (short and long acting?) (Urotensin I)	Short-acting: 8 amino acids + carbohydrate?	Kobayashi et al. (1968); Lederis (1972); Ootani and Yasumasu (personal communication)
Teleost visceral smooth muscle-contracting (urinary bladder, intestine, oviduct, sperm duct) = ? eel hypertensive = ? eel lymph heart-contracting (Urotensin II)	Peptide: MW < 1000	Chan et al. (1969); Lederis et al. (1971); Chan (1971); Lederis (1970, 1971); Berlind (1972b)
Branchial and renal (goldfish) Na$^+$ uptake (Urotensin III)	Not neurohypophysial peptide	Maetz et al. (1964)
Hydrosmotic (toad bladder) (Urotensin IV)	Probably arginine vasotocin	Lacanilao (1969, 1972)

carp *Cyprinus carpio*, and to the eel *Anguilla japonica*). Two of these factors affect smooth muscle. The first factor appears to have the following actions: urinary bladder-contracting (in *Salmo gairdnerii*) (Lederis, 1970; Lederis et al., 1971), sperm duct-contracting (in *Gillichthys*) (Berlind, 1972b), oviduct-contracting (in *Lebistes reticulatus*) (Lederis, 1971) and probably teleost-hypertensive (in *Anguilla*) (Chan et al., 1969). This factor probably also stimulates the caudal lymph hearts of the eel (Chan, 1971). The second 'kinetic' factor is hypotensive in the rat and can be separated by column chromatography from the first factor (Kobayashi et al., 1968; Lederis, 1972). Ootani and Yasumasu (1971, personal communication) have evidence for two such hypotensive factors, one slow-acting and the other fast-acting. Extensive pharmacological and preliminary chemical studies indicate that the kinetic factors are different from any known neurohypophysial hormone. The molecular weight of the bladder-contracting and the eel-hypertensive factor(s) is less than 1000. A third factor is a hydrosmotic principle; it is indistinguishable from arginine vasotocin in its action, its chromatographic ability, its sensitivity to enzymes and other inactivating agents, and its pharmacological profile (Lacanilao, 1969, 1972). Only small amounts are present in the urophysis, and the possibilities that it is taken up by neurosecretory terminals from the blood or by dendritic processes from the cerebrospinal fluid cannot be ruled out.

It should be pointed out that the bladder-contracting activity (and sperm duct-contracting activity) and the hydrosmotic activity are associated with true neuro-hormones of the caudal system. Their release from the urophysis can be demonstrated *in vitro* in response to raising the K$^+$ concentration of the medium and thus depolarizing the membranes of the neurosecretory terminals (simulating the effects of impulse condition). Thus, these factors can be considered as representing the secretory products (*ergo* hormones) of the caudal system (Berlind, 1972a). However, except for the caudal lymph hearts, no target organs of urotensins have been definitively established on a physiological basis. Accordingly, for the time being the activities described must be regarded only as pharmacological indicators of the caudal neurohormones.

b. What is the nature of the secretory process? Although it has been known for a long time that the staining affinities of the caudal system are different from those of the anterior preoptic-neurohypophysial system (the caudal neurons and the urophysis are essentially unstained by paraldehyde fuchsin, chrome hematoxylin, etc.), the electron microscopist has consistently been impressed by the similarity of the two systems in regard to their ultrastructural properties. Elementary neurosecretory granules, perikaryal organelle participation in their formation, axon terminals and exocytic activity, are indistinguishable in the two systems (*cf.* Fridberg and Bern, 1968; Bern, 1969).

Ultracentrifugation studies have demonstrated that the bladder-contracting activity is associated with the elementary granules (Lederis *et al.*, 1971), and preliminary data indicate that the hydrosmotic activity is also. The arginine vasotocin considered responsible for this latter activity is present in such small quantities—20 picograms per *Gillichthys* urophysis—that the staining and cytochemical properties of the caudal neurosecretory material would presumably be unaffected by its presence.

The osmiophilic neurosecretory granule could consist of polymerized hormonal peptides of low molecular weight, or of such peptides bound to carrier-protein(s). Gel electrophoresis reveals the presence of two proteins unique to the urophysis (not seen in the spinal cord or in the neurohypophysis), which are candidates for the carrier-protein role (urophysin) (Berlind *et al.*, 1972). These proteins are prominent in disc electrophoretograms of the granule fraction obtained by ultracentrifugation. Bladder-contracting activity has not been directly associated with them (most often this activity appears to lie between the two bands). The significance of these special proteins remains unknown, but their occurrence raises a series of interesting biological possibilities relevant to the transport and release of urophysial neurohormones.

c. What is the function of the caudal system? As indicated above, pharmacologically established activities of urophysial extracts and even the isolation of specific factors do not necessarily delineate the physiological contribution of this neuroendocrine apparatus. Chan (1971) did find a correlation between the amount of stainable secretion and the activity of "lymph heart-stimulating substance" in the eel urophysis (both were depleted as a result of hemorrhage). Suggestive changes in the amount of bladder-contracting activity in salmon *(Oncorhynchus tshawytscha)* relative to migration, and hence to reproductive activity, have been encountered (Lederis, personal communication). Extreme osmotic stress (direct transfer of *Gillichthys* from sea water to fresh water) causes changes in the specific urophysial proteins and in hydrosmotic factor content, but not in the bladder-contracting activity (Berlind *et al.*, 1972).

A function in osmoregulation or in vascular regulation (the latter indirectly influencing osmoregulation) is certainly possible, as is a role in reproductive physiology.

These are the same activities also being investigated in attempts to elucidate the functions of the neurohypophysial octapeptides in fishes (*cf.* Perks, 1969; Heller, 1972; Sawyer, 1972). Nevertheless, except for the presence of small amounts of arginine vasotocin-like material in urophysomes, there is no basis for regarding the urophysis as an auxiliary neurohypophysis.

I have deliberately avoided raising other possibilities that have been suggested from time to time regarding urophysial function. They have been summarized recently (Bern, 1969; Lederis, 1970). Such disputed actions as buoyancy regulation or caudal mobility control may still need further consideration. In any case, the data available should be sufficient to stimulate considerable physiological and biochemical research on the function and nature of the caudal neurosecretory system and its urotensins.

SUMMARY

There are two separable cranial (hypothalamic) neurosecretory systems in vertebrates, one originating in the preoptic (and homologous) nuclei and the other in the lateral tuberal (and equivalent) nuclei. The latter are exclusively concerned with adeno-hypophysial control, generally through the agency of a median eminence neurohemal area and a portal vascular link. However, in teleosts the median eminence is at most residual, and there is a specialized system of neurosecretory innervation (of various types) of adenohypophysial cells. Innervation of the adenohypophysis, especially of the pars intermedia, occurs in other vertebrates as well. Some hypophysiotropic control systems differ among the several vertebrate groups. Nothing definitive is known about the chemistry of non-mammalian hypophysiotropins.

A caudal neurosecretory system is probably present in all fish groups except cyclostomes and lungfishes, although the urophysis is characteristic only of teleosts. The function of this system is still unknown, but principles with smooth muscle-contracting, hypotensive and hydrosmotic effects are located in and released from the urophysis. The hydrosmotic effect is probably due to arginine vasotocin; the other factors, although peptidic, are not related to neurohypophysial octapeptides. Proteins unique to the urophysis (urophysins?) can be demonstrated and undergo changes in response to certain stimuli. An increasing amount of pharmacological information on urophysial principles is available, but the physiology of the system remains essentially unknown.

ACKNOWLEDGEMENTS

I am indebted to Mr. Richard S. Nishioka and Dr. David Zambrano for their contributions to the discussion of cranial neurosecretory systems; to Professor Karl Lederis, Professor Irving I. Geschwind, Dr. Allan Berlind, Dr. Flor Lacanilao, Dr. Donald Johnson, Mr. Robert Gunther and Mr. Richard Nishioka for their contributions to the discussion of the caudal neurosecretory system; and to Mrs.

References p. 94

Emily Reid for the preparation of Fig. 1. Research referred to from the author's laboratory was aided by U.S. National Science Foundation Grant GB-23033.

REFERENCES

BALL, J. N., BAKER, B. I., OLIVEREAU, M. AND PETER, R. E. (1972) Investigations on hypothalamic control of adenohypophysial functions in teleost fishes, *Gen. comp. Endocr.*, Suppl. 3.

BAUMGARTEN, H. G., FALCK, B. AND WARTENBERG, H. (1970) Adrenergic neurons in the spinal cord of the pike *(Esox lucius)* and their relation to the caudal neurosecretory system. *Z. Zellforsch.*, **107**, 479–498.

BELENKY, M. A., KONSTANTINOVA, M. S. AND POLENOV, A. L. (1970) On neurosecretory and adrenergic fibers in the intermediate lobe of the hypophysis in albino mice. *Gen. comp. Endocr.*, **15**, 185–197.

BERLIND, A. (1972a) Teleost caudal neurosecretory system: I. Release of urotensin II from isolated urophyses. *Gen. comp. Endocr.*, in press.

BERLIND, A. (1972b) Teleost caudal neurosecretory system: III. Sperm duct contraction induced by urophysial material. *J. Endocrinol.*, 52, 567–574.

BERLIND, A., LACANILAO, F. AND BERN, H. A. (1972) Teleost caudal neurosecretory system: II. Effects of osmotic stress on urophysial proteins and active factors. *Comp. Biochem. Physiol.*, in press.

BERN, H. A. (1969) Urophysis and caudal neurosecretory system. In *Fish Physiology, Vol. II*, W. S. HOAR AND D. J. RANDALL (Eds.), Academic Press, New York, pp. 399–418.

CHAN, D. K. O. (1971) The urophysis and the caudal circulation of teleost fish. *Mem. Soc. Endocrinol.*, **19**, 391–412.

CHAN, D. K. O., CHESTER JONES, I. AND PONNIAH, S. (1969) Studies on the pressor substances of the caudal neurosecretory system of teleost fish: Bioassay and fractionation. *J. Endocr.*, **45**, 151–160.

CHAN, D. K. O. AND HO, M. W. (1969) Pressor substances in the caudal neurosecretory system of teleost and elasmobranch fishes. *Gen. comp. Endocr.*, **13**, 498.

FERNHOLM, B. (1972) Neurohypophysial-adenohypophysial relations in hagfish. *Gen. comp. Endocr.*, Suppl. 3, in press.

FRIDBERG, G. AND BERN, H. A. (1968) The urophysis and the caudal neurosecretory system of fishes. *Biol. Rev.*, **43**, 175–199.

HAYASHIDA, T. AND LAGIOS, M. D. (1969) Fish growth hormone: A biological, immunochemical, and ultrastructural study of sturgeon and paddlefish pituitaries. *Gen. comp. Endocr.*, **13**, 403–411.

HELLER, H. (1972) The effect of neurohypophysial principles on the female reproductive tract of lower vertebrates. *Gen. comp. Endocr.*, Suppl. 3, in press.

HENDERSON, N. E. (1969) Structural similarities between the neurohypophyses of brook trout and tetrapods. *Gen. comp. Endocr.*, **12**, 148–153.

JASINSKI, A. (1969) Vascularization of the hypophyseal region in lower vertebrates (cyclostomes and fishes). *Gen. comp. Endocr.*, Suppl. 2, 510–521.

JASINSKI, A. AND GORBMAN, A. (1966) Hypothalamo-hypophysial vascular and neurosecretory links in ratfish, *Hydrolagus colliei. Gen. comp. Endocr.*, **6**, 476–490.

JØRGENSEN, C. B. (1968) Central control of adenohypophysial functions. In *Perspectives in Endocrinology*, E. J. W. BARRINGTON AND C. B. JØRGENSEN (Eds.), Academic Press, New York, p. 469.

KNIGGE, K. M. AND SCOTT, D. E. (1970) Structure and function of the median eminence. *Amer. J. Anat.*, **129**, 223–244.

KOBAYASHI, H. AND MATSUI, T. (1969) Fine structure of the median eminence and its functional significance. In *Frontiers in Neuroendocrinology*, W. F. GANONG AND L. MARTINI (Eds.), Oxford Univ. Press, London, p. 46.

KOBAYASHI, H., MATSUI, T. AND ISHII, S. (1970) Functional electron microscopy of the hypothalamic median eminence. *Int. Rev. Cytol.*, **29**, 281–381.

KOBAYASHI, H., MATSUI, T., HIRANO, T., IWATA, T. AND ISHII, S. (1968) Vasodepressor substance in the fish urophysis. *Annot. Zool. japon.*, **41**, 154–158.

KOBAYASHI, H. AND UEMURA, H. (1972) The neurohypophysis of the hagfish, *Eptatretus burgeri. Gen. comp. Endocr.*, Suppl. 3, in press.

LACANILAO, F. J. (1969) Teleostean urophysis: Stimulation of water movement across the bladder of the toad *Bufo marinus. Science*, **163**, 1326–1327.

LACANILAO, F. J. AND BERN, H. A. (1972) The urophysial hydrosmotic factor of fishes. III. Survey of fish caudal spinal cord regions for hydrosmotic activity. *Proc. Soc. exp. Biol. (N.Y.)*, in press.

LACANILAO, F. J. (1972) The urophysial hydrosmotic factor of fishes. I and II. *Gen. comp. Endocr.*, in press.

LAGIOS, M. D. (1968) Tetrapod-like organization of the pituitary gland of the polypteriformid fishes, *Calamoichthys calabaricus* and *Polypterus palmas*. *Gen. comp. Endocr.*, **11**, 300–315.

LAGIOS, M. D. (1970) The median eminence of the bowfin, *Amia calva* L. *Gen. comp. Endocr.*, **15**, 453–463.

LAGIOS, M. D. (1972) Evidence for a hypothalamo–hypophysial portal vascular system in the coelacanth *Latimeria chalumnae*. *Gen. comp. Endocr.*, **18**, 73–82.

LEDERIS, K. (1972) Active substances in the caudal neurosecretory system of bony fishes. *Mem. Soc. Endocrinol.*, **18**, 465–484.

LEDERIS, K. (1972) Recent progress in research on the urophysis. *Gen. comp. Endocr.*, Suppl. 3, in press.

LEDERIS, K., BERN, H. A., NISHIOKA, R. S. AND GESCHWIND, I. I. (1971) Some observations on biological and chemical properties and subcellular localization of urophysial active principles. *Mem. Soc. Endocrinol*, **19**, 413–433.

MAETZ, J., BOURGUET, J. ET LAHLOUH, B. (1964) Urophyse et osmorégulation chez *Carassius auratus*. *Gen. comp. Endocr.*, **4**, 401–414.

MEURLING, P. (1967a) The vascularization of the pituitary in elasmobranchs. *Sarsia*, **28**, 1–104.

MEURLING, P. (1967b) The vascularization of the pituitary in *Chimaera monstrosa* (Holocephali). *Sarsia*, **30**, 83–106.

NAYAR, S. AND PANDALAI, K. (1963) Pars intermedia of the pituitary gland and integumentary colour changes in the garden lizard, *Calotes versicolor*. *Z. Zellforsch.*, **58**, 837–845.

PERKS, A. M. (1969) The neurohypophysis. In *Fish Physiology, Vol. 1*, W. S. HOAR AND D. J. RANDALL (Eds.), Academic Press, New York, p. 112.

RODRÍGUEZ, E. M. AND GIMENEZ, A. (1972) Comparative aspects of nervous control of pars intermedia. *Gen. comp. Endocr.*, Suppl. 3, in press.

RODRÍGUEZ, E. M. AND LAPOINTE, J. (1970) Light and electron microscopic study of the pars intermedia of the lizard, *Klauberina riversiana*. *Z. Zellforsch.*, **104**, 1–13.

RODRÍGUEZ, E. M., VEGA, J. A. AND LAMALFA, J. A. (1970) The different origins of the neurosecretory hypothalamo–hypophysial tracts of the toad *Bufo arenarum* Hensel. *Gen. comp. Endocr.*, **14**, 248–255.

SAENKO, I. I. (1970) Caudal neurosecretory system in sturgeons. *Doklady Akad. Nauk SSSR, Otd. Biol.*, **194**, 218–221.

SAWYER, W. H. (1972) Neurohypophysial hormones and water and sodium excretion in the African lungfish. *Gen. comp. Endocr.*, Suppl. 3, in press.

SCHALLY, A. V. AND KASTIN, A. J. (1972) Hypothalamic releasing and inhibiting hormones. *Gen. comp. Endocr.*, Suppl. 3, in press.

SCHARRER, B. (1972) Comparative aspects of neuroendocrine communication. *Gen. comp. Endocr.*, Suppl. 3, in press.

TIXIER–VIDAL, A. AND GOURDJI, D. (1972) Cellular aspects of the control of prolactin secretion in birds. *Gen. comp. Endocr.*, Suppl. 3, in press.

ZAMBRANO, D. (1972) Innervation of the teleost pituitary. *Gen. comp. Endocr.*, Suppl. 3, in press.

ZAMBRANO, D., NISHIOKA, R. S. AND BERN, H. A. (1972) The innervation of the pituitary gland of teleost fishes. Its origin, nature and significance. In *Brain–Endocrine Interaction. Median Eminence Structure and Function*, K. M. KNIGGE, D. E. SCOTT AND A. WIENDL (Eds.), S. Karger, Basel, p. 50.

DISCUSSION

KNOWLES: I would like to refer to some recent studies with the electron microscope showing that in some primitive reptiles there seems to be a barrier of ependymal end feet between the neurosecretory fibers and the blood vessels. Apparently the neurosecretory fibers don't in effect empty their content directly in the blood vessels. Could you make a comment on this point?

BERN: I can't make any comment, only suggest that the diffusion of material could still occur and could still be responsible for the control mechanisms.

SWAAB: Did you make any observations in living animals after destruction of the urophyseal system?

BERN: Yes, but it is a very unhappy kind of experimental technique. Urophysectomies are not difficult to do by cautery for example or by the very sophisticated technique of chopping the tail off. It was necessary to perform that sophisticated operation because the second generation of this system is very rapid. Even when you remove the cells of origin and the urophysis, the posterior ependymal elements give rise to a new caudal neurosecretory apparatus.

STOECKART: Why do some groups of vertebrates have a caudal neurosecretory system and others not?

BERN: I do not have the slightest idea, because I don't know what it really is doing in those vertebrates which do have a caudal neurosecretory system. All these activities that we have been painfully demonstrating here are really not saying anything about the physiology of the system. It is nice to have something that regulates blood pressure, but it is very unlikely that the effectors from this system are particularly important because there are all kinds of other factors involved in blood pressure. It is very difficult for me to get out of my mind the picture of these fantastically, richly innervated neurons. There must be some very finely modulated function.

GANONG: You showed in one of your diagrams that monoaminergic neurons participate in axo-axonal contacts on neurosecretory cells. This would be a significant finding in view of the fact that mono-amines participate in axo-axonal synapses.

BERN: Not only that monoaminergic neurons were doing this kind of thing but also cholinergic neurons.

GANONG: So this is an established example of an axo-axonal synapse of an aminergic neuron.

Hypothalamic Mechanisms Controlling Pituitary Function

BÉLA HALÁSZ

2nd Department of Anatomy, University Medical School, Budapest (Hungary)

It is generally accepted that anterior pituitary function is controlled by the central nervous system, first of all by the hypothalamus. Further, there is no doubt that environmental factors (light, smell, temperature, sound etc; for details see Everett, 1964) as well as various internal stimuli have a great influence on the adenohypophysis. Some of them are essential for normal pituitary function. Depending on the way of action, internal stimuli are of two types, neural and humoral. Among the neural impulses, those arising from the genital tract are of special significance. This is clearly indicated by the facts that in the rabbit the rupture of the Graafian follicles occurs in response to copulation, and that in the rat mechanical or electrical stimulation of the cervix of the uterus causes pseudopregnancy (Long and Evans, 1922; Shelesnyak, 1931). The humoral factors best-known are the hormones. Removal of the gonads, adrenals or thyroid gland results in an increase in pituitary gonadotrophic (GTH), adrenocorticotrophic (ACTH) or thyrotrophic hormone (TSH) secretion, and an excess of the peripheral hormones inhibits pituitary GTH, ACTH and TSH production, respectively (negative feedback). There is evidence that also a positive feedback of these hormones might exist, at least in the control of the gonadotrophic function. Several years ago it has been demonstrated that small amounts of œstrogen increase luteinizing hormone (LH) output from the pituitary (Hohlweg, 1934) and progesterone induces ovulation (Everett and Sawyer, 1949). Apart from the feedback action of the peripheral hormones (external feedback), there is some indication that also trophic hormones themselves would influence anterior pituitary function (internal feedback, see Szentágothai *et al.*, 1968).

It is clear that external and internal neural stimuli exert their influence on the anterior lobe through the central nervous system. It seems very likely that also the hormonal feedback is mediated, at least in part, via neural elements. This idea was first raised by Hohlweg and Junkmann (1932), who did not find castration cells in the pituitaries transplanted under the kidney capsule. Therefore, they suggested that the gonadal hormones influence gonadotrophic functions by way of a hypothetical sexual center located somewhere in the brain. Flerkó and Szentágothai (1957) furnished the first experimental evidence for their view that sexual steroid-sensitive structures exist in the brain. They demonstrated that a small fragment of the ovary, when implanted into the anterior hypothalamus, inhibits gonadotrophic activity. Concerning the site of the trophic hormone feedback action, it is assumed that neural elements are involved in these events, since pituitary tissue or ACTH placed into the

References p. 111

This view is first of all consistent with the morphology of the median eminence region. A large number of nerve endings are present in the surface zone of the median eminence (zona palisadica) (Fig. 2). Under the electron microscope, many axon endings intermingled with some ependymal and glial processes and end feet can be seen in this layer. The axon endings contain numerous small synaptic-like vesicles, about 200–700 Å in size, as well as bigger so-called dense-core vesicles, the diameter of which varies between 500 Å–1300 Å, the majority showing a diameter between 700–900 Å. The large neurosecretory granules, most of them measuring 1500 Å–2100 Å, which are characteristic of the supraoptico- and paraventriculo-hypophysial tracts, do not occur in this layer (Szentágothai and Halász, 1964; Monroe, 1967; Akmayev, 1969). These latter granules are exclusively present in the internal or fibrous layer of the median eminence, where the fibers of the mentioned tracts do pass. The nervous tissue of the median eminence is separated from the blood vessels of the portal system by a thin tissue interspace. Between an extremely delicate outer membrane of the median eminence and the basement membrane of the capillaries there is a connective tissue space of 1–2 μ in width. The capillaries of the portal system are lined by a fenestrated endothelium.

The neurovascular theory of adenohypophysial control contains two main assumptions:

1. Some substances are produced in the hypothalamus which are essential for the pituitary.

2. The material is transported to the anterior lobe by the portal system.

The data accumulated in the last, nearly 25 years support unequivocally both assumptions, and thus favor the neurovascular hypothesis.

1. Hypothalamic hypophysiotrophic releasing and inhibiting factors

It has been shown by several authors that hypothalamic extracts have a direct effect on pituitary function. Such an action was first demonstrated on ACTH secretion (Saffran and Schally, 1955; Guillemin and Rosenberg, 1955). The active principle has been named corticotropic releasing factor (CRF). Further studies suggested that hypothalamic extracts contain also substances which influence the secretion of other pituitary hormones. It has been reported that hypothalamic extracts stimulate the release of pituitary thyroid-stimulating hormone (TSH) (Shibusawa et al., 1956a, b; Schreiber et al., 1961; Guillemin et al., 1962), luteinizing hormone (LH) (McCann et al., 1960; Campbell et al., 1961; Nikitovitch-Winer, 1962), follicle-stimulating hormone (FSH) (Igarashi and McCann, 1964) and growth hormone (GH) (Franz et al., 1962; Deuben and Meites, 1964). These substances have been called TSH-releasing factor (TRF), LH-releasing factor (LRF), FSH-releasing factor (FRF) and GH releasing factor (GRF), respectively. Beside the factors mentioned, there is evidence that the hypothalamus produces a substance which exerts a tonic inhibitory effect on prolactin release (prolactin-inhibiting factor, PIF) (Pasteels, 1961a, b, 1962; Meites et al., 1962; Talwalker et al., 1963).

The first observations on the existence of hypothalamic releasing and inhibiting substances have been corroborated in various laboratories by *in vivo* as well as *in vitro* studies (see McCann and Dhariwal, 1966; Schally *et al.*, 1968a; McCann and Porter, 1969).

The functional significance of these factors is underlined by the fact that concentration of the substances in the hypothalamus varies in connection with changes in pituitary function. It has been shown, among others, that during the sexual cycle of female rats there is a fluctuation in hypothalamic LRF content (Ramirez and Sawyer, 1965; Chowers and McCann, 1965). Suckling or oestradiol treatment, beside influencing prolactin secretion, cause a decrease in PIF activity of the hypothalamus (Ratner and Meites, 1964). Hypothalamic CRF activity shows a similar diurnal rhythm as pituitary ACTH secretion. The daily peak of CRF concentration in the hypothalamus is 3 h earlier than the daily corticosterone peak in the blood (David–Nelson and Brodish, 1969; Hiroshige *et al.*, 1969). Thyroidectomy results in an increase in hypothalamic TRF and pituitary TSH content (Sinha and Meites, 1965–66). There is more GRF in the hypothalamus of young rats (30-day-old) than in old ones (2-year-old) (Pecile *et al.*, 1965).

It appears that the hypothalamic hypophysiotrophic substances are responsible for both the structural as well as functional maintenance of the cells of the anterior lobe. If the pituitary is disconnected from the hypothalamus, by transplanting it under the kidney capsule or into the anterior ocular chamber, its structure becomes dedifferentiated being composed mainly of chromophobe cells while its hormone secretion is markedly reduced (Cutuly, 1941; Cheng *et al.*, 1949; McDermott *et al.*, 1950; Fortier, 1951; Harris and Jacobsohn, 1952; Siperstein and Greer, 1956; Goldberg and Knobil, 1957; Nikitovitch-Winer and Everett, 1959). Normal histology as well as the function of the dedifferentiated pituitary graft under the renal capsule can be restored by retransplanting the anterior lobe under the median eminence (Nikitovitch-Winer and Everett, 1958, 1959). Hypothalamic extracts reactivate cytologically and functionally 8–67-day-old renal pituitary autografts, if the extracts are infused continuously into the renal artery for periods of 7–36 days (1–3 fragments/day) (Evans and Nikitovitch-Winer, 1969). These findings are consistent with the view that the hypothetical hypothalamic substances exert a trophic influence on the pituitary cells. Concerning the function of the anterior lobe it seems very likely that the action of the hypothalamic substances is not only limited to the release of the trophic hormones, but that they might also stimulate hormone synthesis. This is indicated by the significant increase of pituitary TSH (Sinha and Meites, 1966; Mittler *et al.* 1969), ACTH (Uemura, 1968), FSH (Jutisz and de la Llosa, 1967), LH (Jutisz *et al.*, 1967) and GH content (Symchowicz *et al.*, 1966; Schally *et al.*, 1968b), if *in vitro* hypothalamic extract or the appropriate releasing factor is added to the medium. Intracarotically administered median eminence extract causes a two to five fold increase in pituitary ACTH content (Vernikos-Danellis, 1965).

It is not known at present whether separate trophic and 'releasing' factors are produced by the hypothalamus, or only the latter ones, which, beside influencing hormone synthesis and release, might also exert a trophic effect on the anterior lobe.

Regarding the mechanism of action of the hypothalamic mediators on the pituitary the reader is referred to the excellent work of Geschwind (1969).

The hypothalamic neurohormones appear to be small polypeptides. The chemical structure of TRF has been recently discovered (Burgus et al., 1969; Schally et al., 1970). It is 2-pyrrolidone-5-carboxylyl-histidyl-prolyl-amide (Burgus and Guillemin, 1970). Purification, isolation and identification of the chemical structure of the other factors is in progress (McCann and Porter, 1969; Burgus and Guillemin, 1970).

2. Releasing and inhibiting factors in the portal blood

By collecting blood coming from the transected pituitary stalk it has been demonstrated that this exhibits LRF (Fink et al., 1966, 1967; Fink, 1967; Kamberi et al., 1969), FRF (Kamberi et al., 1970a), TRF, GRF (Wilber and Porter, 1970), CRF (Porter, 1970), and PIF (Kamberi et al., 1970b) activity. According to Harris (1970) LRF is present in the portal blood during all phases of the sexual cycle except oestrus, and electrical stimulation of the hypothalamus causes an increase in LRF activity of this blood.

It should be mentioned that in the peripheral blood of intact animals the presence of these substances has not been demonstrated as yet. This was only possible under special experimental circumstances, such as following hypophysectomy, when presumably the releasing factors are released in larger amounts from the hypothalamus (CRF: Schapiro et al., 1956; Eik-Nes and Brizzee, 1958; Brodish and Long, 1962; LRF: Nallar and McCann, 1965; FRF: Negro-Vilar et al., 1968; GRF: Krulich and McCann, 1966; Müller et al., 1967; TRF: Redding and Schally, 1969; PIF: Chen et al., 1970). If the medial basal hypothalamus is destroyed, the releasing or inhibiting activity of the peripheral blood of the hypophysectomized animals is not evident, suggesting the hypothalamic origin of the active principles.

II. FIRST CONTROL LEVEL. THE RELEASING AND INHIBITING FACTORS-PRODUCING ELEMENTS AND THEIR ROLE IN PITUITARY CONTROL

There is still a complete lack of any direct information about the site of production of the releasing and inhibiting factors. The indirect information available seems to indicate that this function might be limited to a special part of the hypothalamus.

By implanting anterior pituitary tissue into various hypothalamic and extra-hypothalamic regions of the brain it was found that structure and function of the pituitary graft is maintained only when it is placed in the medial basal hypothalamus (Halász et al., 1962, 1965; Flament-Durand, 1965). Pituitaries situated in this region contain numerous basophile, periodic acid–Schiff (PAS)-positive cells, whereas in grafts outside this area these cells are not evident. Since the basophile cells appear to be most sensitive to hypothalamic connections—the presence or absence of eosinophile cells depends on blood thyroxine levels rather than on direct hypothalamic connections (Halász et al., 1963)—the occurrence of this cell type was used as a criterion to

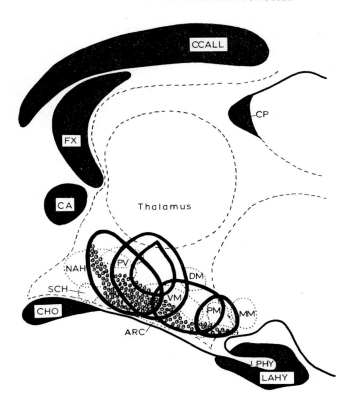

Fig. 3. The location of the hypophysiotrophic area of the hypothalamus. –––––, Outline of third ventricle; ......, mid-sagittal projection of main hypothalamic nuclei; ▬▬, outlines of five relatively midline pituitary grafts; ○○ PAS-positive basophile cells. ARC, arcuate nucleus; CA, anterior commissure; CCALL, corpus callosum; CHO, optic chiasm; CP, posterior commissure; DM, dorsomedial nucleus; FX, fornix; LAHY, anterior lobe of hypophysis; LPHY, posterior lobe of hypophysis; MM, medial mamillary nucleus; NAH, anterior hypothalamic nucleus; PM, premamillary nucleus; PV, paraventricular nucleus; SCH, suprachiasmatic nucleus; VM, ventromedial nucleus. From Halász et al., 1962.

map the extension of the hypothalamic region being capable of maintaining normal pituitary cytology. Fig. 3 shows the extent of this area which reaches down ventralward from the paraventricular nuclei to the optic chiasma and extends caudalward as far as to the mamillary region. In the rat brain, the lateral extent of the area is 0.5–1.0 mm from the midline. This region has been called the hypophysiotrophic area (HTA). The area includes the arcuate nuclei, the ventral part of the anterior periventricular nuclei, the medial part of the retrochiasmatic region and the median eminence.

Gonadotrophic hormone secretion of the pituitary graft is normal only if it is placed into this HTA. In this case nearly normal cycles reappear after a shorter or longer time interval following implantation, and the ovaries of such animals contain ripe follicles and fresh corpora lutea; in male rats spermiogenesis and spermiohistogenesis is well maintained. If the grafts are outside the HTA, the gonads are atrophic.

References p. 111

TSH, ACTH and growth hormone secretion by the pituitary impants is also significantly better preserved if the graft is located in the HTA than when it is outside this
region.

In accordance with the findings mentioned it has been reported that only the extracts
made of the medial basal hypothalamus exhibit LRF (McCann, 1962), FRF (Wata-
nabe and McCann, 1968) and CRF activity (Vernikos-Danellis, 1964).

These data strongly suggest that the hypothalamic substances essential for the
structural and functional maintenance of the anterior lobe might be produced and
released by the HTA.

This view fits well with the morphology of the HTA. It is known that the axons
of the neurons in the area turn in a ventral or ventromedial direction and form the
fine-calibered tubero-hypophysial (Laruelle, 1934; Spatz, 1951; Nowakowski, 1951;
Martinez, 1960) or tubero-infundibular tract (Szentágothai, 1962, 1964; Akmayev,

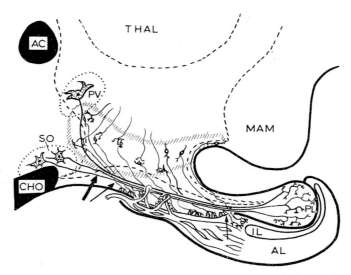

Fig. 4. Diagram illustrating the tubero-infundibular and the supraoptico- and paraventriculo-
hypophysial tract. Thin arrows indicate proximal and distal ends of the zona palisadica containing
the nerve terminals of the tubero-infundibular tract. Larger nerve fibers (thick arrow) are those
of the supraoptico- and paraventriculo-hypophysial tract, which can be traced to the neurohypophysis.
Hatched zone in the diagram indicates the HTA which corresponds to the localization of the nerve
cells giving rise to the tubero-infundibular tract. AC, anterior commissure; AL, anterior lobe; CHO,
optic chiasm; IL, intermediate lobe; MAM, mamillary body; PL, posterior lobe; PV, paraventricular
nucleus; SO, supraoptic nucleus; THAL, thalamus. Dashed line indicates outlines of 3rd ventricle.
By courtesy of Szentágothai, 1964.

1969). The fibers of this tract terminate mainly in the surface zone of the median
eminence and in the proximal part of the pituitary stalk. A much smaller number of
nerve endings of this pathway can be found around the capillary loops of the median
eminence (Fig. 4). Thus, it appears that the neurons in the HTA have their endings in
the region where the hypothalamic releasing and inhibiting factors are supposed to
be released.

Further support to the assumption that the HTA is the site of production of the hypophysiotrophic substances has been furnished by observations showing that axons of nerve cells outside this area do not terminate in the surface zone of the median eminence (Réthelyi and Halász, 1970). In these studies, various hypothalamic areas were partially or totally separated from the brain by means of a stereotaxically manipulated bayonet-shaped knife designed by us (Halász and Pupp, 1965), and the zona palisadica of the median eminence and pituitary stalk was examined for secondary degeneration of axon terminals under the electron microscope. If the medial basal hypothalamus, including the suprachiasmatic area, was disconnected from the rest of the brain, degenerated nerve endings did not occur in the palisade zone. Axon degeneration, however, was observed, if any part of the medio-basal hypothalamic area was separated from the median eminence or became necrotic.

When considering the morphology of the hypophysiotrophic area it should be mentioned that the ependymal and glial elements in this region are of a peculiar type having their end feet in the zona palisadica. It has been proposed by several authors (Löfgren, 1961; Leveque and Hofkin, 1961; Leveque et al., 1966; Vigh et al., 1963; Kumar, 1968; Knowles and Kumar, 1969) that these cells might be somehow involved in the control of pituitary hormone secretion (for details see Knowles in this volume).

If the assumption is accepted that the hypophysiotrophic factors would be produced in the medial basal hypothalamus, the question arises whether there are separate regions inside this area that manufacture the various substances or whether a diffuse representation exists in it.

Mess and coworkers (1966) lesioned three different regions of the HTA in rats, the suprachiasmatic area, the region of the paraventricular nuclei, and the area of the arcuate and ventromedial nuclei, and measured the content of the various releasing factors in the median eminence. After destruction of the suprachiasmatic, arcuate and ventromedial regions, the LRF content of the extracts was decreased. Electrolytic lesions in the paraventricular area resulted in a decrease in FRF content. TRF content of the extracts was decreased after all three kinds of lesions. Schneider et al. (1969) detected significant LRF activity in extracts of the suprachiasmatic region. Large amounts of LRF are present in the median eminence following surgical isolation of the arcuate region. In contrast, FRF activity of median eminence extracts is markedly reduced after a similar operation (Tima, 1971). These findings seem to suggest that LRF might be produced in the suprachiasmatic and arcuate region and FRF in the paraventricular area, whereas the whole HTA would be involved in TRF production. A diffuse representation of TRF production has also been proposed by D'Angelo et al. (1964). On the contrary, Flament-Durand and Desclin (1968) assume—on the basis of intrahypothalamic pituitary implantation studies—that TRF is produced only in the supra- and retrochiasmatic part of the HTA. There is now much evidence supporting the view that CRF production is restricted to the median eminence region (see Halász, 1969).

As, so far, information seems insufficient, we feel that any definite proposition regarding the precise localization of the structures producing various releasing factors inside the hypophysiotrophic area should wait till more data are available.

References p. 111

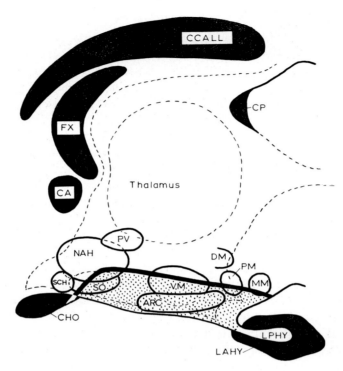

Fig. 5. Schematic drawing of the experimental situation in the animals with complete deafferentation of the HTA. The area cut around (dotted region) is in contact with the pituitary but is disconnected from other parts of the brain as indicated by the heavy line. For abbreviations see legend to Fig. 3. From Halász and Pupp, 1965.

The findings obtained in animals with a neurally isolated medial basal hypothalamus (Fig. 5) seem to indicate that the HTA does not need the influence of other nervous structures to produce and release the releasing factors. This is shown by the following observations. In male rats, gonadotrophic hormone secretion is fairly well maintained after the interruption of all neural connections with the hypothalamic region mentioned (Halász and Pupp, 1965; Halász *et al.*, 1967a; Voloschin *et al.*, 1968). Testicular weight and histology are nearly normal. There is no gonadal atrophy in female rats after such an operation, but pituitary FSH and LH secretion appear to be seriously altered (Halász and Pupp, 1965; Halász and Gorski, 1967; Palka *et al.*, 1969). These animals are not able to ovulate, their ovaries are usually polyfollicular and do not contain fresh corpora lutea. Isolation of the medial basal hypothalamus does not cause any decrease in basal ACTH secretion (Halász *et al.*, 1967b, c; Greer and Rockie, 1968; Voloschin *et al.*, 1968; Palka *et al.*, 1969; Makara *et al.*, 1970), but, on the contrary, secretion increases after the operation (Halász *et al.*, 1967b, c; Greer and Rockie, 1968). We found elevated pituitary ACTH and plasma corticosterone levels 4 weeks following complete deafferentation of the region. As indicated by the thyroid epithelial cell height, ^{131}I uptake and the biological half-life of thyroidal ^{131}I tests, interruption of the neural connections to the medial basal hypothalamus results in a moderate decrease in basal TSH activity only (Halász et al., 1967a). Young rats grow fairly well after isolation of the hypophysiotrophic area (Halász, 1968) indicating the maintenance of pituitary GH secretion under such conditions.

On the basis of the above cited observations it may be concluded that the medial basal hypothalamus is not merely the final center in the hypothalamic control of the anterior pituitary, which only transforms and forwards the influence of other nervous structures to the anterior lobe, but that this area represents a separate level in the hypothalamic control of the adenohypophysis. Generally speaking, it appears that the structure of the pituitary gland as well as the basal secretion of the trophic hormones is maintained to a great extent by the HTA.

As mentioned above, interruption of the neural connections of the medial basal hypothalamus interferes with pituitary gonadotrophic function in the female, but not in the male. This difference is probably related to the fact that pituitary FSH and LH secretion is tonic in the male and cyclic in the female (see Flerkó, 1968). It therefore seems likely that the medial basal hypothalamus is responsible for tonic gonadotrophic hormone secretion, while cyclic release depends on neural afferents to the area.

There is much evidence suggesting that the neurons of the hypophysiotrophic area are sensitive to target gland hormones as well as to trophic hormones. Small amounts of oestrogen or androgen implanted into the arcuate region cause gonadal atrophy (Lisk, 1960, 1962; Davidson and Sawyer, 1961a, b) and prevent the development of the post-castration changes in the pituitary (Kanematsu and Sawyer, 1963, 1964; Lisk, 1963; Ramirez et al., 1964). Individual neurons in the HTA accumulate oestradiol (Stumpf, 1968; Attramadal, 1970) and show a pattern of uptake and retention of [^{3}H]oestradiol that is similar to the pattern found in other oestrogen-sensitive structures such as the uterus and vagina (McGuire and Lisk, 1969). Corticoids, placed into the medial basal hypothalamus, result in a decrease in hypothalamic CRF and pituitary ACTH content (Chowers et al., 1967), reduce adrenal weight and corticosteroid secretion (Endrőczi et al., 1961; Chowers et al., 1963; Bohus and Endrőczi, 1964; Corbin et al., 1965), and inhibit compensatory hypertrophy of the remaining adrenal following unilateral adrenalectomy (Davidson and Feldman, 1963). It seems very likely that the hormone-sensitive nervous elements are sensitive to local increase as well as to local decrease of sexual- and corticosteroid hormone levels. In the case of thyroid hormones, however, the nerve cells probably react only on a local decrease of the hormonal level and not on its increase (Reichlin, 1966).

The neurons in the HTA appear to be sensitive to target gland hormones in the absence of neural afferents. This is shown by the findings that, after neural isolation of the area, unilateral adrenalectomy is followed by the compensatory hypertrophy of the remaining adrenal (Halász et al., 1967b), gonadectomy results in increased pituitary LH secretion and formation of castration cells in the anterior lobe (Halász and Gorski, 1967; Maric and Nikitovitch-Winer, 1967), while thiouracil treatment causes a significant rise in TSH secretion (Halász et al., 1967a).

Concerning trophic hormone sensitivity of the HTA, it has been reported that small amounts of LH implanted into the median eminence region result in a decrease in pituitary LH secretion (David *et al.*, 1966; Corbin, 1966; Ojeda and Ramirez, 1969). FSH placed into the medial basal hypothalamus of adult female rats reduces hypothalamic FRF and pituitary FSH levels (Corbin and Story, 1967). In prepuberal animals this leads to precocious puberty (Ojeda and Ramirez, 1969). Prolactin implants in the median eminence region cause an increase in hypothalamic PIF and a decrease in pituitary prolactin content (Clemens and Meites, 1968; Mishkinsky *et al.*, 1969). Anterior lobe tissue or ACTH, when implanted in the HTA, inhibits pituitary ACTH secretion (Halász and Szentágothai, 1960; Motta *et al.*, 1965). According to Steiner *et al.* (1969) locally applied ACTH enhances the electrical activity of the arcuate neurons depressed by dexamethasone.

Török (1954, 1962) and Szentágothai *et al.* (1957) observed that a small fraction of the blood which has passed the pars tuberalis and, under certain circumstances, even blood which irrigates some part of the pars distalis by internal vessels of the stalk is drained towards the hypothalamus. The trophic hormones might reach the hypophysiotrophic area by this route.

Thus, it may be assumed that the basic functional level of the HTA is not independent of the internal environment, but is influenced in a feedback fashion by the hormonal levels in the blood.

There is evidence that, in addition to hormones, other substances may also act on the hypophysiotrophic area. In rats with median eminence-pituitary islands ether stress causes increased ACTH secretion (Matsuda *et al.*, 1964; Halász *et al.*, 1967b; Greer and Rockie, 1968; Palka *et al.*, 1969). Greer and Rockie have demonstrated that in such animals the high plasma corticosterone levels, induced by ether, can be decreased to the resting level seen in intact rats by administering pentobarbital. It has been shown that there is a pituitary ACTH response to immobilization (Dunn and Critchlow, 1969; Palka *et al.*, 1969; Feldman *et al.*, 1970), tibia turnique (Greer *et al.*, 1970) and a large dose of formalin (Makara *et al.*, 1970).

The HTA is, however, insufficient by itself to sustain hormone secretion at a normal level. This is evident from the observation that in the animals with an isolated medial basal hypothalamus ovulation is blocked (Halász and Gorski, 1967), the diurnal rhythm in ACTH secretion fails (Halász *et al.*, 1967b, c; Palka *et al.*, 1969), basal TSH secretion is slightly reduced and the pituitary TSH response to propylthiouracil is subnormal (Halász *et al.*, 1967a). It may be assumed that all the pituitary functions that fail or are disturbed after the neural isolation of the HTA are maintained by a second control level.

The first control level is probably a 'closed system' in the sense that, although its inputs are multiple, it has a single output channel, the tubero-infundibular tract ending in the surface zone of the median eminence. This level appears to be primarily involved with the discharge into the portal circulation of the releasing and inhibiting factors.

It has been demonstrated that some neurons in the medial basal hypothalamus contain great amounts of monoamines, primarily dopamine (Carlsson *et al.*, 1962; Fuxe, 1964). The intensity of the monoamine fluorescence in the nerve cells varies among others in connection with the sexual cycle (Fuxe *et al.*, 1967; Hyyppä, 1969; Lichtensteiger, 1968), increases during pregnancy (Hyyppä, 1969). The turnover of the monoamines is enhanced during pregnancy, pseudopregnancy and lactation (Fuxe *et al.*, 1969). If a small amount of reserpine causing local depletion of monoamines is implanted into the medial basal hypothalamus this results in pseudopregnancy (Van Maanen and Smelik, 1967, 1968).

These and several other observations suggest that the monoamines in the HTA might play a role in the control of the anterior pituitary, primarily in the regulation of gonadotrophic function. Fuxe and Hökfelt (1969) assume that, in the median eminence, the monoaminergic neurons form axo-axonic synapses with the releasing and inhibiting factors-producing nerve cells. Thus the monoamine system would influence (enhancing or inhibiting) the release of the hypophysiotrophic substances. This assumption is supported by the finding that dopamine, when injected into the third ventricle, causes LRF and FRF release (Schneider and McCann, 1969; Kamberi *et al.*, 1969, 1970a; for details see Fuxe and Hökfelt, 1969).

III. THE SECOND CONTROL LEVEL AS A MODULATOR OF THE STRUCTURES PRODUCING THE HYPOTHALAMIC NEUROHORMONES

The neural elements outside the medial basal hypothalamus that participate in the control of the anterior lobe constitute, collectively, the second control level. These structures include several hypothalamic nuclei and extrahypothalamic regions, such as the whole limbic system and all its primary and secondary connections, the mesencephalon, etc.

There is ample evidence that the elements of this second control level exert stimulatory as well as inhibitory influences on trophic hormone secretion. Generally speaking, it appears that the amygdaloid complex, the septum, the preoptic area and certain ill-defined mesencephalic regions are primarily excitatory, while the hippocampus and probably some other mesencephalic structures are mainly inhibitory (for details see Davidson, 1966; Flerkó, 1966; Mangili *et al.*, 1966; Meites, 1966; Reichlin, 1966). The neurogenic stimulus causing the ovulatory surge of LH in the rat probably arises from the preoptic area, although other areas might be involved as well. It has been demonstrated that animals in which the anterior, lateral and superior connections of the preoptic area were bilaterally interrupted, leaving the region in contact with the HTA only, did ovulate. Conversely, disconnection of the preoptic region from the HTA blocked ovulation up to 100% (Köves and Halász, 1970; Kaasjager *et al.*, 1971).

The second control level receives and integrates the environmental as well as the internal neural stimuli influencing anterior pituitary function. In addition, it appears that the elements of this level are also hormone sensitive. The preoptic region, septum, amygdaloid complex, hippocampus show a selective uptake of labelled estrogen or testosterone (Michael, 1964; Attramadal, 1964, 1970; Kato and Villee, 1967; Pfaff, 1968a, b, c; Stumpf, 1968; Stumpf and Sar, 1969, 1971; McEven and Pfaff, 1970; Tuohimaa, 1970). Corticosteroids implanted into the hippocampus or midbrain reticular formation inhibit basal pituitary ACTH secretion (Corbin *et al.*, 1965; Slusher, 1966). Bohus *et al.* (1968) reported that cortisol when placed into the midbrain, amygdala or basal septal region depresses, whereas in the hippocampus it enhances pituitary ACTH response to stress. Thus, it may be assumed that the second control system is influenced not only by pure neural pathways, but also by the hormone levels in the blood suggesting that the control function of these structures is a highly integrated one.

Concerning localization of the control functions of the various trophic hormones there are probably no special cell groups, *i.e.* 'centers', which control distinct functions, but rather functional patterns might exist. The second control level can be envisaged as a kind of computer which, according to a number of built-in programs, elaborates the solution for each actual situation on the basis of a large body of information partly stored, partly flowing in continuously through neural and humoral

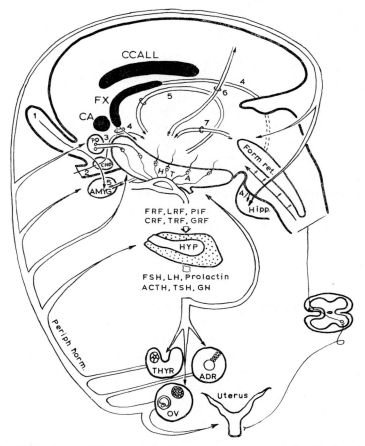

Fig. 6. A simplified scheme of the neural double control system regulating the anterior pituitary. 1. Olfactory system; 2. optic nerve and tract; 3. preoptico-tuberal tract; 4. fornix, medial cortico-hypothalamic tract; 5. stria terminalis; 6. connections between cerebral cortex and hypothalamus. ADR, adrenal; AMYG, amygdala complex; FORM RET, reticular formation; HIPP, hippocampal complex; HTA, hypophysiotrophic area; HYP, hypophysis; OV, ovary; P, portal system; PERIPH HORM, peripheral hormones; PO, medial preoptic nucleus; THYR, thyroid gland. For other abbreviations see legend to Fig. 3.

channels. The 'results' are then distributed over a number of 'print-out' channels. The second control level is, in contrast to the first level, an 'open' system with a wealth of efferent connections.

When taking into account that the nerve terminals in the surface zone of the median eminence arise exclusively from neurons in the HTA, and that fibers of other origin do not terminate in this zone, it is close at hand to assume that the neural structures outside the HTA do not act directly on the anterior lobe but might exert their influence via the HTA exclusively.

The second control level probably modulates the synthesis and release of the hypothalamic releasing and inhibiting substances produced by the HTA.

Fig. 6 summarizes the mechanisms controlling the anterior pituitary.

SUMMARY

The data available suggest that there are two levels in the neural control of the anterior pituitary. The first level is situated in the medial basal hypothalamus. It is termed 'hypophysiotrophic area' (HTA). It seems likely that this region produces the hypothalamic releasing and inhibiting substances that regulate anterior pituitary function and are carried by the portal circulation to the pituitary cells. Probably, this area can maintain the basal secretion of the anterior lobe hormones by itself. Part of the feedback action of the peripheral hormones and of the trophic hormones, as well as the action of some other substances appear to be exerted on this region. The second control level comprises neural structures outside the HTA, such as other hypothalamic regions, the limbic system, the midbrain, etc. This level controls normal pituitary function, among others cyclic release of the trophic hormones. Environmental as well as internal neural stimuli influencing pituitary hormone secretion are integrated at this level. The neural elements of this system appear to be hormone-sensitive and thus might react to changes in the actual levels of peripheral hormones in the blood. The second control level exerts stimulatory as well as inhibitory effects on the adenohypophysis, presumably acting via the HTA.

REFERENCES

AKMAYEV, I. G. (1969) Morphological aspects of the hypothalamic–hypophyseal system. I. Fibers terminating in the neurohypophysis of mammals. *Z. Zellforsch.*, **96**, 609–624.

ATTRAMADAL, A. (1964) Distribution and site of action of oestradiol in the brain and pituitary gland of the rat following intramuscular administration, Proc. 2nd Int. Congr. Endocrin., Amsterdam, *Excerpta med. int. Congr. Ser.*, **83**, 612–616.

ATTRAMADAL, A. (1970) Cellular localization of ³H-oestradiol in the hypothalamus. An autographic study in male and female rat. *Z. Zellforsch.*, **104**, 572–581.

BOHUS, B. AND ENDRÖCZI, E. (1964) Effect of intracerebral implantation of hydrocortisone on adrenocortical secretion and adrenal weight after unilateral adrenalectomy. *Acta physiol. Acad. Sci. hung.*, **25**, 11–19.

BOHUS, B., NYAKAS, CS. AND LISSÁK, K. (1968) Involvement of suprahypothalamic structures in the hormonal feedback action of corticosteroids. *Acta physiol. Acad. Sci. hung.*, **34**, 1–8.

BRODISH, A. AND LONG, C. N. H. (1962) ACTH-releasing hypothalamic neurohumor in peripheral blood. *Endocrinology*, **71**, 298–306.

BURGUS, R., DUNN, T. F., DESIDERIO, D. ET GUILLEMIN, R. (1969) Structure moléculaire du facteur hypothalamique hypophysiotrope TRF d'origine ovine: mise en évidence par spectrométrie de masse de la séquence PCA-His-Pro-NH$_2$, *C.R. Acad. Sci. (Paris)*, **269**, 1870–1873.

BURGUS, R. AND GUILLEMIN, R. (1970) Hypothalamic releasing factors. *Ann. Rev. Biochem.*, **39**, 499–526.

CAMPBELL, H. J., FEUER, G., GARCIA, J. AND HARRIS, G. W. (1961) The infusion of brain extracts into the anterior pituitary gland and the secretion of gonadotrophic hormone. *J. Physiol. (Lond.)*, **157**, 30P–31P.

CARLSSON, A., FALCK, B. AND HILLARP, N. A. (1962) Cellular localization of brain monoamines. *Acta physiol. scand.*, **56**, Suppl. 196, 1–28.

CHEN, C. L., AMENOMORI, Y., LU, K. H., VOOGT, J. L. AND MEITES, J. (1970) Serum prolactin levels in rats with pituitary transplants or hypothalamic lesions. *Neuroendocrinology*, **6**, 220–227.

CHENG, C. P., SAYERS, G., GOODMAN, L. S. AND SWINYARD, C. A. (1949) Discharge of ACTH from transplanted pituitary tissue. *Amer. J. Physiol.*, **159**, 426–432.

CHOWERS, I., CONFORTI, N. AND FELDMAN, S. (1967) Effects of corticosteroids on hypothalamic cortic otropin releasing factor and pituitary ACTH content. *Neuroendocrinology*, **2**, 193–199.

CHOWERS, I., FELDMAN, S. AND DAVIDSON, J. M. (1963) Effects of intrahypothalamic crystalline steroids on acute ACTH secretion. *Amer. J. Physiol.*, **205**, 671–673.

CHOWERS, I. AND MCCANN, S. M. (1965) Content of luteinizing hormone releasing factor and luteinizing hormone during the estrous cycle and after changes in gonadal steroid titers. *Endocrinology*, **76**, 700–708.

CLEMENS, J. A. AND MEITES, J. (1968) Inhibition by hypothalamic prolactin implants on prolactin secretion, mammary growth and luteal function. *Endocrinology*, **82**, 878–881.

CORBIN, A. (1966) Pituitary and plasma LH of ovariectomized rats with median eminence implants of LH. *Endocrinology*, **78**, 893–896.

CORBIN, A., MANGILI, G., MOTTA, M. AND MARTINI, L. (1965) Effect of hypothalamic and mesencephalic steroid implantations on ACTH feedback mechanism. *Endocrinology*, **76**, 811–818.

CORBIN, A. AND STORY, J. C. (1967) 'Internal' feedback mechanism: response of pituitary FSH and of stalk–median eminence follicle stimulating hormone-releasing factor to median eminence implants of FSH. *Endocrinology*, **80**, 1006–1012.

CUTULY, E. (1941) Autoplastic grafting of anterior pituitary in male rats. *Anat. Rec.*, **80**, 83–97.

D'ANGELO, S. A., SNYDER, J. AND GRODIN, J. M. (1964) Electrical stimulation of the hypothalamus: simultaneous effects on the pituitary-adrenal and thyroid systems of the rat. *Endocrinology*, **75**, 417–427.

DAVID, M. A., FRASCHINI, F. AND MARTINI, L. (1966) Control of LH secretions: role of a 'short' feedback mechanism. *Endocrinology*, **78**, 55–60.

DAVID-NELSON, M. A. AND BRODISH, A. (1969) Evidence for a diurnal rhythm of corticotrophin releasing factor (CRF) in the hypothalamus. *Endocrinology*, **85**, 861–866.

DAVIDSON, J. M. (1966) Control of gonadotropin secretion in the male. In *Neuroendocrinology*, *Vol. I.*, L. MARTINI AND W. F. GANONG (Eds.), Academic Press, New York and London, p. 565.

DAVIDSON, J. M. AND FELDMAN, S. (1963) Cerebral involvement in the inhibition of ACTH secretion by hydrocortisone. *Endocrinology*, **72**, 936–946.

DAVIDSON, J. M. AND SAWYER, C. H. (1961a) Effects of localized intracerebral implantation of oestrogen on reproductive function in the female rabbit. *Acta endocr. (Kbh.)*, **37**, 385–393.

DAVIDSON, J. M. AND SAWYER, C. H. (1961b) Evidence for a hypothalamic focus of inhibition of gonadotropin by androgen in the male. *Proc. Soc. exp. Biol. (N.Y.)*, **107**, 4–7.

DEUBEN, R. R. AND MEITES, J. (1964) Stimulation of pituitary growth hormone release by a hypothalamic extract *in vitro*. *Endocrinology*, **74**, 408–414.

DUNN, J. AND CRITCHLOW, V. (1969) Pituitary-adrenal response to stress in rats with hypothalamic islands. *Brain Research*, **16**, 395–403.

EIK-NES, K. B. AND BRIZZEE, K. R. (1958) Some aspects of corticotrophin secretion in the trained dog. I. The presence of a corticotrophin releasing factor in the blood stream of dogs shortly after hypophysectomy. *Acta endocr. (Kbh.)*, **29**, 219–223.

ENDRÖCZI, E., LISSÁK, K. AND TEKERES, M. (1961) Hormonal feedback regulation of pituitary–adrenocortical activity. *Acta physiol. Acad. Sci. hung.*, **18**, 291–299.

EVANS, J. S. AND NIKITOVITCH-WINER, M. B. (1969) Functional reactivation and cytological restoration of pituitary grafts by continuous local intravascular infusion of median eminence extracts. *Neuroendocrinology*, **4**, 83–100.

EVERETT, J. W. (1964) Central neural control of reproductive functions of the adenohypophysis. *Physiol. Rev.*, **44**, 373–431.

EVERETT, J. W. AND SAWYER, C. H. (1949) A neural timing factor in the mechanism by which progesterone advances ovulation in the cyclic rat. *Endocrinology*, **45**, 581–595.

FELDMAN, S., CONFORTI, N., CHOWERS, I. AND DAVIDSON, J. M. (1970) Pituitary-adrenal activation in rats with medial basal hypothalamic islands. *Acta endocr. (Kbh.)*, **63**, 405–414.

FINK, G. (1967) Nature of luteinizing hormone releasing factor in hypophysial portal blood. *Nature (Lond.)*, **215**, 159–161.

FINK, G., NALLAR, R. AND WORTHINGTON, W. C., JR. (1966) Determination of luteinizing hormone releasing factor (LRF) in hypophysial portal blood. *J. Physiol. (Lond.)*, **183**, 20P–21P.

FINK, G., NALLAR, R. AND WORTHINGTON, W. C., JR. (1967) The demonstration of luteinizing hormone releasing factor in hypophysial portal blood of pre-oestrous and hypophysectomized rats. *J. Physiol. (Lond.)*, **191**, 407–416.

FLAMENT–DURAND, J. (1965) Observations on pituitary transplants into the hypothalamus of the rat. *Endocrinology*, **77**, 446–454.

FLAMENT–DURAND, J. AND DESCLIN, L. (1968) A topographical study of a hypothalamic region with a 'thyrotrophic' action. *J. Endocr.*, **41**, 531–539.

FLERKÓ, B. (1966) Control of gonadotropin secretion in the female. In *Neuroendocrinology, Vol. I.*, L. MARTINI AND W. F. GANONG (Eds.), Academic Press, New York, London, p. 613.

FLERKÓ, B. (1968) Hypothalamic control of hypophyseal gonadotrophic function. In *Hypothalamic Control of the Anterior Pituitary*, J. SZENTÁGOTHAI, B. FLERKÓ, B. MESS AND B. HALÁSZ (Eds.), Akadémiai Kiadó, Budapest, p. 249.

FLERKÓ, B. AND SZENTÁGOTHAI, J. (1957) Oestrogen sensitive nervous structures in the hypothalamus. *Acta endocr., (Kbh.)*, **26**, 121–127.

FORTIER, C. (1951) Dual control of adrenocorticotropin release. *Endocrinology*, **49**, 782–788.

FRANZ, J., HASELBACH, C. H. AND LIBERT, O. (1962) Studies on the effect of hypothalamic extracts on somatotrophic pituitary function. *Acta endocr. (Kbh.)*, **41**, 336–350.

FUXE, K. (1964) Cellular localization of monoamines in the median eminence and infundibular stem of some mammals. *Z. Zellforsch.*, **61**, 710–724.

FUXE, K. AND HÖKFELT, T. (1969) Catecholamines in the hypothalamus and the pituitary gland. In *Frontiers in Neuroendocrinology, 1969*, W. F. GANONG AND L. MARTINI (Eds.), Oxford Univ. Press, New York, London, Toronto, p. 47.

FUXE, K., HÖFKELT, T. AND NILSSON, O. (1967) Activity changes in the tubero-infundibular dopamine neurons of the rat during various states of the reproductive cycle. *Life Sci.*, **6**, 2057–2061.

FUXE, K., HÖFKELT, T. AND NILSSON, O. (1969) Factors involved in the control of the activity of the tubero-infundibular dopamine neurons during pregnancy and lactation. *Neuroendocrinology*, **5**, 257–270.

GESCHWIND, E. (1969) Mechanism of action of releasing factors. In *Frontiers in Neuroendocrinology, 1969*, W. F. GANONG AND L. MARTINI (Eds.), Oxford Univ. Press, New York, London, Toronto, p. 389.

GOLDBERG, R. C. AND KNOBIL, E. (1957) Structure and function of intraocular hypophysial grafts in the hypophysectomized male rat. *Endocrinology*, **61**, 742–752.

GREEN, J. D. AND HARRIS, G. W. (1947) The neurovascular link between the neurohypophysis and adenohypophysis. *J. Endocr.*, **5**, 136–146.

GREER, M. A., ALLEN, C. F., GIBBS, F. P. AND GULLICKSON, C. (1970) Pathways at the hypothalamic level through which traumatic stress activates ACTH secretion. *Endocrinology*, **86**, 1404–1409.

GREER, M. A. AND ROCKIE, C. (1968) Inhibition by pentobarbital of ether induced ACTH secretion in the rat. *Endocrinology*, **83**, 1247–1252.

GUILLEMIN, R. AND ROSENBERG, B. (1955) Humoral hypothalamic control of anterior pituitary: A study with combined tissue cultures. *Endocrinology*, **57**, 599–607.

GUILLEMIN, R., YAMAZAKI, E., JUTISZ, M. ET SAKIZ, E. (1962) Présence dans un extrait de tissus hypothalamiques d'une substance stimulant la sécrétion de l'hormone hypophysaire thyréotrope (TSH). Première purification par filtration sur le Sephadex. *C.R. Acad. Sci. (Paris)*, **255**, 1018–1020.

HALÁSZ, B. (1968) The role of the hypothalamic hypophysiotrophic area in the control of growth hormone secretion. In *Growth Hormone*, A. PECILE AND E. E. MÜLLER (Eds.), Proc. First Internat. Symp., Milan, Italy, September 11–13, 1967. *Excerpta med. int. Congr. Ser.* **158**, p. 204.

McCann, S. M., Taleisnik, S. and Friedman, H. M. (1960) LH-releasing activity in hypothalamic extracts. *Proc. Soc. exp. Biol. (N.Y.)*, **104**, 432–434.

McDermott, W. V., Fry, E. G., Brobeck, J. R. and Long, C. N. H. (1950) Release of adrenocorticotrophic hormone by direct application of epinephrine to pituitary grafts. *Proc. Soc. exp. Biol. (N.Y.)*, **73**, 609–610.

McEven, B. S. and Pfaff, D. W. (1970) Factors influencing sex hormone uptake by rat brain regions. I. Effects of neonatal treatment, hypophysectomy and competing steroid on estradiol uptake. *Brain Research*, **21**, 1–16.

McGuire, J. L. and Lisk, R. D. (1969) Localization of oestrogen receptors in the rat hypothalamus. *Neuroendocrinology*, **4**, 289–295.

Meites, J. (1966) Control of mammary growth and lactation. In *Neuroendocrinology, Vol. I*, L. Martini and W. F. Ganong (Eds.), Academic Press, New York, London, p. 669.

Meites, J., Talwalker, P. K. and Ratner, A. (1962) Evidence for a prolactin-inhibiting factor in rat hypothalamic tissue. *Program 44th Endocrine Soc., Chicago*, p. 19.

Mess, B., Fraschini, F., Motta, M. and Martini, L. (1966) The topography of the neurons synthesizing the hypothalamic releasing factors. *Excerpta med. int. Congr. Ser.*, **132**, 1004–1013.

Michael, R. P. (1964) The selective accumulation of oestrogen in the neural and genital tissues of the cat. *Proc. 1st Intern. Congr. Hormonal Steroids*, Milan, 1962, Academic Press, New York, 457–469.

Mishkinsky, J., Nir, I. and Sulman, F. G. (1969) Internal feedback of prolactin in the rat. *Neuroendocrinology*, **5**, 48–52.

Mittler, J. C., Redding, T. W. and Schally, A. V. (1969) Stimulation of thyrotropin (TSH) secretion by TSH-releasing factor (TRF) in organ cultures of anterior pituitary, *Proc. Soc. exp. Biol. (N.Y.)*, **130**, 406–409.

Monroe, B. G. (1967) A comparative study of the ultrastructure of the median eminence, infundibular stem and neural lobe of the hypophysis of the rat. *Z. Zellforsch.*, **76**, 405–432.

Motta, M., Mangili, G. and Martini, L. (1965) A 'short' feedback loop in the control of ACTH secretion. *Endocrinology*, **77**, 392–395.

Müller, E. E., Arimura, A., Saito, T. and Schally, A. V. (1967) Growth hormone releasing activity in plasma of normal and hypophysectomized rats. *Endocrinology*, **80**, 77–81.

Nallar, R. and McCann, S. M. (1965) Luteinizing hormone-releasing activity in plasma of hypophysectomized rats. *Endocrinology*, **76**, 272–275.

Negro-Vilar, A., Dickerman, E. and Meites, J. (1968) FSH releasing factor activity in plasma of rats after hypophysectomy and continuous light. *Endocrinology*, **82**, 939–944.

Nikitovitch-Winer, M. B. (1962) Induction of ovulation in rats by direct intrapituitary infusion of median eminence extracts. *Endocrinology*, **70**, 350–358.

Nikitovitch-Winer, M. and Everett, J. W. (1958) Functional restitution of pituitary grafts retransplanted from kidney to median eminence. *Endocrinology*, **63**, 916–930.

Nikitovitch-Winer, M. and Everett, J. W. (1959) Histologic changes in grafts of rat pituitary on the kidney and upon re-transplantation under the diencephalon. *Endocrinology*, **65**, 357–368.

Nowakowski, H. (1951) Infundibulum und Tuber cinereum der Katze. *Dtsch. Z. Nervenheilk.*, **165**, 201–239.

Ojeda, S. R. and Ramirez, V. D. (1969) Automatic control of LH and FSH secretion by short feedback circuits in immature rats. *Endocrinology*, **84**, 786–797.

Palka, Y., Coyer, D. and Critchlow, V. (1969) Effects of isolation of medial basal hypothalamus on pituitary–adrenal and pituitary–ovarian functions. *Neuroendocrinology*, **5**, 333–349.

Pasteels, J. L. (1961a) Sécrétion de prolactine par l'hypophyse en culture de tissus. *C.R. Soc. Biol, (Paris)*, **253**, 2140–2142.

Pasteels, J. L. (1961b) Premiers résultats de culture combinée *in vitro* d'hypophyse et d'hypothalamus, dans le but d'en apprécier la sécrétion de prolactine. *C.R. Soc. Biol. (Paris)*, **253**, 3074–3075.

Pasteels, J. L. (1962) Élaboration par l'hypophyse humaine en culture de tissus d'une substance le jabot de Pigeon. *C.R. Soc. Biol. (Paris)*, **254**, 4083–4085.

Pecile, A., Müller, E., Falconi, G. and Martini, L. (1965) Growth hormone releasing activity of hypothalamic extracts at different ages. *Endocrinology*, **77**, 241–246.

Pfaff, D. W. (1968a) Autoradiographic localization of radioactivity in rat brain after injection of tritiated sex hormones. *Science*, **161**, 1355–1356.

Pfaff, D. W. (1968b) Autoradiographic localization of testosterone-^{3}H in the female rat brain and estradiol-^{3}H in the male rat brain. *Experientia (Basel)*, **24**, 958–959.

PFAFF, D. W. (1968c) Uptake of ^{3}H-estradiol by the female rat brain. An autoradiographic study. *Endocrinology*, **82**, 1149–1155.

PORTER, J. C. (1969) Hypophysiotropic hormones in portal vessel blood. In *Hypophysiotrophic Hormones of the Hypothalamus: Assay and Chemistry*, J. MEITES (Ed.), Proceedings of the Workshop Conference, Tucson, Ariz. 1969. Williams and Wilkins, Baltimore, p. 282.

RAMIREZ, V. D., ABRAMS, R. M. AND MCCANN, S. M. (1964) Effect of estradiol implants in the hypothalamo-hypophysial region of the rat on the secretion of luteinizing hormone. *Endocrinology*, **75**, 243–248.

RAMIREZ, V. D. AND SAWYER, C. H. (1965) Fluctuations in hypothalamic LH-RF (luteinizing hormone-releasing factor) during the rat estrous cycle. *Endocrinology*, **76**, 282–289.

RATNER, A. AND MEITES, J. (1964) Depletion of prolactin-inhibiting activity of rat hypothalamus by estradiol or suckling stimulus. *Endocrinology*, **75**, 377–382.

REDDING, T. W. AND SCHALLY, A. V. (1969) Studies on the thyrotropin-releasing hormone (TRH) activity in peripheral blood. *Proc. Soc. exp. Biol. (N.Y.)*, **131**, 420–425.

REICHLIN, S. (1966) Control of thyrotropic hormone secretion. In *Neuroendocrinology, Vol. I*, L. MARTINI AND W. F. GANONG (Eds.), Academic Press, New York, London, p. 445.

RÉTHELYI, M. AND HALÁSZ, B. (1970) Origin of the nerve endings in the surface zone of the median eminence of the rat hypothalamus. *Exp. Brain Res.*, **11**, 145–158.

SAFFRAN, M. AND SCHALLY, A. V. (1955) Release of corticotrophin by anterior pituitary tissue *in vitro*. *Canad. J. Biochem. Physiol.*, **33**, 408–415.

SCHALLY, A. V., ARIMURA, A., BOWERS, C. Y., KASTIN, A. J., SAWANO, S. AND REDDING, T. W. (1968a) Hypothalamic neurohormones regulating anterior pituitary function. *Recent Progr. Hormone Res.*, **24**, 497–588.

SCHALLY, A. V., FOLKERS, K., BOWERS, C. Y., ENZMANN, F., BØLER, J., NAIR, R. M. G. AND BARRETT, J. F. (1969) The structure of porcine thyrotropin-releasing-hormone (TRH). In *Hypophysiotrophic Hormones of the Hypothalamus; Assay and Chemistry*, J. MEITES (Ed.), Proceedings of the Workshop Conference, Tucson, Ariz., 1969. Williams and Wilkins, Baltimore, p. 226.

SCHALLY, A. V., MÜLLER, E. E. AND SAWANO, S. (1968b) Effect of porcine growth hormone-releasing factor on the release and synthesis of growth hormone *in vitro*. *Endocrinology*, **82**, 271–276.

SCHAPIRO, S., MARMORSTON, J. AND SOBEL, H. (1956) Pituitary stimulating substance in brain blood of hypophysectomized rat following electric shock 'stress'. *Proc. Soc. exp. Biol. (N.Y.)*, **91**, 382–386.

SCHNEIDER, H. P. G., CRIGHTON, D. B. AND MCCANN, S. M. (1969) Suprachiasmatic LH-releasing factor. *Neuroendocrinology*, **5**, 271–280.

SCHNEIDER, H. P. G. AND MCCANN, S. M. (1969) Possible role of dopamine as transmitter to promote discharge of LH-releasing factor. *Endocrinology*, **85**, 121–132.

SCHREIBER, V., ECKERTOVA, A., FRANZ, Z., KOČI, J., RYBÁK, M. AND KMENTOVÁ, V. (1961) Effect of a fraction of bovine hypothalamic extract on the release of TSH by rat adenohypophysis *in vitro*. *Experientia (Basel)*, **17**, 264–265.

SHELESNYAK, M. C. (1931) Induction of pseudopregnancy in the rat by means of electrical stimulation. *Anat. Rec.*, **49**, 179–183.

SHIBUSAWA, K., SAITO, S., NISHI, K., YAMAMOTO, T., ABE, CH. AND KAWAI, T. (1956a) Effects of thyrotrophin releasing principle (TRF) after section of the pituitary stalk. *Endocr. jap.*, **3**, 151–157.

SHIBUSAWA, K., SAITO, S., NISHI, K., YAMAMOTO, T., TOMIZAWA, K. AND ABE, C. (1956b) The hypothalamic control of the thyrotroph-thyroidal function. *Endocr. jap.*, **3**, 116–124.

SINHA, D. K. AND MEITES, J. (1965–66) Effects of thyroidectomy and thyroxine on hypothalamic concentration of 'thyrotropin releasing factor' and pituitary content of thyrotropin in rats. *Neuroendocrinology*, **1**, 4–14.

SINHA, D. AND MEITES, J. (1966) Stimulation of pituitary thyrotropin synthesis and release by hypothalamic extract. *Endocrinology*, **78**, 1002–1006.

SIPERSTEIN, E. R. AND GREER, M. A. (1956) Observation on the morphology and histochemistry of the mouse pituitary implanted in the anterior eye chamber. *J. nat. Cancer Inst.*, **17**, 569–599.

SLUSHER, M. A. (1966) Effects of cortisol implants in the brainstem and ventral hippocampus on diurnal corticosteroid levels. *Exp. Brain. Res.*, **1**, 184–194.

SPATZ, H. (1951) Neues über die Verknüpfung von Hypophyse und Hypothalamus. *Acta neuroveg. (Wien)*, **3**, 1–49.

STEINER, F. A., RUF, K. AND AKERT, K. (1969) Steroid-sensitive neurones in rat brain: anatomical localization and responses to neurohumours and ACTH. *Brain Research*, **12**, 74–85.

In this pursuit of the natural experiment Ernst Scharrer—I will limit myself to vertebrate physiology—concentrated his attention on diverse species throughout the vertebrates, seeking from a comparative analysis to derive some functional clue from the curious features of his so-called 'secretory' neurones. He attempted to correlate what he interpreted as secretory cycles with different endocrine states. This form of essentially speculative analysis was near success in the early forties, when Von Gaupp, on pathological, and Palay (a student of the Scharrers), on morphological grounds, suggested that it was in fact down the nerves of the supraopticohypophyseal system that posterior-pituitary principles passed into the infundibular process of the neurohypophysis. Bargmann (1949), using the chrome-alum-haematoxylin technique (CAH), reached the same conclusion on far stronger cytological evidence, and with Ernst Scharrer, who had been influenced by curious accumulations seen by Drager (1950), derived from the cut pituitary stalk of the snake, postulated (Bargmann and Scharrer, 1951) the definitive theory.

The question arises now as to what extent we have succeeded, in the intervening years, in setting up experiments capable of testing these initial and brilliant speculations. We have in fact advanced far less than might be thought from reading the blackboard physiology to which this field seems absurdly susceptible.

No attempt will be made to labour the definition of 'neurosecretion', beyond the statement that here we are concerned primarily with cells resembling neurones whose principal occupation appears to be the secretion of a hormone. In the HNS oxytocin, vasopressin and substances such as neurophysin are derived from the supraoptic and paraventricular nuclei (SON and PVN), most of whose fibres end on blood vessels in the neurohypophysis, and in particular in the infundibular process; other substances, certainly dopamine (DA), originate in the tubero-infundibular nuclei (TIN), whose nerve fibres end primarily in the peripheral zone of the median eminence. The source and mode of secretion of other pharmacological agents found in the floor of the third ventricle are unknown; and the same is true of the Release Factors (Hormones).

Our main concern here is to consider four categories of cell, any of which might be thought likely to play a role in the formation and transference of those release-factors or hormones which have been extracted from the neurohypophysis. These four categories are, first the neurones whose fibres pass to the region; second, its interstitial cells, most of which are probably neuroglial; third, the ependyma of the region; and fourth, the cells of pars tuberalis and pars intermedia. These tissues, as well as numerous vessels and their associated pericytes and fibrocytes, form the samples containing very many hundreds of thousands of cells from which pharmacological extracts are made; we must bear in mind the heterogeneity of such samples.

The glandular sheath of the neurohypophysis, namely, pars intermedia and pars tuberalis

Little is as yet known of the function of *pars tuberalis*, the glandular part of the adenohypophysis which partially ensheaths the median eminence.

With regard to *pars intermedia*, it is accepted that this contains cells which secrete melanin stimulating hormone (MSH) and Purves (1966) observes that such cells, in species lacking a definitive pars intermedia, must be distributed elsewhere in the adenohypophysis.

The role of neurosecretory fibres in the control of pars intermedia is largely at the *speculative* stage, although pharmacological evidence certainly points towards this form of control and indeed suggests that we should not dismiss the possibility that similar mechanisms play a part in modifying other aspects of adenohypophyseal function. The evidence centres on the facts, first, that MSH shares the structure of ACTH; and second, that the tripeptide release factor (Pro-Leu-Gly-NH$_2$) which inhibits the secretion of MSH, has part of the structure of oxytocin (Schally, 1971).

Schally's discovery certainly bears out the possibility of the neurosecretory control of MSH release. The *anatomical* pathways by which this could occur are evident in particular in fishes, where the close apposition of neural with glandular elements often involves more than the meta-adenohypophysis, that is, that part of the pituitary which is normally identified with the pars intermedia of higher vertebrates (Dodd and Kerr, 1963). The mechanism of this form of neurosecretory innervation is still obscure. Knowles and Anand Kumar (1969) have speculated on secretory-motor and inhibitor roles for neurosecretory fibres apposed to different poles of single glandular cells in elasmobranchs. It is tempting, in the light of Enemar and Falck's (1965) observations on the frog to suppose that these fibres are in part aminergic, in part peptidergic.

In mammals, too, secretory fibres have been observed by electron microscopy entering pars intermedia, for example by Ziegler (1963). The same is probably true in man, although here evidence is confined to light microscopy. The 'intermediate zone' of the adult human is represented in part by groups of basophil cells within the substance of the infundibular process, cells which Morris *et al.* (1956) showed to contain MSH.

Experimental evidence, however, on the functional significance of this innervation is scanty, and confined to lower vertebrates (Etkin, 1941; Enemar and Falck, 1965; Meurling *et al.*, 1969). Further evidence of this kind will be of value, for we may well have underestimated the importance of the secretory innervation of the adenohypophysis—this for three reasons: first, in a wide variety of mammals nerve fibres have been identified passing into pars tuberalis and pars intermedia; second, the adenohypophyseal sheath of the neurohypophysis often includes a junctional region between the tuberal, distal and intermediate parts, and this has yet to be specifically analysed pharmacologically: it could well, for example, possess substances such as ACTH. Third, in the light, in particular, of the work of Hortense and Etienne Legait (1962), it may well be that the function of pars intermedia is not confined to the secretion of MSH. The curious manner in which [^{35}S]methionine accumulated only in the lateral wing of the rat pars intermedia, struck me as conforming with this hypothesis (Sloper *et al.*, 1960): for MSH contains methionine, and I had anticipated its accumulation throughout pars intermedia.

The Legaits correlated, especially in the rat, morphological changes in the secretory neurones of the HNS with corresponding changes in pars intermedia. Such changes, they showed, occurred following a wide range of physiological stresses, ranging from

able to show marked differences between stressed and normal animals. Yet our experiments were of tentative value in that we found it difficult to take into account the alterations in the volume of the grossly enlarged nuclear regions.

Now these latter observations, in that they involved the photometric comparison of sections of control and stressed animal taken from a single paraffin block, overcame one of the biggest technical problems in photometry, namely variation in section-thickness. When one appreciates that this particular precaution has yet to be taken by others in this field; that the CAH technique probably demonstrates Nissl substance, which itself alters in distribution in stressed animals; and that the aldehyde fuchsin technique picks up inclusions which probably represent lysosomes, it will be realised that attempts to quantitate minor variations in the cytological distribution of neurosecretory material have been of rather limited value. This is not to deny that in grossly stressed animals one can virtually empty the entire system of protein-bound cystine, but to emphasise the difficulty of performing definitive experiments on a system composed of very elongated cells which show considerable plasticity.

(c) Can the direction of flow of neurohormone be demonstrated experimentally? With the CAH method, Hild and Zetler (1953) showed that CAH-NSM, vasopressin and oxytocin accumulated on the hypothalamic side of lesions in the tractus hypophyseus; we showed that the same was true of cystine-rich NSM, and now Uttenthal and his collaborators (1971) have established that neurophysin-II accumulates in the same manner. On the other hand, such disturbances in flow have yet, in vertebrates, to be demonstrated *in vivo*. Moreover, there remains the possibility that in some fibres flow could be centripetal (Collin, 1928).

2. Dynamic investigation of neurosecretion

The use of radioisotopes was introduced into the study of neurosecretion with a view to elucidating the dynamics of the process. We postulated that following the subarachnoid injection of [^{35}S]cysteine there should be early a high uptake in the SON and PVN, and only later a high uptake in the infundibular process. Following the injection of [^{35}S]methionine, which the vasopressor and oxytocic octapeptides lack, we postulated the same early nuclear region uptake, but no late posterior pituitary uptake.

Our experiments, first reported at Lund in 1957, were the first to provide dynamic evidence of the Bargmann–Scharrer theory of neurosecretion.

Our early technical problems are of interest, for they tend to have been overlooked by successive and most recent workers in the field of neurosecretion. Thus, in 1956 we were tempted to work with the radioactivity of tissue samples as well as autoradiographs. The great limitation of the first technique is the difficulty of localising the radioisotope. This particularly applies to the posterior lobe of the pituitary, samples of which necessarily include pars intermedia. It would, incidentally, be preferable nowadays to use a less penetrant isotope than ^{35}S, in order to facilitate its intracellular localisation. Nishioka *et al.* (1970) have recently achieved just this, using L-[^{3}H]-cystine. It is essential that the same technique be applied to the ligatured tractus hypophyseus. I would add that it is better to use cysteine than cystine, in that the latter, although easier to obtain, is insoluble at neutrality. This is especially important if one plans a subarachnoid injection. In fact, we only obtained good and repeatable delayed uptake of radioisotope in the infundibular process, if we injected labelled cysteine into the subarachnoid space, that is, into the CSF. This point was overlooked by Sachs (1960) in his early attempts to biosynthesise labelled vasopressin with the aid of our technique, although he achieved success when he administered labelled cysteine into the ventricles. Probably for the same reason, Goslar and Schulze (1958) and Ford and Hirschman (1958) failed to demonstrate delayed uptake of radioisotope in the posterior pituitary.

It was the accumulation of isotope in this region 5 h and longer after injection which allowed us to suggest in 1957, first, that we might have biosynthesised labelled hormone; and second, that this possibly flowed down the tractus hypophyseus at the rate of a millimeter or so an hour. Our assumptions have been corroborated in terms of vasopressor activity by Sachs; and most recently in terms of the synthesis of the neurophysins by Burford et al. (1971) in Bristol, and Norström and Sjöstrand (1971) in Gothenburg.

Nevertheless, the limitations of our early autoradiographic observations must be stressed. In the first place, they were made by light microscopy and they *could* be explained in terms of the passage of labelled polypeptides into the nerve-endings of the posterior pituitary by some other route than the tractus hypophyseus. This is the less likely, now that Desclin and Flament Durand (1963) have demonstrated the accumulation of radioisotope, using the same technique, on the hypothalamic side of the severed pituitary stalk of the rat; and Norström et al. (1971) have shown that colchicine, which possibly inhibits axoplasmic flow, blocks the accumulation of labelled neurohypophyseal proteins in the posterior lobe of the pituitary. Secondly, our evidence that the isotope demonstrated in the posterior pituitary was present in neurohormone was necessarily indirect.

Third, the term 'late uptake' was used with some reservation. What we did was merely to claim that, in terms of grain-counts, the amount of radioisotope in the infundibular process differed from that in an overlying part of the hypothalamus, relatively devoid of neuronal cell-bodies. Despite these shortcomings, our experiments had this merit, that they failed to invalidate the theory of neurosecretion. Their significance was greatly strengthened by Sachs' work. Definitive cytophysiological experiment, however, will require that such work is performed at the ultrastructural level, in conjunction with autoradiography, and the immunofluorescent localisation of, for example, neurophysin-II.

3. Ultrastructural analysis of neurosecretion

In the '50's and early '60's, the view persisted that the presence of optically demonstrable NSM was a measure of the secretory activity of the HNS. Observations on the variability of the NSM content of the median eminence of long hypophysectomised human subjects, led me early in 1956 to question this, and to suggest that large accumulations of NSM, as found in the infundibular process, were a measure not of activity but of the secretory reserve of the system. For a pathologist, there were three corol-

of DA. They themselves note that we must assume that this secretory activity has preceded any possible pharmacological effect at the nerve ending. Such experiments have led them to suggest that DA-secreting neurones modify pituitary gonadotrophic activity by influencing the secretion of Release or Inhibitory Factors. Interestingly enough, it was by a rather similar technique that Pellegrino de Iraldi and Etcheverry (1967) demonstrated a measurable increase in 800–1000 Å granules within nerve endings of the median eminence, granules which they therefore regarded as vehicles of DA.

Rather similar experiments by Zambrano and De Robertis (1966, 1968) were concerned with the effects of castration of the rat on the numbers of electron-dense vesicles (800–1300 Å in diameter) in normal cell-bodies in the arcuate nuclei, and in nerve-endings in the palisade zone of the median eminence. These findings certainly suggest the participation of such vesicles in the secretion of GRF.

Their earlier investigations of 1966 in stressed rats had suggested that high secretory activity in the supraoptic nucleus was characterised by a number of features, some already suspected or documented by light microscopy. These include (Fig. 1):

(1) Nuclear and nucleolar enlargement;
(2) A diminution in the number of neurosecretory vesicles in the perikaryon;
(3) An increase in the size of the Golgi apparatus;
(4) An increase in the size of the granular endoplasmic reticulum;
(5) An increase in the size and number of lysosomes.

Their inferences are probably correct, but need to be corroborated by detailed quantitative studies. The underlying difficulty is the obviously irregular distribution of inclusions in the cytoplasm of secretory neurones, and again the fact that a cell 30 micra in diameter requires nearly 500 sections of 600 Å thickness for its survey.

In particular, while nuclear and nucleolar enlargement are obvious enough by light microscopy (see Ortmann, 1951), NSV are not uniform in distribution. The area, too, occupied by the Golgi apparatus and endoplasmic reticulum will be very difficult to measure. Moreover, in the light of Edström and Eichner's findings (1960), changes in the ribosomal content of the endoplasmic reticulum probably reflect dispersal. The fine filaments Zambrano and De Robertis observed in stressed animals are interesting and merit further study.

As for lysosomes, it is nice to speculate on a correlation between lysosomal activity and active secretion, but this has not been confirmed in terms of acid phosphatase activity by the quantitative cytochemistry of Jongkind (1967, 1969). There is, in this respect, incidentally, urgent need for ultrastructural studies which can extend the brilliant observations of Jongkind and his collaborators here in Amsterdam. Their work, which centres on the light-microscopical estimation of the distribution of thymidine diphosphate dihydrolase (TTPase) is much the most satisfactory yet accomplished in the field of the enzyme histochemistry of neurosecretion. TTPase, a Golgi zone enzyme, and glucose 6-phosphate hydrogenase, a pentose-shunt enzyme, have been shown to increase markedly in the perikarya of dehydrated rats. Jongkind links their activity with the RNA content of the perikarya and thus with protein synthesis.

Now the alterations in the perikarya so far analysed in dehydrated rats have also been seen in the perikarya of the SON of rats suffering from the congenital diabetes insipidus (Orkand and Palay, 1967), a disease carefully analysed by Valtin (*e.g.* 1967). These neurones show, as it were, a frustration-hypertrophy, in that they form no vasopressin; the changes seen correspond fairly closely with the work-hypertrophy elicited by saline administration or dehydration. A similar hypertrophy has, moreover, been seen by Orkand and Palay in the axoplasm and endings of affected neurones in the neurohypophysis. Unfortunately, however, these features, like those seen in dehydrated rats, have yet to be quantitated.

4. Nuclear regions from which the nerve-endings of the median eminence and infundibular process are derived

Reference has already been made to the current tendency to separate in terms of function the upper and lower parts of the neurohypophysis, and to the fact that, in terms of the regions drained by portal vessels, such a distinction is overarbitrary. It is indisputable that most of the nerve endings with infundibular process are derived from the SON and PVN, but it is denied that any of the fibres ending in the median eminence have a similar origin.

One of the arguments put forward lies in the claim that this region, although traversed by the tractus hypophyseus, lacks any innervation by fibres derived from the SON and PVN. Pharmacological evidence on this point is scanty, but Kobayashi and his co-workers (1970) have noted that the amount, for example, of vasopressin in the median eminence, is more than can be accounted for in terms of that contained by the tractus hypophyseus. Morphological evidence corroborates this, in that it has repeatedly been noted that there is some NSM, whether demonstrated by stains or cytochemical technique, in the peripheral zone of the median eminence. Now this could be present in deviant fibres which continue back from the peripheral zone and down to the tractus hypophyseus; this, however, seems unlikely, the more so because in pituitary-stalk-sectioned animals the peripheral zone becomes rich in NSM and, incidentally, in vasopressin and oxytocin.

The effect of pituitary stalk section can be explained in two ways which are not mutually exclusive, namely, first in terms of the growth into the peripheral zone of collateral nerve fibres derived from interrupted fibres in the tractus hypophyseus: or second, in terms of the assumption of a 'storage' rather than merely 'secretory' role by pre-existing secretory fibres passing from the SON and PVN into the peripheral zone of the median eminence. This second explanation would account for the relative paucity of endings that contain NSM in the median eminence of the normal subject.

Whatever the explanation, one thing is clear, namely that these cystine-rich nerve endings in the residual median eminence of hypophysectomised subjects are derived from magnocellular neurones, some few of which survive in the SON, and many of which survive in the caudal parts of the PVN (Sloper and Adams, 1956). If therefore the majority of the endings rich in NSM found in the residual median eminence do reflect the growth of collaterals from injured fibres, then it must be accepted that many unmyelinated fibres can survive interruption, presumably if perikaryon, site of injury

Zambrano, D. and De Robertis, E. (1966) The secretory role of the supraoptic neurons in the rat. A structural–functional correlation. *Z. Zellforsch.*, **73**, 414–431.

Zambrano, D. and De Robertis, E. (1967) Ultrastructure of the hypothalamic neurosecretory system in the dog. *Z. Zellforsch.*, **81**, 264–282.

Zambrano, D. and De Robertis, E. (1968) Ultrastructural changes of the neurohypophysis of the rat after castration. *Z. Zellforsch.*, **86**, 14–25.

Ziegler, B. (1963) Licht- und elektronmikroskopische Untersuchungen an Pars intermedia und Neurohypophyse der Ratte. *Z. Zellforsch.*, **59**, 486–506.

DISCUSSION

Swaab: In using the cystein technique you showed that radioactivity may be found in the posterior lobe some 9 to 10 hours after injection. Jones and co-workers using tyrosine as a marker found that oxytocin and vasopressin are accumulating within one to two hours in the posterior lobe. Would you mind to comment on this difference?

Sloper: I think it is a question of how many animals you kill. It was obvious that we found a peak at about 10 hours. You have to remember that it is a very time-consuming experiment. There is one point however, the moment you find material, it probably has arrived there much earlier than one is able to demonstrate by autoradiography.

Swaab: But Jones and co-workers looked at earlier stages too, *e.g.*, after 2 hours, 4 hours, 6 hours, but they did not find any.

Sloper: Well, I can't answer that question, because I don't remember the specific technique being used.

Bern: The radioautographic work of the type you perform is at best preliminary. There is not any evidence of accumulation of radioactive material in axon terminals until about 2 hours. If one looks at axon terminals in the thirsting rat after the administration of tritiated cystein one gets something that one can observe and count after 2 hours but not before. Pickering's biochemical data agree with this finding. We are interested in using this technique in trying to answer some other questions such as whether there is axonal synthesis or taking up of material in the terminals.

Dreifuss: Has local synthesis in the terminals been excluded and have retrogade changes been described after stalk section in nuclei other than the supraoptic and paraventricular nuclei?

Sloper: One may attack this problem with the technique of intracarotid and arachnoidal injection and use radioactive methionine. Then one could try to demonstrate a high uptake of material in the axonal terminal, as compared to the cell body. I think this would entail sections of both methods in direct comparison. The investigations and results with the isolated pituitary stalk argue against any local synthesis.

   With regard to your second point about retrogade degeneration following human hypophysectomy or stalk ligature, this results in heavy bleeding and tissue destruction. There are often widespread lesions in the hypothalamus. These ascending hemorrhagic lesions in the hypothalamus are probably due to poor drainage into the hypothalamic capillaries. As a pathologist I have been struck again and again by the extent of the necrosis that can follow lesions anywhere in the system.

Dreifuss: The paper of Palay you referred to concerned the electron microscopy of paraventricular neurons. Have they found specific neurosecretory granules? This would of course be important to the concept of the two-neuron system, one producing oxytocin, the other vasopressin.

Sloper: I cannot really remember that point. I have not looked at the paraventricular nucleus myself either.

Smelik: There are many advantages and disadvantages of the fluorescence method. Without any pharmacological means you can visualize a monoaminergic system. I trust the specificity of it, although it is still very difficult to make a difference between dopamine and noradrenaline. All drugs or treatments which deplete catecholamines will cause the disappearance of fluorescence. I hesitate to believe that it is possible, for instance, as Fuxe did, to determine the turn-over rate of these neurons by blocking synthesis by some drug and then looking at the rate of depletion or disappearance of fluorescence. This brings up the most difficult thing, namely whether it would be possible to quantify the method. Several people including Fuxe himself use now a more objective method. There is another problem about how to measure the mean amount of light which you see in the field. Several people are planning to develop a sort of scanner which will scan the field, but you need a computer attached to it. Then it may be possible to make some quantifications.

GANONG: How good is the evidence that there is no synthesis in the axonal endings? If there is synthesis what we are looking at is a release of an amine in the synaptic cleft. If we get depletion with a particular drug so much the better and if we don't get it, that does not mean the release has changed.

SLOPER: We don't know enough about this and experiments of the type of Dr. Fuxe are very difficult.

SCHARRER: I would like to make a remark following Dr. Ganong's: You know you can deplete the posterior pituitary beautifully by a thirsting experiment but in respect to the oxytocin content under conditions of use or disuse you cannot deplete these neurons.

SLOPER: In animals giving a response to osmotic stress you find changes in a large area, but much more in the supraoptic region.

BBB, blood–brain barrier; NSO, supraoptic nucleus; Aff, afferent fiber connections; +, excitatory synaptic input; −, inhibitory synaptic input; ?, an unknown entity. (Modified from *Brain Research*, **23**, 1970 by courtesy of the Elsevier Publ. Co., Amsterdam).

References p. 157

of the amygdala, areas generally considered primary olfactory cortex, failed to release vasopressin from the neurohypophysis in the monkey (Hayward and Smith, 1963; Hayward, 1972). In other adjacent portions of the amygdaloid nuclear complex less directly connected to olfactory input (Nauta, 1963; Nauta and Haymaker, 1969), the medial, basal, accessory basal and lateral nuclei, electrical stimulation in the conscious monkey did elicit an antidiuretic response with decrease in free water clearance without change in osmolal or inulin clearances (Hayward and Smith, 1963). Other sites of descending pathways in the limbic forebrain area found to release vasopressin from the neurohypophysis in the unanesthetized monkey include the uncus of the hippocampus, the olfactory tubercle, the diagonal band of Broca, the ventral amygdala–hypothalamic pathway and the medial forebrain bundle (Hayward and Smith, 1963, 1964). In these same experiments, sites in the middle and inferior temporal gyri (neocortex), temporal pole and periamygdaloid cortex failed to release ADH. Other workers using cat and rabbit found similar results (see Rothballer, 1966; Hayward, 1972). Those workers studying the dog found vasopressin release from excitation of the anterior cingulate and prepyriform cortex (see Rothballer, 1966; Hayward, 1972). In view of the known influence of "emotional stress" and conditional factors on release of vasopressin (Verney, 1947; Harris, 1960; Corson, 1966; Heller and Ginsburg, 1966) and the proposed association of limbic forebrain areas with "behavior" (see Nauta, 1963; Hayward, 1972), it is perhaps not surprising that electrical stimulation of the amygdala and some of its subcortical connections should provide excitatory synaptic input to the supraoptic neurons. While the exact meaning of such a connection remains obscure at the moment, the pathways involved probably include a direct bisynaptic route from amygdala to the perinuclear zone dorsal to the supraoptic nucleus (Nauta, 1963; Raisman, 1966; Nauta and Haymaker, 1969), as well as less direct neural and humoral routes (see Hayward, 1972).

The detailed *intra-hypothalamic* connections between these ascending and descending neural pathways funneling into the region of the supraoptic nucleus and the local perinuclear zone interneuronal circuitry are not well known. Studies of specific chemical pathways indicate that a direct adrenergic and cholinergic synaptic input acts on supraoptic cells (Shute and Lewis, 1966; Rechardt, 1969). Electron microscopical and histochemical studies indicate a double population of supraoptic neurons with axo-dendritic, axo-somatic and axo-axonal endings with at least three types of synaptic vesicles (Rechardt, 1969). The poor impregnation of supraoptic neurons with silver techniques (Szentágothai *et al.*, 1968) has made analysis of interneuronal connections difficult. On the basis of physiological studies in monkeys, we proposed two types of "osmosensitive" interneurons lying in the perinuclear zone dorsal to the supraoptic nucleus (Fig. 1; Hayward and Vincent, 1970; Vincent and Hayward, 1970). Whether such a group of interneurons is involved in other input mechanisms to the supraoptic neurons from limbic forebrain and midbrain areas is not known at present. While the studies of Woods *et al.* (1966) on the deafferented hypothalamus, the so-called hypothalamic island, indicated that the supraoptic nuclei and a small bit of surrounding hypothalamus connected to the neurohypophysis are all the neural tissue necessary for "*osmometric*" control of vasopressin release and water balance, the integration of supraoptic neuronal activity with the *non-osmotic* bodily functions requires intact ascending and descending neural pathways.

CEREBROSPINAL FLUID INPUT TO SUPRAOPTIC NEURONS

Intraventricular ions. Changes produced by the choroid plexus in the chemical composition of the cerebrospinal fluid can alter the extracellular fluid composition of the supraoptic neurons and activate periventricular "osmoreceptors". The diffusion barrier for passage of larger molecules ($> 2000 \, M_r$) between blood–brain and blood–CSF (Brightman *et al.*, 1970) does not exist between the third ventricular CSF and the hypothalamus (Feldberg and Myers, 1963; Davson, 1967; Myers and Veale, 1970) and other periventricular nervous tissue (Fenstermacher *et al.*, 1970). Intraventricular injections of ions have been used as a tool to study body temperature regulation (Myers and Veale, 1970) and the "osmoreceptor" regulation of drinking behavior, neurohypophysial hormone release (Olsson, 1969; Andersson and Eriksson, 1971) and sodium excretion by the kidney (Mouw and Vander, 1970; Andersson and Eriksson, 1971). The basic controversy as to the nature of the blood–brain barrier (see Pappenheimer, 1970; Yudilevich and DeRose, 1971) and the recent discrepancies between "osmometric" release of ADH via intracarotid and intraventricular routes of administration of hypertonic solutions (Andersson and Eriksson, 1971; Eriksson *et al.*, 1971) suggested to these workers that Verney's "osmoreceptors" may actually be sodium sensitive elements (intracellular sodium levels) in close connection with the third ventricular cerebrospinal fluid. Under this hypothesis, changes in CSF sodium produced by the choroid plexus under physiological conditions of dehydration or hydration would be detected by these periventricular "sodium detectors". The detection signal would then be transmitted to supraoptic neurons for regulation of ADH, to neural mechanisms for drinking and for regulation of renal sodium secretion and renin release (Mouw and Vander, 1970; Andersson and Eriksson, 1971). These workers suggest that the blood–brain barrier to sodium, urea and sucrose (Davson, 1967) prevents these substances from entering the perineuronal spaces of the supraoptic nucleus and perinuclear zone (Olsson, 1969; Andersson and Eriksson, 1971; Eriksson *et al.*, 1971) as demanded by the "osmoreceptor" theory of Verney (see Verney, 1947; Jewell and Verney, 1957; Hayward and Vincent, 1970; Vincent and Hayward, 1970; Hayward, 1972). While the capillaries of the supraoptic nucleus have tight junctions of the blood–brain barrier type (Rechardt, 1969; Brightman *et al.*, 1970), electron microscopic studies show intimate contacts between the neurons and capillaries with glial swelling and increased distance between neurosecretory cells and capillaries during dehydration in rats (Rechardt, 1969). These findings support the hypothesis of Pappenheimer (1970) and Yudilevich and DeRose, 1971) that the blood–brain barrier for ions and other smaller molecules involves resistance through capillary inter-endothelial slits of 10–15 Å with active transport and facilitated diffusion by glial processes. In the supraoptic nucleus and perinuclear zone, a region with the richest capillary bed in the brain (Finley, 1939; Daniel, 1966), local factors, such as

and not merely modulate a pre-existing impulse traffic", and also that "they do not have any other function as well, *e.g.* that of a synapse or an interneurone". While these studies of Cross and Green (1959) and Joynt (1964) seemed to support the concept of a specific "osmoreceptor" of Verney in the perinuclear zone of the supra-optic nucleus, other workers (Koizumi *et al.*, 1964) found "osmosensitive" cells in the immediate vicinity of the supraoptic nucleus of the anesthetized cat which did respond to afferent stimuli from leg nerves and to electrical stimulation of cingulate gyrus, motor cortex, prefrontal cortex and cerebellar cortex.

In an attempt to resolve some of these differences in the definition of an "osmo-sensitive" cell and to further differentiate the forebrain "osmoreceptors" of Verney and Sawyer, we (Hayward and Vincent, 1970; Vincent and Hayward, 1970) studied single cells in the anterior hypothalamus of the conscious monkey with our chronic recording and intracarotid injection techniques (Hayward, 1969a, b; Findlay and Hayward, 1969; Hayward and Vincent, 1970). We found two basic types of "osmo-sensitive" cells in the anterior hypothalamus of the conscious monkey: the "*specific*" "osmosensitive" cells distributed in the supraoptic nucleus (NSO) and the immediate perinuclear zone (PNZ) and responding exclusively to intracarotid hypertonic sodium chloride and not to sensory stimuli; the "*non-specific*" "osmosensitive" cells, distributed widely throughout the antero-lateral hypothalamus–preoptic area, and responding to both osmotic and sensory stimuli (Fig. 1). We consider that these latter "non-specific" "osmosensitive" cells probably belong to the olfactory–limbic forebrain "osmoreceptors" of Sawyer and respond to behavioral aspects of body water balance and supraoptic neuronal control (Hayward, 1972).

Within the category of the "specific" "osmoreceptors" we found two patterns of response to intracarotid hypertonic solutions: (1) cells located in the *supraoptic nucleus* (NSO) which responded to an osmotic stimulus with a "biphasic" discharge; (2) cells in the perinuclear zone (PNZ) of the supraoptic nucleus which responded to an osmotic stimulus with a "monophasic" discharge (Fig. 1). We consider that the former, "biphasic" cells, are the neuroendocrine cells of this system and the latter, "monophasic" cells, are the forebrain "osmoreceptors" of Verney (Hayward and Vincent, 1970; Vincent and Hayward, 1970). We further speculate that the "osmo-receptors" of Verney, which are single neural elements, receive their primary input across the blood–brain barrier of the dense capillary bed of the supraoptic region via changes in ionic concentration and osmotic pressure of the carotid arterial blood. In some unknown way this arterial blood causes changes in the firing rate of these central receptors (see discussion in this paper in earlier section: CSF Input: intra-ventricular ions, page 149). The forebrain "osmoreceptors" of Verney may provide excitatory axo-somatic synaptic drive to the supraoptic neurons (Fig. 1). In addition the supraoptic neurons also may receive excitatory axo-dendritic and inhibitory axo-axonal synaptic input from the forebrain "osmoreceptors" of Sawyer, from cholinergic and adrenergic pathways and from other unknown sites (Fig. 1; Hayward and Vincent, 1970; Vincent and Hayward, 1970; Hayward, 1972). We account for the "biphasic" excitatory–inhibitory sequence of the supraoptic neurons by a system of postulated recurrent collaterals with or without an interposed inhibitory inter-neuron (a neuroendocrine "Renshaw cell") as seen in Fig. 1 (Vincent and Hayward, 1970). Other workers have also found evidence for such collateral inhibition in these magnocellular neuroendocrine cells (Kandel, 1964; Kelly and Dreifuss, 1970; Yamashita *et al.*, 1970). This excitatory–inhibitory sequence must be of considerable importance for the release of vasopressin. Such intermittent interruption of a sustained excitatory synaptic drive (osmotic, pain, limbic, etc.) on the supraoptic cells could provide a finely tuned control for the blood levels of vasopressin. In view of the short half-life (T½ = 3–4 min) of vasopressin in the blood of the monkey (Lauson, 1967) and the short refractory period of osmoreceptors and neuroendocrine cells (less than 1 min, Hayward and Vincent, 1970), such a minute-to-minute control is possible. The quanta of vasopressin released into the bloodstream by such an excitatory–inhibitory sequence of these neurosecretory cells may produce a pulsatile pattern of plasma vasopressin oscillations (Vincent and Hayward, 1970).

Carotid blood hormone levels. The levels of various "hormones" in the carotid arterial blood can produce profound effects on supraoptic neuronal activity and the release of vasopressin from the neurohypophysis (Harris, 1960; Heller and Ginsburg, 1966; Barker *et al.*, 1971b). At present there is no evidence of a "short" feedback loop (negative or positive) whereby *arginine vasopressin* might have a direct influence on the supraoptic neurons or neurohypophysial release mechanisms. Presumably the blood–brain barrier for vasopressin (Vorherr *et al.*, 1968) restricts its action to the median eminence and neurohypophysis where such a barrier for peptide molecules is absent (Brightman *et al.*, 1970; Knigge and Scott, 1970). *Angiotensin II* is the octapeptide end product of ionic and vascular changes in the juxtaglomerular apparatus of the renal cortex via renin, renin substrate and angiotensin I (Vander, 1967), which may be involved in supraoptic neuronal–neurohypophysial activity. Blood volume reduction, body sodium depletion and intraventricular hyponatremic infusions (Vander, 1967; Mouw and Vander, 1970) lead to an increased production of renin and subsequently angiotensin II. Angiotensin II can release vasopressin from the neurohypophysis (Bonjour and Malvin, 1970) and cause increased drinking (Fitzsimmons and Simons, 1969; Andersson and Eriksson, 1971) and enhanced sodium excretion by the kidney (Andersson and Eriksson, 1971). Vasopressin, via a negative feedback loop, can decrease renin release in the sodium-depleted, conscious dog (Tagawa *et al.*, 1971). Further work is needed to determine the *site of stimulation* of ADH release by angiotensin II. Is there a non-specific release by angiotensin of transmitters in the median eminence; a specific release of transmitters at the supraoptic neurons; does this octapeptide release vasopressin directly from the neurosecretory terminals in the infundibular process? Whatever physiological role angiotensin II plays in the regulation of ADH during changes in blood volume and osmolality is currently unknown. In the possible indirect mechanisms of vasopressin release secondary to electrical stimulation of brain stem and limbic structures in the conscious monkey (Hayward and Smith, 1963, 1964; Hayward, 1972), angiotensin II stimulation of vasopressin release (Bonjour and Malvin, 1970), secondary to renal vasoconstriction, due

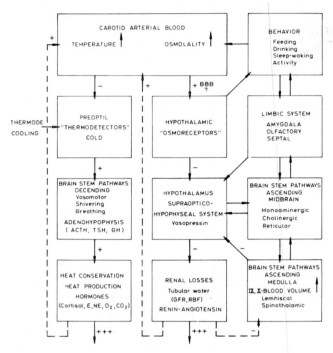

Fig. 2. Summary diagram of some of the hypothalamic input pathways to supraoptic neurons following preoptic cooling and central cold diuresis in the unanesthetized monkey. Three negative feedback loops are diagrammed: (1) preoptic thermodetector–thermoregulatory–blood temperature loop (left column, dashed line); (2) Osmoreceptor–supraoptic nuclear complex–blood osmolality loop (middle column, dashed line); (3) volume receptor (high and low pressure) IX, X–solitario–supraoptic pathway–blood volume loop (right column). Preoptic cooling opens the thermoregulatory feedback loop and triggers a sequence of autonomic, behavioral and endocrine events which culminate in the inhibition of supraoptic neurons and inhibition of vasopressin release. BBB, blood–brain barrier; ACTH, adrenocorticotropin; TSH, thyrotropin; GH, growth hormone; E, epinephrine; NE, norepinephrine; GFR, glomerular filtration rate; RBF, renal blood flow; IX, glossopharyngeal nerve; X, vagus nerve.

to hypoxia or directly due to brain stimulation (Hayward and Baker, 1968b; Hayward, 1972) should be included.

Hydrocortisone can elevate the threshold for osmotic release of vasopressin from the neurohypophysis with apparently little change in the response to nicotine (see Share, 1969). At present it is not known whether this action of hydrocortisone is via an expansion of blood volume with the consequential interaction of "volume receptor" inhibition and "osmoreceptor" excitatory drives on the supraoptic neurons (Fig. 2; Share, 1969; Johnson *et al.*, 1970) or whether a more direct action occurs at the level of the forebrain "osmoreceptors" or supraoptic neurons (see Hayward, 1972). *Estrogen* injected systemically is accumulated by supraoptic neurons (Stumpf, 1970) and alterations in body water balance and thresholds for vasopressin release occur in relation to states of increased estrogen secretion, *i.e.*, estrous cycle, menstrual cycle and pregnancy (Harris, 1960; Heller and Ginsburg, 1966). Whether estrogen and progesterone act directly or indirectly on the supraoptic neurons, neurohypophysis or drinking behavior is not known.

Carotid blood temperature. A strong linkage exists between body water regulation and thermoregulation. Exposure to cold and hot environments can change the amounts of salt and water excreted by the kidney. In monkey (Hayward and Baker, 1968a) and man (Segar and Moore, 1968), for example, cooling inhibits and warming excites ADH release. In the dog and rat "cold diuresis" has primarily a renal basis (see Hayward and Baker, 1968a), while cooling in the goat excites ADH release (Olsson, 1969), an effect opposite to that seen in monkey and man. There is at least one possible explanation for these contradictions in the supraoptic neuronal response to thermal stress: the major anatomical differences between species that underlie the mode by which the carotid arterial blood regulates hypothalamic temperature (Hayward and Baker, 1969). In the *internal carotid species*, monkey, man and rabbit, the temperature of the arterial blood is the same in the body core and in the hypothalamic arteries (Hayward *et al.*, 1966; Hayward, 1967; Baker and Hayward, 1967a; Hayward and Baker, 1968b, 1969). These species have large areas of relatively bare, exposed skin and tend to rely on cutaneous vasomotor defenses for conservation or dissipation of heat with inevitable, concomitant and associated shifts in blood volume (Fig. 2; see Hayward and Baker, 1968a; Segar and Moore, 1968). The primates are also adapting to an upright posture which further sensitizes the "volumetric" homeostatic systems, including vasopressin release (Segar and Moore, 1968; Share, 1969). In the *carotid rete species*, cat, dog, sheep and goat, the temperature of the hypothalamic arterial blood varies, depending upon two simultaneous events: evaporative heat loss from the upper respiratory passages and head and the circulation of the carotid arterial blood through the counter-current heat exchanger "rete mirable" on its way to the hypothalamus (Baker and Hayward, 1967b, 1968; Hayward, 1968; Hayward and Baker, 1969; Baker, 1971). The preoptic thermoreceptors receive arterial blood at a different temperature than the body core (spinal cord) thermoreceptors receive (Bligh, 1966; Hayward and Baker, 1969; Jessen and Simon, 1971). The carotid rete species are generally heavily furred and depend primarily upon upper respiratory vasomotor defences, particularly panting (Hayward, 1968; Baker and Hayward, 1968; Baker, 1971), for conservation or dissipation of heat with probably little associated change in blood volume. The horizontally aligned cat, dog, sheep and goat certainly do not share the primates' need for specific mechanisms for regulating blood volume against gravity. None of these generalizations should oversimplify the problems of comparing one species with another; it is only a necessary reminder that preoptic cooling in the monkey inhibits ADH release (Hayward and Baker, 1968a) whereas preoptic cooling in the goat excites ADH release (Olsson, 1969), and that preoptic thermodetectors in the dog receive a thermal input different from the thermal input to the body core (spinal cord) thermoreceptors (Hayward, 1968; Jessen and Simon, 1971).

That the ADH inhibition and increased free water clearance found in the lightly

References p. 157

clothed sitting or supine human exposed to a cool environment (Suzuki *et al.*, 1967; Segar and Moore, 1968) is the result of a shift of blood to central venous sites and activation of intrathoracic blood volume receptors and vagally mediated inhibition of supraoptic neurons has been proposed by several workers (Segar and Moore, 1968; Share, 1969). Whether the endocrine changes associated with "cold diuresis" augment inhibition of supraoptic neurons is not known (Suzuki *et al.*, 1967).

In order to duplicate the phenomenon of man's "cold diuresis", we cooled the preoptic area in the conscious monkey and produced a sequence of behavioral, autonomic and endocrine responses, including the expected ADH inhibition and increased free water clearance (Hayward and Baker, 1968a). Cooling the preoptic field by 2 °C produced a behavioral arousal, restlessness and shivering, an elevation of arterial blood pressure and a rapid rise in arterial blood temperature (Hayward and Baker, 1968a). When arterial blood temperature reached a plateau at + 2 °C, the increased urine flow, free water clearance, decreased urine osmolality with no change in inulin, PAH or osmolal clearances indicated a vasopressin release inhibition. In Fig. 2 we see that preoptic cooling activates the following: (1) a descending chain of sympathetic neurons leading to peripheral cutaneous vasoconstriction (Hayward and Baker, 1968a) and to an increased production of epinephrine and norepinephrine (Andersson *et al.*, 1964); (2) shivering (Hayward and Baker, 1968a); (3) increased adenohypophysial secretion of ACTH, TSH and GH (Andersson *et al.*, 1964; see Hayward, 1972). All of these events contribute to increased heat production and heat conservation with a rapid rise in arterial blood temperature which reaches a plateau due to negative feedback of preoptic, brain stem or spinal thermoreceptors (Bligh, 1966; Jessen and Simon, 1971).

The rising level of plasma osmolality (301 $\pm$ 2 to 306 $\pm$ 4 mOsm/kg) during water diuresis suggests that inhibitory input dominates "osmoreceptor" excitation in the supraoptic neurons (Fig. 2). The major physiological event inhibiting supraoptic neurons during preoptic cooling is probably an ascending barrage of impulses arising from intrathoracic "volume receptors" traveling along the vagal nerves, tractus solitarius and its nucleus and synaptic relays in the dorsal tegmental nucleus via the mamillary peduncle to the supraoptic nucleus (Fig. 2; Morest, 1961, 1967; Nauta, 1963; Rothballer, 1966; Hayward and Baker, 1968a; Segar and Moore, 1968; Share, 1969; Nauta and Haymaker, 1969; Hayward, 1971). Intrathoracic blood volume increases during peripheral or central cooling because of peripheral veno- and vaso-constriction. The blood shifts from peripheral to central venous sites (Share, 1969). While the available evidence supports this concept of the primary mechanisms and pathways involved in "cold diuresis", full elucidation of the neural pathways remains to be demonstrated.

Adjunctive mechanisms leading to inhibition of supraoptic neurons and inhibition of vasopressin release from the neurohypophysis and "cold diuresis", shown in Fig. 2, include: (1) elevated levels of circulating (and brain?) catecholamines (Andersson *et al.*, 1964; Suzuki *et al.*, 1967; Barker *et al.*, 1971b); (2) elevated plasma levels of hydrocortisone (see Share, 1969; Suzuki *et al.*, 1967; Hayward, 1972); (3) possible depressed levels of angiotensin II (Bonjour and Malvin, 1970); (4) inhibition of drinking (Andersson *et al.*, 1964; Sundsten, 1969).

SUMMARY

The supraoptic neurons receive a diverse input from neural, CSF and vascular routes. These magnocellular neuroendocrine cells lie strategically positioned in the antero-lateral hypothalamus to receive synaptic input from ascending, reticular and chemical, and descending, olfactory and limbic, pathways as well as intrahypothalamic connections. The cerebrospinal fluid of the third ventricle is intimately connected with the extracellular fluid space of the supraoptic neurons which undoubtedly plays a crucial but poorly understood role in regulation of these neuroendocrine cells. A dual set of forebrain "osmoreceptors", the "osmoreceptors" of Verney and the "osmoreceptors" of Sawyer, are involved in regulation of osmotic input to supraoptic neurons. The "osmoreceptors" of Sawyer, located in the olfactory bulb, olfactory tubercle, preoptic area and amygdala, relate to non-specific and behaviorally related factors of supraoptic neurons. The "osmoreceptors" of Verney, located in the peri-nuclear zone of the supraoptic nucleus, provide the major osmotic input to supraoptic neurons. Of the adjunctive non-osmotic factors regulating supraoptic neuronal activity, blood volume, blood temperature and blood hormone levels are important. "Cold diuresis" in primates involves primarily "volume receptor" inhibition of supraoptic neurons with humoral and behavioral events of secondary importance. I anticipate that in the future this group of hypothalamic neurons will continue to provide our greatest insight into central neurosecretory activities related to hypothalamic input mechanisms, particularly with the use of intracellular recording (Kandel, 1964; Oomura *et al.*, 1970) and radioimmunoassay for vasopressin (Oyama *et al.*, 1970).

ACKNOWLEDGEMENTS

Supported in part by the Ford Foundation and U.S. Public Health Service Grants NS-05638 and Fellowship NS-02277.

I thank Mrs. R. Lawrence for valuable technical assistance and the illustration division of the Nobel Institute for Neurophysiology, Karolinska Institutet, Stockholm, Sweden, for aid with the Figures.

REFERENCES

ANDERSSON, B. AND ERIKSSON, L. (1971) Conjoint action of sodium and angiotensin on brain mechanisms controlling water and salt balances. *Acta physiol. scand.*, **54**, 191–192.
ANDERSSON, B., GALE, C. C. AND SUNDSTEN, J. W. (1964) Preoptic influences on water intake. In *Thirst, Proc. First Internat. Symposium on Thirst in the Regulation of Body Water*, M. J. WAYNER (Ed.), Pergamon Press, Oxford, pp. 361–377.
BAKER, M. A. (1971) Brain cooling during thermal panting in the cat. *Anat. Rec.*, **169**, 270–271.

BAKER, M. A. AND HAYWARD, J. N. (1967a) Autonomic basis for the rise in brain temperature during paradoxical sleep. *Science*, **157**, 1586–1588.

BAKER, M. A. AND HAYWARD, J. N. (1976b) Carotid rete and brain temperature of cat. *Nature (Lond.)*, **216**, 139–141.

BAKER, M. A. AND HAYWARD, J. N. (1968) The influence of the nasal mucosa and the carotid rete upon hypothalamic temperature in sheep, *J. Physiol. (Lond.)*, **198** 561–579.

BARKER, J. L., CRAYTON, J. W. AND NICOLL, R. A. (1971a) Supraoptic neurosecretory cells: autonomic modulation. *Science*, **171**, 206–207.

BARKER, J. L., CRAYTON, J. W. AND NICOLL, R. A. (1971b) Supraoptic neurosecretory cells: adrenergic and cholinergic sensitivity. *Science*, **171**, 208–209.

BEYER, C. AND SAWYER, C. H. (1969) Hypothalamic unit activity related to control of the pituitary. In *Frontiers in Neuroendocrinology*, W. F. GANONG AND L. MARTINI (Eds.), Oxford Univ. Press, New York, pp. 255–287.

BLIGH, J. (1966) Thermosensitivity of the hypothalamus and thermoregulation in mammals. *Biol. Rev.*, **41**, 317–367.

BONJOUR, J. P. AND MALVIN, R. L. (1970) Stimulation of ADH release by the renin-angiotensin system. *Amer. J. Physiol.*, **218**, 1555–1559.

BRIGHTMAN, M. W., REESE, T. S. AND FEDER, N. (1970) Assessment with the electronmicroscope of the permeability to peroxidase of cerebral endothelium and epithelium in mice and sharks. In *Capillary Permeability. The Transfer of Molecules and Ions Between Capillary Blood and Tissue. Alfred Benzon Symposium II*, C. CRONE AND N. A. LASSEN (Eds.), Academic Press, New York, pp. 483–490.

CORSON, S. A. (1966) Conditioning of water and electrolyte excretion. *Publ. Ass. Res. nerv. ment. Dis.*, **43**, 140–198.

CROSS, B. A. AND GREEN, J. D. (1959) Activity of single neurones in the hypothalamus: effect of osmotic and other stimuli. *J. Physiol. (Lond.)*, **148**, 554–569.

CROSS, B. A. AND SILVER, I. A. (1966) Electrophysiological studies on the hypothalamus. *Brit. med. Bull.*, **22**, 254–260.

DANIEL, P. M. (1966) The blood supply of the hypothalamus and pituitary gland. *Brit. med. Bull.*, **22**, 202–208.

DAVSON, H. (1967) *Physiology of the Cerebrospinal Fluid*. Little, Brown, Boston.

DYBALL, R. E. J. (1971) Oxytocin and ADH secretion in relation to electrical activity in antidromically identified supraoptic and paraventricular units. *J. Physiol. (Lond.)*, **214**, 245–256.

ERIKSSON, L., FERNANDEZ, O. AND OLSSON, K. (1971) Central regulation of ADH release in the conscious goat, *Acta physiol. scand.*, Meeting Scand. Physiol. Soc., 21A (Abstract).

EULER, C. VON (1953) A preliminary note on slow hypothalamic "Osmo-potentials". *Acta physiol. scand.*, **29**, 133–136.

FELDBERG, W. AND MYERS, R. D. (1963) A new concept of temperature regulation by amines in the hypothalamus. *Nature (Lond.)*, **200**, 1325.

FENSTERMACHER, J. D., RALL, D. P., PATLAK, C. S. AND LEVIN, V. A. (1970) Ventriculo-cisternal perfusion as a technique for analysis of brain capillary permeability and extracellular transport. In *Capillary Permeability. The Transfer of Molecules and Ions Between Capillary Blood and Tissue, Alfred Benzon Symposium II*, C. CRONE AND N. A. LASSEN (Eds.), Academic Press, New York, pp. 483–490.

FINDLAY, A. L. R. AND HAYWARD, J. N. (1969) Spontaneous activity of single neurones in the hypothalamus of rabbits during sleep and waking. *J. Physiol. (Lond.)*, **201**, 237–258.

FINLEY, K. H. (1939) Angio-architecture of the hypothalamus and its peculiarities. *Publ. Ass. Res. nerv. ment. Dis.*, **20**, 286–309.

FITZSIMMONS, J. T. AND SIMONS, B. J. (1969) The effect on drinking in the rat of intravenous infusion of angiotensin given alone or in combination with other stimuli of thirst. *J. Physiol. (Lond.)*, **203**, 45–57.

HARRIS, G. W. (1947) The innervation and actions of the neurohypophysis: an investigation using the method of remote-control stimulation. *Phil. Trans. B*, **232**, 385–441.

HARRIS, G. W. (1960) Central control of pituitary secretion. *Handbook Physiology, Sect. I, Neurophysiology*, **2**, 1007–1038.

HAYWARD, J. N. (1967) Cerebral cooling during increased cerebral blood flow in the monkey. *Proc. Soc. exp. Biol. (N.Y.)*, **124**, 555–557.

HAYWARD, J. N. (1968) Brain temperature regulation during sleep and arousal in the dog. *Exp. Neurol.*, **21**, 201–212.

HAYWARD, J. N. (1969a) Hypothalamic single cell activity during the thermo-regulatory adjustments of sleep and waking in the monkey. *Anat. Rec.*, **163**, 197.

HAYWARD, J. N. (1969b) Brain temperature and thermosensitive nerve cells in the monkey. *Trans. Amer. neurol. Ass.*, **94**, 157–159.

HAYWARD, J. N. (1972) The amygdaloid nuclear complex and mechanisms of release of vaso-pressin from the neurohypophysis. In *Neurobiology of the Amygdala*, B. E. ELEFTHERIOU (Ed.), Plenum Press, New York.

HAYWARD, J. N. AND BAKER, M. A. (1968a) Diuretic and thermoregulatory responses during pre-optic cooling in the monkey. *Amer. J. Physiol.*, **214**, 843–850.

HAYWARD, J. N. AND BAKER, M. A. (1968b) The role of the cerebral arterial blood in the regulation of brain temperature in the monkey. *Amer. J. Physiol.*, **215**, 389–403.

HAYWARD, J. N. AND BAKER, M. A. (1969) A comparative study of the role of the cerebral arterial blood in the regulation of brain temperature in five mammals. *Brain Research*, **16**, 417–440.

HAYWARD, J. N. AND SMITH, W. K. (1963) Influence of limbic system on neurohypophysis. *Arch. Neurol. (Chic.)*, **9**, 171–177.

HAYWARD, J. N. AND SMITH, W. K. (1964) Antidiuretic response to electrical stimulation in brain stem of the monkey. *Amer. J. Physiol.*, **206**, 15–20.

HAYWARD, J. N. AND VINCENT, J. D. (1970) Osmosensitive single neurones in the hypothalamus of unanesthetized monkeys. *J. Physiol. (Lond.)*, **210**, 947–972.

HAYWARD, J. N., SMITH, E. AND STUART, D. G. (1966) Temperature gradients between arterial blood and brain in the monkey, *Proc. Soc. exp. Biol. (N.Y.)*, **121**, 547–551.

HELLER, H. AND GINSBURG, M. (1966) Secretion, metabolism and fate of the posterior pituitary hormones. In *The Pituitary Gland, Vol. 3*, G. W. HARRIS AND B. T. DONOVAN (Eds.), Butterworths, London, pp. 330–373.

JESSEN, C. AND SIMON, E. (1971) Spinal cord and hypothalamus as core sensors of temperature in the conscious dog, III. Identity of function. *Pflügers Arch. ges. Physiol.*, **324**, 205–216.

JEWELL, P. A. AND VERNEY, E. B. (1957) An experimental attempt to determine the site of neuro-hypophysial osmoreceptors in the dog. *Phil. Trans. B*, **240**, 197–324.

JOHNSON, J. A., ZEHR, J. E. AND MOORE, W. W. (1970) Effects of separate and concurrent osmotic and volume stimuli on plasma ADH in sheep. *Amer. J. Physiol.*, **218**, 1273–1280.

JOYNT, R. J. (1964) Functional significance of osmosensitive units in the anterior hypothalamus. *Neurology, (Minneap.)*, **14**, 584–590.

KAMBERI, I. A., MICAL, R. S. AND PORTER, J. C. (1971) Effect of anterior pituitary perfusion and intraventricular injection of catecholamines on FSH release. *Endocrinology*, **88**, 1003–1011.

KANDEL, E. R. (1964) Electrical properties of hypothalamic neuroendocrine cells. *J. gen. Physiol.*, **47**, 691–717.

KELLY, J. S. AND DREIFUSS, J. J. (1970) Antidromic inhibition of identified rat supraoptic neurones. *Brain Research*, **22**, 406–409.

KOIZUMI, K., ISHIKAWA, T. AND BROOKS, C. MC. (1964) Control of activity of neurones in the supra-optic nucleus. *J. Neurophysiol.*, **27**, 878–892.

KNIGGE, K. M. AND SCOTT, D. E. (1970) Structure and function of the median eminence. *Amer. J. Anat.*, **129**, 223–244.

KUMAR, T. C. A. AND KNOWLES, F. G. W. (1967) A system linking the third ventricle with the pars tuberalis of the rhesus monkey. *Nature (Lond.)*, **215**, 54–55.

LAUSON, H. D. (1967) Metabolism of antidiuretic hormones, *Amer. J. Med.*, **42**, 713–744.

MEHLER, W. H., FEFERMAN, M. E. AND NAUTA, W. J. H. (1960) Ascending axon degeneration following anterolateral cordotomy. *Brain*, **83**, 718–750.

MOREST, D. K. (1961) Connexions of the dorsal tegmental nucleus (DTN) in rat and rabbit. *J. Anat. (Lond.)*, **95**, 229–246.

MOREST, D. K. (1967) Experimental study of the projections of the nucleus of the tractus solitarius and area postrema. *J. comp. Neurol.*, **130**, 277–300.

MOUW, D. R. AND VANDER, A. J. (1970) Evidence for brain Na receptors controlling renal Na excretion and plasma renin activity. *Amer. J. Physiol.*, **219**, 822–832.

MYERS, R. D. AND VEALE, W. L. (1970) Body temperature: possible ionic mechanisms in the hypo-thalamus controlling the set point. *Science*, **170**, 95–97.

NAUTA, W. J. H. (1963) Central nervous organization and the endocrine motor system. In *Advances in Neuroendocrinology*, A. V. NALBANDOV (Ed.), Univ. Illinois Press, Urbana, pp. 5–21.

NAUTA, W. J. H. AND HAYMAKER, W. (1969) Hypothalamic nuclei and fiber connections. In *The*

Hypothalamus, W. Haymaker, E. Anderson and W. J. H. Nauta (Eds.), Thomas, Springfield, Ill., pp. 136–209.

Norström, A. and Sjöstrand, J. (1971) Axonal transport of proteins in the hypothalamo-neuro-hypophysial system of the rat. *J. Neurochem.*, **18**, 29–39.

Olsson, K. (1969) Studies on central regulation of secretion of antidiuretic hormone (ADH) in the goat. *Acta physiol. scand.*, **77**, 465–474.

Oomura, Y., Ono, T. and Ooyama, H. (1970) Inhibitory action of the amygdala on the lateral hypothalamic area in rats. *Nature (Lond.)*, **228**, 1108–1110.

Oyama, S. N., Kagan, A. and Glick, S. M. (1970) Radioimmunoassay study of urinary vasopressin during hydration and dehydration. *Program 52nd Meeting of the Endocrine Society*, St. Louis, Mo., 691 pp.

Pappenheimer, J. R. (1970) Transport of HCO$_3$ between brain and blood. In *Capillary Permeability. Transfer of Molecules and Ions Between Capillary Blood and Tissue. Alfred Benzon Symposium II*, C. Crone and N. A. Lassen (Eds.), Academic Press, New York, pp. 454–458.

Raisman, G. (1966) Neural connexions of the hypothalamus. *Brit. med. Bull.*, **22**, 197–201.

Rechardt, L. (1969) Electron microscopic and histochemical observations on the supraoptic nucleus of normal and dehydrated rats. *Acta physiol. scand.*, **329**, 1–79.

Rosendorf, C. and Cranston, W. I. (1971) Effects of intrahypothalamic and intraventricular nor-epinephrine and 5-hydroxytryptamine on hypothalamic blood flow in the conscious rabbit. *Circulat. Res.*, **28**, 492–502.

Rothballer, A. B. (1966) Pathways of secretion and regulation of posterior pituitary factors. *Publ. Ass. Res. nerv. ment. Dis.*, **43**, 86–131.

Sachs, H., Fawcett, P., Takabatake, Y. and Portanova, R. Biosynthesis and release of vaso-pressin and neurophysin. *Recent Progr. Hormone Res.*, 25 (1969) 447–492.

Sawyer, C. H. and Fuller, G. R. (1960) Electroencephalographic correlates of reflex activation of the neurohypophysial antidiuretic mechanism. *Electroenceph. clin. Neurophysiol.*, **12**, 83–93.

Sawyer, C. H. and Gernandt, B. E. (1956) Effects of intracarotid and intraventricular injections of hypertonic solutions on electrical activity of the rabbit brain. *Amer. J. Physiol.*, **185**, 209–216.

Segar, W. E. and Moore, W. W. (1968) The regulation of antidiuretic hormone release in man. I. Effects of change in position and ambient temperature on blood ADH levels. *J. Clin. Invest.*, **47**, 2143–2151.

Share, L. (1969) Extracellular fluid volume and vasopressin secretion. In *Frontiers in Neuroendo-crinology*, W. F. Ganong and L. Martini (Eds.), Oxford Univ. Press, London, (1966) pp. 183–210.

Shute, C. C. D. and Lewis, P. R. (1966) Cholinergic and monoaminergic pathways in the hypo-thalamus. *Brit. med. Bull.*, **22**, 221–226.

Sloper, J. C. (1966) Hypothalamic neurosecretion. *Brit. med. Bull.*, **22**, 209–215.

Stumpf, W. E. (1970) Estrogen neurons and estrogen-neuron systems in the periventricular brain. *Amer. J. Anat.* **129**, 207–218.

Sundsten, J. W. (1969) Alterations in water intake and core temperature in baboons during hypo-thalamic thermal stimulation. *Ann. N.Y. Acad. Sci.*, **157**, 1018–1029.

Suzuki, M., Tonoue, T., Matsuzaki, S. and Yamamoto, K. (1967) Initial response of human thyroid, adrenal cortex and adrenal medulla to acute cold exposure. *Canad. J. Physiol. Pharmacol.*, **45**, 423–432.

Szentágothai, J., Flerkó, B., Mess, B. and Halász, B. (1968) *Hypothalamic Control of the Anterior Pituitary*, 3rd ed., Akademiai Kiadó, Budapest, pp. 25–106.

Tagawa, H., Vander, A. J., Bonjour, J. P. and Malvin, R. L. (1971) Inhibition of renin secretion by vasopressin in unanesthetized sodium-deprived dogs. *Amer. J. Physiol.*, **220**, 949–951.

Vander, A. J. (1967) Control of renin release. *Physiol. Rev.*, **47**, 359–382.

Verney, E. B. (1947) The antidiuretic hormone and the factors which determine its release. *Phil. Trans. B.*, **135**, 25–106.

Vincent, J. D. and Hayward, J. N. (1970) Activity of single cells in the osmoreceptor-supraoptic nuclear complex in the hypothalamus of the waking rhesus monkey. *Brain Research*, **23**, 105–108.

Vorherr, H., Bradbury, N. W. B., Haghoughi, N. and Kleeman, C. R. (1968) Antidiuretic hormone in cerebrospinal fluid during exogenous and endogenous changes in its blood levels. *Endocrinology*, **83**, 246–250.

Winterstein, H. (1961) The actions of substances introduced into the cerebrospinal fluid and the problem of intracranial receptors. *Pharmacol. Rev.*, **13**, 71–107.

Woods, J. W., Bard, P. and Bleier, R. (1966) Functional capacity of the deafferented hypothalamus:

water balance and response to osmotic stimuli in the decerebrate cat and rat. *J. Neurophysiol.*, **29**, 751–767.

YAGI, K. T., AZUMA, T. AND MATSUDA, K. (1966) Neurosecretory cells capable of conducting impulses in rats. *Science*, **154**, 778–779.

YAMASHITA, H., KOIZUMI, K. AND BROOKS, C. McC. (1970) Electrophysiological studies of neurosecretory cells in the cat hypothalamus. *Brain Research*, **20**, 462–466.

YUDILEVICH, D. L. AND DEROSE, N. (1971) Blood-brain transfer of glucose and other molecules measured by rapid indicator dilution. *Amer. J. Physiol.*, **220**, 841–846.

DISCUSSION

MAITI: I don't have much experience on this subject, but we have performed some experiments on dogs, in which we recorded electrical activity from the paraventricular and supraoptic nuclei. The interpretation of the results depends to some extent on the type of anaesthesia. I would like to ask you three questions:

1. did you find a specific stimulus that increases the electrical activity of one of these nuclei or of the amygdalar complex;
2. we analysed the action of oestrogen on the interstitial elements of the brown fat tissue and we found some specific effects in normal and ovariectomized animals. Do you believe that these mechanisms also play a role in the supraoptic nucleus;
3. do you think that the baroreceptors in the carotid sinus have also some efferent connections to endocrine nuclei?

HAYWARD: My answer to your first question is the following: We have not made recordings in the amygdala and supraoptic nuclei at the same time. So I can't answer your questions as to whether specific changes occur in our animals simultaneously. As to your other questions we have no specific data on these mechanisms.

MAITI: Domino and co-workers performed some experiments under di-ethyl-ether-anaesthesia in which they found hypersynchronous activity in the various nuclear complexes, suggesting that there may be some connections.

HAYWARD: I think there are certainly pathways between the amygdala and the vicinity of the supraoptic nucleus in the monkey, at least as described by Nauta. Recently, at the Munich conference, somebody discussed recordings from antidromically identified supraoptic neurones in the rabbit. With spontaneous arousal or with induced arousal from limbic stimulation it has been found that inhibition occurs in the supraoptic nucleus. The work of Backer and Nichol is also of importance. They showed that upon stimulation of the carotid sinus nerve and the vagus nerve excitation occurs of identified supraoptic neurons. One has to be careful if one has arousal in an animal, whether anaesthetized or unaesthetized, because there are also changes in the systemic arterial blood pressure. Changes in blood pressure in turn could lead to an inhibitory effect on the supraoptic neurons, because the two systems that control the supraoptic nucleus are the osmoreceptor system and the blood volume receptor system. If you have changes in the blood pressure with synchronous waves in the amygdala, then in turn by a feedback effect one could influence the supraoptic nuclei.

To come back to your second question: the oestrogen effect on the supraoptic nucleus. There is very little known about these effects. We know from radioautographic work of Stumpf that oestrogen is localized in the supraoptic nucleus to some degree, not perhaps as much as in the paraventricular. The work of Zuckermann on the effects of oestrogen in primates on waterbalance is suggestive, but we have no direct physiological effects in relation to supraoptic function.

As far as your third question is concerned: Scharrer has done a great deal of work in this area. The problem is that if you stimulate a nerve that carries both excitatory and inhibitory functionally fibres, it is difficult to sort out the exact mechanism. With changes in blood volume the situation occurs that if you have a decrease in blood volume you may find a release of a hormone, but if you have an increase in blood volume or blood pressure you may have an inhibition of the hormone release. So it is very difficult to work out all of the variables.

SWAAB: Can I make a short comment on the effect of oestrogen on the supraoptic nucleus? We used

162

enzymatic parameters for the hormone synthesis in the supraoptic and paraventricular nuclei. We found an enzyme activity of a certain degree in metoestrus control rats. After castration or ovariectomy these parameters increased indicating an increase in hormone synthesis in the supraoptic and paraventricular nuclei. After giving oestrogen to those animals that lowered the gonadotropic hormone levels it also decreased the enzymatic parameters. If, however, we gave to the ovariectomized animals estradiolbenzoate the enzymatic parameters rose again. Oestrogens apparently did not have any direct effect upon the supraoptic nucleus, but they were indirectly affecting via gonadotropic hormone levels. If the gonadotropic levels are high like after castration or ovariectomy, the synthetic activity of posterior lobe hormones is high; if the gonadotropic hormones are low like in dioestrus or after injection of estradiol benzoate, the production of posterior lobe hormones is low.

SLOPER: Could you specify your parameters?

SWAAB: We used two kind of parameters, one histochemical and one microchemical parameter, which are indicators of the enzymes of the Golgi apparatus. The Golgi apparatus of the supraoptic nucleus is increasing in size during activation under various experimental conditions. The enzyme we studied is TPP-ase, which is specific for the Golgi apparatus.

HAYWARD: I just want to know how you interpret these results. Is this a general effect in the hypothalamus or is it specific for the supraoptic and paraventricular nucleus?

SWAAB: It is indeed specific for those two nuclei.

Hypothalamic Inputs: Methods, and Five Examples

A. L. R. FINDLAY

Physiological Laboratory, Cambridge CB2 3EG (Great Britain)

The multiplicity of functions performed by the hypothalamus (in which we will include the preoptic area) has been a recurring theme of this and other recent meetings. The adequate performance of these functions demands the provision of information mediated through other parts of the nervous system, through the bloodstream or, possibly, the cerebrospinal fluid.

I. CLASSIFICATION ACCORDING TO NATURE OF INPUT

At the outset, it seems worthwhile to try to list and classify the enormous array of known hypothalamic input mechanisms. The evidence for the existence of many of the mechanisms listed is beyond dispute; a few are more controversial. The references given are to reviews or research papers, mostly fairly recent, which themselves contain more extensive bibliographies. They are intended only as suggestions for suitable starting points in a coverage of the literature.

A. BLOOD-BORNE STIMULI

1. *Hormones.* Oestrogen, progesterone, testosterone (Pfaff, 1971b); cortisol, ACTH (De Wied and Weijnen, 1970); thyroxine (Reichlin, 1966); TSH, growth hormone, FSH, LH, prolactin (Motta *et al.*, 1969).

2. *Other blood-borne substances.* Glucose (Brown and Melzack, 1969); oxygen, carbon dioxide (Cross and Silver, 1963; Baccelli *et al.*, 1965); angiotensin (Fitzsimons, 1970, 1972; and this chapter); pyrogens (Eisenman, 1969); amino-acids, free fatty acids (Glick, 1969).

3. *Other properties of blood.* Temperature (Hellon, 1967; Hammel, 1968); osmotic pressure (Hayward, 1972).

B. CEREBROSPINAL FLUID-BORNE STIMULI

Possibly melatonin and other substances (Knowles, 1972; Wolstenholme and Knight, 1971).

C. NEURALLY MEDIATED STIMULI

1. *Classification according to transmitter released.* Acetylcholine, noradrenaline, serotonin, plus other unidentified transmitters (Shute, 1970; Fuxe and Hökfelt, 1969).

References p. 184

2. *Classification according to site of origin of afferent neurone* (Nauta, 1963; Raisman, 1966, 1970; Raisman and Field, 1971a). The afferent pathways listed below are almost all complemented by hypothalamic efferent pathways passing along similar routes. A two-way interaction thus takes place between the hypothalamus and most of the structures from which it receives nervous input.

(a) Brain stem. Components include the following:

(i) Inputs related to the mamillary nuclei. Ascending fibres in the "mamillary peduncle" from midbrain areas such as the dorsal and deep tegmental nuclei.

(ii) Afferent components of the medial forebrain bundle to the lateral hypothalamus from midbrain areas such as the ventral and dorsal tegmental nuclei. Some of these fibres are cholinergic (Shute, 1970) or catecholaminergic.

(iii) Afferent components of the periventricular system; that is, fibres originating in the periaqueductal grey matter of the midbrain and terminating mainly in the medial regions of the posterior hypothalamus (Sutin, 1966).

(iv) Fibres originating in cell bodies in the pons and medulla which pass to the hypothalamus via the ventral tegmental area of the midbrain. These fibres represent the main source of the huge networks of noradrenaline-containing terminals in the hypothalamus (Fuxe and Hökfelt, 1969).

(b) Limbic system and associated areas. This projection system is notable for its size, and for the fact that the nature of the transmitters released at the fibre terminations is entirely unknown. Components include:

(i) The ventral amygdalo-fugal pathway fibres which arise from all levels of the pyriform cortex and from the basolateral amygdaloid nuclear group. The fibres supply the whole extent of the medial forebrain bundle, having specific terminations at the premamillary level of the lateral hypothalamus in two cell masses—the "nuclei gemini".

(ii) The stria terminalis which arises principally in the corticomedial group of amygdaloid nuclei, though some fibres may be from the basolateral group. Fibres of the stria terminalis terminate in the medial preoptic area, in the medial part of the anterior hypothalamic area, around the ventromedial nucleus (Heimer and Nauta, 1969), and extend back into the medial hypothalamus as far as the ventral premamillary nucleus.

(iii) Fibres originating in the regio superior (principally field CA 1) of the hippocampus which pass through the dorsal fornix; the fibres are largely directed into the postcommissural fornix which passes through the hypothalamus as a relatively compact bundle and terminates in the mammillary nuclei. Fibres of this system are also distributed to the anterior thalamic nuclei, and may also be distributed to perifornical hypothalamic areas.

(iv) Fibres originating in the regio inferior of the hippocampus (principally field CA 3) are distributed through the fimbria, run in the precommissural fornix, and terminate largely in the septum; the more ventral fibres extend further caudally into the medial forebrain bundle where they terminate in the lateral preoptic and anterior hypothalamic regions. The septal terminations are probably mostly on neurones whose axons terminate in the medial forebrain bundle.

(v) Fibres of the medial cortico-hypothalamic tract which originate in a special area of the hippocampus (the prosubiculum). The fibres start by travelling in the ventral tip of the fimbria, but when they reach the anterior commissure they branch medially and run vertically down to reach the dorsal aspect of the suprachiasmatic nucleus. Thence they run caudally along the base of the brain as far as the arcuate nucleus, in the rostral part of which many fibres seem to terminate.

(c) Other sites

(i) The existence of direct retino-hypothalamic connections is a possibility which has been examined by many workers using both conventional and unconventional anatomical methods. Conventional methods have until recently failed to provide evidence for such connections, though connections from the lateral geniculate body to the lateral hypothalamus have been demonstrated by degeneration methods (Szentágothai *et al.*, 1968). Application of the latest degeneration methods to the rat has now, however, provided what seems good proof of the existence of retino-hypothalamic connections, projecting to, amongst other places, the ventromedial and arcuate nuclei (Sousa–Pinto and Castro–Correia, 1970; Sousa–Pinto, 1970). If labelled serotonin precursor is injected into the eye of a rat, radioactivity can be detected in the hypothalamus shortly afterwards (O'Steen and Vaughan, 1968). The radioactive granules are found over and around the periphery of neurones in the lateral hypothalamus and medial forebrain bundle, and bilaterally and more caudally in the arcuate and premamillary nuclei. Such evidence has yet to be established as sure proof of direct anatomical connection.

(ii) Fibres from the globus pallidus to the hypothalamus have been suggested. In the monkey Nauta and Mehler (1966) could find no evidence for their existence, but recently C.C.D. Shute (personal communication) has found evidence of pallido-hypothalamic cholinergic fibres terminating in the lateral hypothalamus of the rat.

(iii) Thalamo-hypothalamic connections pass from the dorsomedial thalamic nucleus to the lateral hypothalamic region in the monkey. These and other possible connections between the two structures probably serve to transmit impulses of limbic and presencephalic reticular origin (Nauta, 1963).

3. *Classification according to nature of stimulus eliciting activity in mediating neurones*

(a) Gustatory (Norgren, 1970).

(b) Olfactory (Pfaff and Gregory, 1971; Cowley and Wise, 1970; and this chapter).

(c) Visual (Wurtman, 1967; Reiter and Fraschini, 1969; Lofts *et al.*, 1970).

(d) Auditory (Feldman and Dafny, 1968; Tamari, 1970).

(e) Exteroceptors, *e.g.* suckling (Tindal and Knaggs, 1970; and this chapter); coitus (this chapter); pain (Cross and Silver, 1966); temperature (Nakayama and Hardy, 1969).

(f) Interoceptors, *e.g.* uterus and cervix stimulation (see this chapter); arterial and venous blood pressure (Share, 1969); medullary, and aortic and carotid body chemoreceptor stimulation (Baccelli *et al.*, 1965); stomach distension (Takaori *et al.*, 1968).

(g) Ill-defined stimuli, *e.g.* stress (Smelik, 1970), sleep-waking state (Findlay and Hayward, 1969; and this chapter); crowding (Brain and Nowell, 1971).

II. CLASSIFICATION ACCORDING TO HYPOTHALAMIC EFFERENT MECHANISMS AFFECTED

A. CONTROL OF PITUITARY HORMONES (Donovan, 1970)
B. TEMPERATURE CONTROL (Hammel, 1968; Cremer and Bligh, 1969)
C. AUTONOMIC NERVOUS SYSTEM CONTROL (Zanchetti, 1970).
D. DRINKING BEHAVIOUR (Fitzsimons, 1972)
E. EATING BEHAVIOUR AND ASSOCIATED GASTROINTESTINAL ACTIVITY (Smith and Brooks, 1970)
F. ATTACK AND DEFENCE BEHAVIOUR (Zanchetti, 1970; De Wied and Weijnen 1970)
G. SEXUAL BEHAVIOUR (Beach, 1970)

METHODS OF INVESTIGATION

It will be realised from the above classification that we will be unable to consider more than a very few of the many sources of information upon which the hypothalamus is dependent. Before discussing specific problems we might first consider the possible strategies which the experimenter may adopt in investigating an input mechanism.

He may be content to treat the hypothalamus as a "black box" and study simply the effect of some suspected input on a function or functions which he knows to be controlled by the hypothalamus. If his interest is in endocrine mechanisms, he may study the effect of the input upon posterior or anterior pituitary gland, or target gland, activity. He may be interested in feedback effects, in which case he will look at the effect of a systemic or local change in hormone concentration upon the hypothalamically controlled endocrine activity. Exteroceptive inputs may be manipulated or stimulation or lesioning of other areas within the C.N.S. may be employed, in order to study respectively the first or subsequent stages in an afferent pathway. Alternatively non-endocrine functions of the hypothalamus may be observed. Since the hypothalamus does not contain the "final common pathway" for such functions as temperature control, sexual behaviour, drinking or eating, it is less easy to be certain that a response to a manoeuvre is due to alteration of activity in a hypothalamic input mechanism, or else to some effect on the pathway over which the hypothalamus controls the peripheral motoneurones. But if, in such cases, the stimulus (say change in temperature, osmotic pressure) is applied directly to the hypothalamus, and a dramatic change in function results, then such a stimulus may well have a physiological effect at the hypothalamic level.

But we cannot be satisfied simply to describe hypothalamic inputs in terms of their effects on outputs (though this is certainly proving to be no mean task). We need to be able to understand the responses of different hypothalamic elements to variations in input. A sound anatomical knowledge of the neural input systems is important.

Careful structural studies can go a long way towards explaining functional phenomena; for example Raisman and Field (1971b) have recently described a structural difference in synaptic arrangements in the preoptic area of male and female rats (these areas have long been known to be functionally different in adults); in female rats, there seem to be more synaptic endings on dendritic spines than there are in males. There is some evidence that dendritic spine synapses tend to be excitatory (Eccles, 1964) and it is tempting to relate this sexual dimorphism to the periodic excitation of LH release which brings about ovulation in female animals, and for the occurrence of which the preoptic area is indispensable. Conventional degeneration methods for tracing of anatomical pathways have long been used, but new methods, particularly for detection of fine terminals, are still being developed—an indication of continuing dissatisfaction with what is currently available. Histochemical methods, principally those identifying noradrenaline, serotonin, dopamine, and acetylcholinesterase, have been used to trace afferent nerve fibres presumed to be acting via specific neurotransmitters. Finally, anatomical methods may be used to describe structural changes occurring in hypothalamic neurones following manipulation of input mechanisms (*e.g.*, depletion of neurosecretory material or subcellular particles in neurosecretory cells following water deprivation or osmotic stress).

Activation of input mechanisms may be expected to cause metabolic changes in hypothalamic neurones. In the investigation of blood-borne substances suspected of influencing hypothalamic activity, it is important to demonstrate that the substance can gain access to hypothalamic neurones. The substance may be labelled with a radioactive isotope and administered systemically. Uptake of the substance by the brain and other tissues may be assessed by autoradiography or by examining appropriate tissue fragments for their uptake of radioactivity (Pfaff, 1971b). Incorporation of radioactive protein precursor may be used to assess changes in protein synthesis by hypothalamic neurones (Ter Haar, 1972). Cellular RNA content, cell respiration and other metabolic variables may also be studied.

Evidence of activation of hypothalamic input mechanisms may be obtained by measuring the content or turnover of neurotransmitter substances (particularly noradrenaline) and studying the effect of stimuli on these variables. Changes in rates of neurotransmitter release may be followed by use of the push-pull cannula technique, whereby small samples of intracranial fluid may be removed for analysis.

But it is probably changes in the electrical activity which tell us most about how input mechanisms act on the hypothalamus (see reviews by Cross and Silver, 1966; Beyer and Sawyer, 1969). We will begin with what we might call "mass activity" measurements. These include evoked potentials (Malliani *et al.*, 1965), electroencephalographic activity, slow potential (DC) shifts and "multi-unit" activity. These methods have in common the problem that they fail to recognise the individuality of neurones, but rely rather on the assumption that neurones of a similar kind are aggregated in small areas; but they are valuable in the initial stages of study of an input mechanism, particularly in that they indicate the areas which would be most profitably examined with more refined methods. The multi-unit method is useful in supplying some information, however unclear, on the activity of small neurones which are at present incapable of being studied individually with available methods; it does however have problems. A constant difficulty in many forms of electrophysiology is the separation of signal from noise. Where large well-defined action potentials are recorded, the identification of the signal is not difficult; but the signal recorded during multi-unit recording tends to be only quantitatively but not qualitatively different from instrument noise. Various electronic processing devices have been devised to attempt to extract meaningful "single unit" data from such records, but these devices usually ignore the waxing and waning in size of action potentials recorded, picked up by a stationary electrode from a single neurone. Thus we must accept with caution the results of this method of recording, particularly when they purport to describe the activity of single neurones. To be fair I should mention that the technique has strong backing in some quarters (Beyer and Sawyer, 1969). Brown and Melzack (1969), for example, claim that "it integrates . . . the activity of a population of cells at the recording site and thus provides a more representative picture of neural activity in a region than does the single cell approach". Against this, we should remember that the spectacular advances in our knowledge of sensory processing in, say, the visual system, could not possibly have been achieved with the multi-unit method; in this connection, Brindley (1970) says, "Responses to illumination, recorded with electrodes very large in comparison with nerve cells, have provided a useful means of defining the limits of the cortical receiving area for vision and of investigating the projection of the retina upon it; but they do not take us much further. To understand what the visual cortex does, we must learn how single cells of it respond."

Extracellular recording of single cells in the hypothalamus is most often performed with metal microelectrodes of tip diameter considerably smaller than that used in the recording methods mentioned above. Anaesthetized or paralysed animals have been used in most studies. Extensive mid-brain coagulation has been used as a method of immobilisation, but this is clearly impracticable for studies on ascending input mechanisms. I know of no better introduction to the planning and interpretation of cellular electrophysiological experiments than that of Horridge (1968). "Our descriptions", he says, "are based upon the technique of sampling hundreds of nerve cells. The action of each is recorded individually to discover how each nerve cell is most readily excited or inhibited. The most effective types of stimulus . . . are then used to construct a theory of how they interact. The theory is compared with the behaviour of the whole animal, and the integrative activity of the nervous system may thereby be explained. The theory of interaction must of course be compatible with the actual anatomical connexions of the nerve fibres".

Spontaneous activity is usually first observed, and then the effects of changes in the activity of some input mechanism or mechanisms are noted. A full description of the activity of a nerve cell involves more than simply its mean firing rate; the inter-spike interval histogram is but one of the many other methods which may be used to characterise the details of the pattern of spike generation (Perkel *et al.*, 1967). Similarly the assessment of what constitutes a response to a stimulus is no easy matter (Werner and Mountcastle, 1963; Horridge, 1968; Pfaff, 1971a). Identification of recorded cells is important. Cells of the supraoptic and paraventricular nuclei (Dyball, 1971) and of the tubero-infundibular system (Harris *et al.*, 1971) can be identified by antidromic stimulation of their axons, which should be confirmed where possible by use of the collision technique whereby a stimulus is triggered by a naturally occurring spike, and the stimulus-evoked spike collides with and is cancelled by the orthodromic spike. In other cases cells may be identified only by histological methods, though it may prove possible to extend the antidromic method to hypothalamic neurones which send axons to relatively remote parts of the brain.

Input mechanisms differ in the latency and duration of the effect which they have on hypothalamic neurones. Some stimuli may cause responses with a very short latency and time course, and the post-stimulus histogram is a suitable method for the analysis of data in such cases. At the other extreme, some mechanisms may take hours or days to exert their effects. In such cases it may be necessary to study the spontaneous activity of one group of cells in the pre-treatment condition and compare it with that of a second group of cells in the post-treatment condition.

Electrophysiological study of the effects of blood-borne stimuli raises problems of specificity; their action may be direct upon hypothalamic neurones, or may be via an action on some non-hypothalamic sensor mechanism which relays its activity to the hypothalamus, and perhaps to many other places as well. The stimulus may bring about a change in the cortical EEG, and there is good evidence for a close correspondence between a change in cortical EEG and a change in hypothalamic unit activity. Such a change may be stimulus-induced or may arise spontaneously, and may be seen both in conscious (Findlay and Hayward, 1969) and anaesthetised (Lincoln, 1969b) animals. It is therefore of great importance that the EEG be recorded during unit recording experiments, and that EEG-related changes in unit activity be rejected when proof is being sought for specifically hypothalamic input mechanisms (Lincoln, 1969a). One approach to the problem is the restriction of the stimulus to the vicinity of the neurones under examination. Local temperature variations, for example, may be achieved by implanted thermodes (though even these may cause widespread EEG changes) (Von Euler and Söderberg, 1957). Local changes in the concentration of certain polarizable chemical substances may be obtained by their electrophoretic application from glass micropipettes to the surface of the neurone from which activity is being recorded; non-polarizable substances may be ejected from similar micropipettes by electro-osmosis or high-pressure injection. Such methods have been used for the study of the effects of neurotransmitters (Bloom *et al.*, 1963; Oomura *et al.*, 1969; Cross *et al.*, 1971), for substances related to the adrenocortical system (Steiner *et al.*, 1969), and by Setler, Williams and myself (see this chapter) for angiotensin. One must of course remember that responses of neurones to substances applied in this way do not prove that these neurones are normally exposed to them physiologically. Another way of demonstrating a direct action of blood-borne substances on hypothalamic neurones involves the separation of the hypothalamus from neural contact with the rest of the brain by a knife cut. Cross and Dyer (1970) have found that the activity of cells in such islands varies with the oestrous cycle, and Feldman and Sarne (1970) have shown them to be affected by circulating cortisol.

Neurally mediated input mechanisms may be stimulated peripherally or centrally while single neurones are being recorded. Central stimulation is normally performed electrically with the result that groups of afferents, probably never normally simultaneously active, may be excited. Thus electrical stimulation of an afferent mechanism is likely to give a rather oversimplified impression of its physiological role. Conversely these afferent pathways may be lesioned. Irreversible lesioning does not readily lend itself to electrophysiological experiments. If the activity is to be studied before and after the lesion, the method is suitable for the study of only one neurone per animal. Reversible cooling lesion techniques could more usefully be combined with hypothalamic unit recording, but such an approach seems so far to have been little used. A third method could usefully be combined with recording of hypothalamic unit activity—the simultaneous recording of unit activity in neurones suspected of supplying afferent input to the hypothalamus. Cross-correlation techniques (Perkel *et al.*, 1967) are now available to detect interdependencies between neurones. This method could provide accurate quantitative data on the degree to which afferent neurones "drive" neurones in the hypothalamus.

Within the last few years it has proved possible to study the activity of neurones in the hypothalamus of conscious animals. Many hypothalamic input mechanisms are polysynaptic, and thus likely to be disrupted by the use of anaesthetics; only with conscious animals can these mechanisms be studied. Two main kinds of methods are employed. In the first, metal electrodes with relatively large (40–65 μm) tip diameters are implanted into fixed positions in the brain. Signals from these electrodes are amplified and, in the hands of some workers, action potentials of fairly constant size several times larger than the noise level can be recorded. Other neurophysiologists, impressed by the ease with which neuronal cell bodies appear to be impaled and damaged by microelectrodes, are sceptical about the claim that action potentials recorded in this way represent recordings from neuronal cell bodies. Myelinated nerve *axons* are, by contrast, more robust; it may be that it is action potentials from these structures which are being seen over the long durations claimed in some of these studies.

The other method for single unit recording in conscious animals involves the use of movable microelectrodes with a tip diameter of the order of 1 μm. Single neurones can more readily be resolved by this method, but the recordings are of limited duration because a violent movement of the animal will result in loss of the cell. Monkeys, which tolerate head fixation, have certain advantages for this kind of work. Another means of overcoming the early loss of cells might be the use of a weightless microelectrode of the kind described by Gualtierotti and Bailey (1968). This method has been used to record from peripheral nerves in frogs under conditions of violent vibration, but has so far not been used on the central nervous system. But unit recording from conscious animals also presents problems of experimental design and interpretation. In these preparations there is a constantly and uncontrollably varying input to the hypothalamus generated not only by the animal's external environment, but also by its own activities (movements, sleep-waking state, etc.). The input channels to the hypothalamus of such animals are thus very noisy. A test stimulus must therefore be very large, or delivered through a pathway with massive hypothalamic connexions in order that the neurones, with their multiplicity of converging inputs, will respond to the test stimulus by a detectable change in activity.

Thus far we have considered exclusively extracellular recordings from hypothalamic neurones. They give us information about a neurone's response to stimuli, *i.e.* its output. If the rate of firing increases, this may be due to an increase in excitatory input or a decrease of inhibitory input or both. Cell silence may mean profound inhibition or simply lack of excitation. Only by intracellular recording from hypo-thalamic neurones can the details of the synaptic mechanisms forming the input to these cells be elucidated. Thalamic neurones are now proving to be susceptible to intracellular recording methods (Frigyesi and Machek, 1971), and we must expect similar studies in the hypothalamus before very long; indeed as this paper was being prepared, Oomura disclosed that his group have successfully recorded intracellularly from lateral hypothalamic neurones (verbal discussion at the IVth International Conference on the Regulation of Food and Water Intake, Cambridge, August, 1971).

EXAMPLES OF HYPOTHALAMIC INPUTS

Angiotensin

Angiotensin II (hereafter called angiotensin) has a number of actions on the nervous system. When injected into the vertebral artery of the rabbit (Rosendorff *et al.*, 1970) or greyhound (Lowe and Scroop, 1969) it causes an increase in blood pressure and heart rate which is significantly greater than that obtained when the same dose is infused into a vein. This central pressor response is markedly reduced by bilateral ablation of the area postrema (Scroop *et al.*, 1971) which is an area devoid of a blood–brain barrier.

Angiotensin reduces the amobarbital sleeping time in rats, produces marked EEG arousal in cats, increases the total brain acetylcholine content in the mouse and the rabbit, increases acetylcholine output from peripheral nerve endings, increases norad-renaline release from the brain (Palaic and Khairallah, 1967), increases the perme-ability of vascular muscle membrane to sodium and probably to calcium (Villamil *et al.*, 1970), and increases acetylcholine output from the cat cerebral cortex, probably due to changes in the release mechanism (see Elie and Panisset, 1970, for details and other references).

Coming to problems more directly related to hypothalamic function, angiotensin has been shown to stimulate ADH release. Intracarotid infusions were more potent in stimulating ADH release in dogs than intravenous infusions in spite of the fact that both routes of infusion resulted in the same elevation of blood pressure; ven-triculocisternal perfusion of an artificial CSF containing angiotensin also caused ADH release (Mouw *et al.*, 1971). These experiments do not localise the precise site in the brain responsive to angiotensin; the authors did however speculate, on the basis of rather slender evidence, that it might be in the paraventricular nuclei.

There is very good evidence that the kidney exerts control over drinking, and that the substance active in stimulating the brain to cause drinking is angiotensin (see

References p. 184

Fitzsimons, 1970, 1972, for reviews). Intracranial injections of relatively small doses (down to 5 ng) of angiotensin reliably elicit drinking in the water-replete rat when applied to the anterior hypothalamus, the medial preoptic area and the septum (including the nucleus accumbens) (Epstein *et al.*, 1970). Monkeys (Setler, 1971), goats (Andersson and Eriksson, 1971) and rabbits (Findlay and Fitzsimons, unpublished data) also drink in response to intracranial angiotensin. The dipsogenic action of angiotensin has been analysed in more detail by Fitzsimons and Setler (1971) using cholinergic and catecholaminergic antagonists. They found that angiotensin-induced drinking depends on the integrity of catecholaminergic neurones in the preoptic region. This finding is in accord with studies on the effects of angiotensin infusion on catecholamine uptake and release in blood vessels. Khairallah *et al.* (1971) concluded that angiotensin inhibits the uptake, and hence the inactivation, of the sympathetic neurotransmitters. On the other hand Hughes and Roth (1971) have provided evidence that an enhancement of noradrenaline release is the consequence of the action of angiotensin.

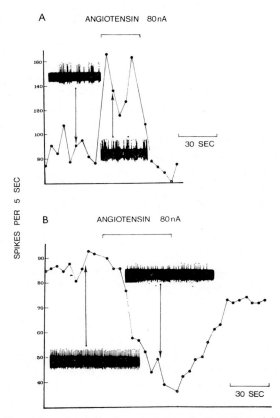

Fig. 1. The effects of iontophoretic application of angiotensin II on the activity of single neurones in (A) the nucleus accumbens septi and (B) the preoptic area. Photographs of cell activity corresponding to periods before and during iontophoresis are shown; the dots adjacent to the photographs are separated by a distance which represents 1 sec of photographed record (Findlay, Setler and Williams, unpublished observations).

We are at present studying the effects in urethane-anaesthetized rats, of ionto-phoretic application of angiotensin to neurones in the areas proven active for the dipsogenic effects of angiotensin (Findlay, Setler and Williams, unpublished data). We do not yet have enough data on all areas, but we have now studied more than twenty cells in the preoptic and neighbouring areas, of which five were inhibited and three were excited after application of angiotensin. All four cells inhibited by angiotensin which were tested with noradrenaline were inhibited by both substances. Examples of records from two cells are given in Fig. 1.

As mentioned above, it is important to demonstrate that a suspected blood-borne input is, in fact, able to gain access to the hypothalamus. In this respect, the evidence with regard to angiotensin is negative. Studies on the fate of injected tritiated angiotensin indicates a concentration of radioactivity in the adrenal glands, kidney, liver and pituitary gland; no part of the brain showed preferential uptake, and the indications were that angiotensin II and/or its metabolites do not readily pass the blood–brain barrier (Osborne et al., 1971).

Further complications to the attractive renal dipsogenic theory for the control of drinking have arisen. Fitzsimons (1971) has shown in rats that intracranial injection, into the angiotensin II-sensitive region, of renin, angiotensin I or synthetic tetra-decapeptide renin substrate (which is converted by renin to angiotensin I) will cause a comparable response. Renin (or another enzyme with identical properties) is present in brain tissue of dogs examined 36 h (Fischer–Ferraro et al., 1971) or twelve days (Ganten et al., 1971) after nephrectomy. Indeed other sites of renin release and production besides the kidney, such as uterus, salivary glands and splanchnic territory have also been suggested (Ganten et al., 1970). It may be that the intracranial injection of angiotensin mimicks the effects not of blood-borne, but of locally released, angiotensin. The control of that local release thus becomes a matter of great significance.

For the time being, the claim that angiotensin is a blood-borne hypothalamic input must be regarded as important, interesting, but not proven.

Olfactory input

The olfactory bulb receives the fibres of the olfactory nerves and projects to the olfactory tubercle, the pyriform cortex and to the corticomedial group of the amygdaloid nuclei. From these areas arise two of the most extensive projections to the hypothalamus, the ventral amygdalo-fugal pathway and the stria terminalis. By these and other routes, it is clear that the olfactory structures of the brain have massive routes of access to the medial and lateral hypothalamus (Raisman, 1966, 1970; Heimer, 1971; Raisman and Field, 1971a).

Olfactory stimuli have clear effects on reproductive endocrine function, which must be mediated by the hypothalamus; some of these are known by the names of those who first described them (Bruce, Lee and Boot, Whitten) (see review by Whitten, 1966). The well-known pregnancy block seen in mice placed in the presence of the odour of strange males (the Bruce effect) has recently been examined in lactating pregnant mice (Bloch, 1971). Implantation is usually delayed during lactation (by an inhibitory action of the suckling stimulus on FSH secretion), but not if the mice were exposed to the odour of a strange male. The odour perhaps induces a secretion of FSH and thus of oestrogen; in the lactating female this endocrine stimulus hastens implantation, but it inhibits nidation in non-lactating animals. Dominic (1966) had earlier ascribed the pregnancy block to lack of prolactin, and this important controversy on the effect of odours on the pituitary will be resolved only by assay of plasma hormone levels in lactating and non-lactating animals exposed to strange males. Pheromonal facilitation of release of ovulation-inducing hormones is also indicated by studies of Zarrow et al. (1970), who showed that PMSG- or HCG-induced ovulation in the immature female mouse is facilitated by exposure to the presence of, but not contact with, an adult male. The effect is not seen if an immature or castrated male is used, or if the olfactory bulbs of the female are removed.

Other evidence shows that exteroceptive factors seem to influence the hormones concerned in lactation. Grosvenor (1965) reported that lactating female rats, when isolated from their young for several hours and then separated from them by only a wire mesh screen, would respond to the presence of their young with a significant depletion of pituitary prolactin stores. Recent work (Mena and Grosvenor, 1971) suggests that olfactory signals from the pups play some part in this phenomenon. The fact that a *release* of prolactin occurs in these circumstances (compared with the inhibition alleged by Dominic to occur in the presence of strange males in the Bruce effect) emphasizes the specificity of these olfactory signals.

In the human, data are obviously less clear. Analyses have been made on the menstrual cycles of students at an American women's college (McClintock, 1971). Amongst room-mates and close friends, there was a statistically significant tendency for increasing synchronisation of menstrual cycles over a six-month period of study. Exposure to common lighting patterns seemed less important than the fact that the members of the group should spend time together, and pheromonal effects offer one possible explanation for the phenomenon.

Certain patterns of behaviour—over which the hypothalamus probably exerts some control—are profoundly altered by changes in olfactory input (see review by Cowley and Wise, 1970). Mating behaviour in the male golden hamster was eliminated by removal of the olfactory bulb (Murphy and Schneider, 1970), whilst a similar operation in female rats abolished copulatory behaviour (Moss, 1971), and in lactating and virgin mice resulted in abolition of maternal behaviour (Gandelman et al., 1971). The urine of female mice contains pheromones which can increase or decrease the aggressive behaviour of isolated males (Mugford and Nowell, 1971). The *anti-aggression* activity of urine was abolished by spaying or injections of testosterone propionate. Urine from spayed mice treated with testosterone actually caused *greater* aggression than that from intact testosterone-treated animals. A series of studies on primate sexual behaviour by Michael and collaborators (1971) has led to the suggestion that a substance or substances (with the suggested name of "copulin") in the vaginal secretions of rhesus monkeys powerfully stimulates male interest in the female and overt sexual behaviour. The substances, produced under the influence of oestrogen, have recently been identified as short-chain aliphatic acids, by combining partitioning and chromatographic procedures with behavioural studies (Michael *et al.*, 1971).

Meanwhile, neurophysiological studies have been proceeding in an attempt to understand the neural mechanisms underlying the variety of endocrine and behavioural reactions to olfactory inputs described above. The situation in invertebrates seems rather clear. For example, in the cockroach, Yamada (1971) has described two patterns of response of single nerve cells in the olfactory lobe. Some cells ("odour generalists") responded to a wide variety of smells, whereas others ("odour specialists") responded specifically to biologically important substances. "Specialist" cells responding specifically to the cockroach sex attractant odour were localized in particular regions of the olfactory lobe. Electrophysiological studies in the olfactory lobe and preoptic area of the male rat have revealed the presence of neurones exhibiting enhanced responses to olfactory stimuli after the injection of testosterone. Particularly interesting is the claim that these effects of testosterone were especially marked when the odour tested was that of female rat urine (Pfaff and Pfaffmann, 1969). Further work (Pfaff and Gregory, 1971) in male rats failed to demonstrate any cells comparable to the "odour specialists" of the cockroach. However, more units in the preoptic area than in the olfactory bulb responded differentially to oestrous compared to ovariectomized female urine odours (Fig. 2), and a high proportion of all units, in the olfactory bulb and preoptic area, responded differently to any given urine odour compared to any given non-urine odour. In female rats, of a strain in which the oestrus cycle can be accelerated by urine odour from normal males, but not from castrated males, neurones in the olfactory bulb, preoptic area and lateral hypothalamus responded to these biologically significant odours. However, no neurones were observed that responded exclusively to urine odours and only a few neurones showed consistently different responses to the odour from normal and castrated males; though other animals when tested behaviourally spent more time sniffing urine from normal males than castrated male urine (Scott and Pfaff, 1970).

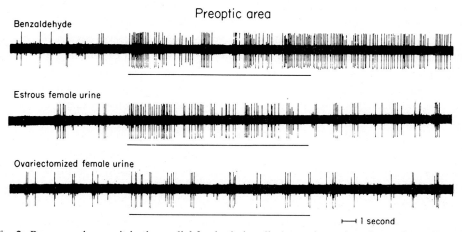

Fig. 2. Responses by a unit in the medial forebrain bundle (preoptic area) to three odours. Benzaldehyde regularly gave the largest responses, and ovariectomized female urine odour the smallest responses from this unit. This unit is an example of those showing differential response magnitude to three odours (from Pfaff and Gregory, 1971).

References p. 184

SLEEP–WAKING STATE

It is, perhaps, rather unorthodox to include sleep–waking state as a hypothalamic input mechanism. It might be objected that sleep is a state involving the whole brain and that input–output relationships cannot be accurately defined. Indeed there are those who claim that the hypothalamus and preoptic area, far from being passively influenced by sleep, are active in bringing about a change in sleep–waking state (Nauta, 1946; Clemente and Sterman, 1963; McGinty and Sterman, 1968). More recent studies have tended to assign primary responsibility for the induction of sleep to structures in the brain stem. A group of serotonin-containing neurones in the mid-brain raphe system are said to induce slow-wave sleep, and neurones in the pons to induce paradoxical sleep (Jouvet, 1967; Frederickson and Hobson, 1970; McCarley and Hobson, 1971).

But initiator or not, the hypothalamus is clearly profoundly influenced by changes in the sleep–waking state. During wakefulness growth hormone is barely detectable in humans except during minor post-prandial rises; but early in sleep, a major rise is seen which is related to the first occurrence of stages III and IV of sleep by EEG criteria (VanderLaan et al., 1970). There are 24-h circadian rhythms (which will normally be entrained to the sleep–waking rest–activity rhythm), of which the most dramatic is that described by Everett and Sawyer (1950): small doses of barbiturate given during the "critical period" between 2 p.m. and 4 p.m. to female rats on the day of pro-oestrus will delay the onset of oestrus for 24 h. The normally rather precise timing of the ovulatory surge of LH release in rats may be the result of facilitation of LH release by progesterone of adrenal origin; thus the LH release mechanism would be entrained to the light–dark rhythm via circadian variations in ACTH release (Feder et al., 1971). Circadian rhythms are, in fact, seen in almost all the variables, which are under hypothalamic control, such as temperature, drinking, eating, and plasma levels of corticosterone and other hormones (Retiene, 1970). All these rhythms are entrained by the 24-h light–dark rhythm, and the hypothalamus is thus described in terms of being a light dependent structure; the avid search for direct retino-hypothalamic nervous connections has resulted from this kind of thinking. But sleep–waking and/or rest–activity cycles (the two are related but not synonymous) are also closely tied to the 24-h pattern of light and dark by mechanisms which we do not understand. The dependence is presumably genetically determined since some species of animal are light-active and some are dark-active. If humans are maintained on a rigid 24-h activity rhythm in total darkness then physiological rhythms (urinary excretion of catecholamines, 17-hydroxycorticosteroid and sodium, and body temperature) are indistinguishable from those seen in normal lighting conditions (Aschoff et al., 1971).

The activity of single neurones in the hypothalamus is greatly influenced by the behavioural state (waking, slow-wave sleep, paradoxical sleep) of the animal. Maximum activity in most, but not all, neurones is seen during paradoxical sleep (Findlay and Hayward, 1969). Many neurones tend to be somewhat more active in waking than in slow-wave sleep, though there is great heterogeneity of cell behaviour (Fig. 3).

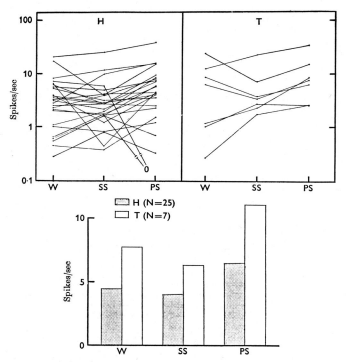

Fig. 3. Spontaneous discharge rates (spikes/sec) of twenty-five hypothalamic (H) and seven extra-hypothalamic (T) cells during waking (W), slow-wave sleep (SS) and paradoxical sleep (PS) in rabbit. Upper row: spontaneous discharge rates on the ordinate (Log. scale) and plots obtained from the same cell during each behavioural state (W, SS, PS) connected along the abscissa. Lower row: mean firing rates (spikes/sec) of the groups of cells during the three states of behaviour. Note the great heterogeneity of cell behaviour (from Findlay and Hayward, 1969).

There are also marked changes in the pattern of firing in certain areas; in the dorsal hypothalamus, neurones display a pattern of high-frequency bursts of spikes separated by quite long intervals, but during wakefulness and paradoxical sleep, the pattern of firing becomes more regular. The large number of cells responsive to sleep-waking state which can be demonstrated contrasts with the rather small number of cells in which Lincoln and Cross (1967) could demonstrate visual sensitivity; though Dafny *et al.* (1965) were able to demonstrate photic sensitivity in more than half the hypothalamic cells studied, they did not observe the EEG of the animals, and thus it is hard to know whether or not the responses were simply non-specific arousal effects.

There seems no clear answer in the literature as to whether, in the case of many of the circadian rhythms of hypothalamic output, the situation can be summarised as:

LIGHT RHYTHM→SLEEP/ACTIVITY RHYTHM→HYPOTHALAMIC→ENDOCRINE,
　　　　　　　　　　　　　　　　RHYTHM　　　　　TEMPERATURE
or　　　　　　　　　　　　　　　　　　　　　　　ETC. RHYTHM.

SLEEP/ACTIVITY RHYTHM←LIGHT RHYTHM→HYPOTHALAMIC→ENDOCRINE,
　　　　　　　　　　　　　　　　RHYTHM　　　　　TEMPERATURE
　　　　　　　　　　　　　　　　　　　　　　　ETC. RHYTHM.

Clearly other causal interactions are possible. We plan to try to investigate the problem by placing rats on "experimental shift work". It will be interesting to see how endocrine and other rhythms adjust to an imposed pattern of activity.

The mammary glands, and particularly the teats, contain receptors sensitive to mechanical stimuli (Findlay, 1966) which are of great importance in influencing the hypothalamic control of oxytocin and prolactin when they are activated by the stimulus of suckling (Fig. 4). Oxytocin release in response to suckling (the milk-

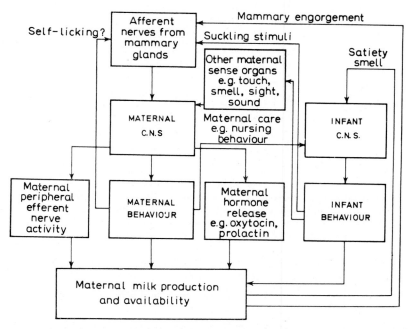

Fig. 4. The principal routes of interaction between mother, maternal lactation and infant. Input from mammary nerves acts via the maternal hypothalamus to affect maternal hormone release and, possibly, maternal behaviour (from Findlay, 1971).

ejection reflex) in the rabbit is abolished by local anaesthesia of the teats (Findlay, 1968). Whilst suckling can clearly be shown to influence release of prolactin from the anterior pituitary gland (Grosvenor and Turner, 1957), it does not appear to be essential for the continuance of lactation in all species (Linzell, 1963). We know something of the quantitative and temporal aspects of hormone release in response to the suckling stimulus. Fuchs and Wagner (1963) showed that suckling of one or two rabbit pups elicited the release of only 1–2 mU of oxytocin in the mother; during suckling of a whole litter, from 50–100 mU were liberated, which corresponds to 10–15 mU per pup; this pattern of reflex response is a good example of spatial summation. Edwardson and Eayrs (1967) described a relationship between the neural stimulus of suckling and the endocrine response of the hypothalamo-pituitary system such that increase in litter size is associated with an overall increase in milk yield up to a limit beyond which the addition of further young to the litter is without effect. Grosvenor and Mena (1971) have shown that a period of time (a refractory period) must elapse after suckling-induced prolactin release before suckling can again effect hormone release. The delay is due not to depletion of pituitary prolactin stores, but to the failure of some central component of the releasing mechanism to respond to stimulation.

The teats of the rabbit are richly innervated, predominantly by unencapsulated sensory nerve endings supplied by unmyelinated fibres (Ballantyne and Bunch, 1966; Cross and Findlay, 1969). Few encapsulated endings were found in the human by Cathcart *et al.* (1948). From the mammary gland, the sensory fibres pass to the spinal cord. Lesions of the cord have been made by various authors in order to ascertain the ascending pathway. Lactation is impaired in the rat by lesions in the lateral funiculi (Eayrs and Baddeley, 1956) and in the rabbit by lesions of the ventrolateral funiculi (Mena and Beyer, 1968). In the goat, on the other hand, lesions of the dorsal funiculi block the milk-ejection reflex (though not lactation) (Tsaekhaev, 1955; Denamur and Martinet, 1959).

Studies on the afferent pathways in the brain stem have mainly been carried out by Tindal and collaborators (see Tindal and Knaggs, 1970, for details, references, and a thoughtful review of the evolutionary aspects of mammary sensory mechanisms). The first studies were performed in the guinea-pig and the rabbit, and involved electrical stimulation in multiple sites in the midbrain and diencephalon, coupled with observation of milk ejection from a lactating mammary gland—a useful index of oxytocin release. Sympathetic-adrenal responses were abolished by brain stem transection at the mid-cerebellar level. Vasopressin, if released, was detected in the later studies by continuous measurement of arterial blood pressure. In the midbrain, milk ejection was evoked by stimulation of the lateral wall of the tegmental region. At the anterior limit of the midbrain, the pathway lies medio-ventral to the medial geniculate body and then diverges, one portion passing forward close to the rostral central grey matter and the other passing medioventrally into the subthalamus. The two pathways merge in the posterior hypothalamus, passing forward to more rostral levels and probably many fibres converge on the paraventricular nuclei, which are thought to be largely responsible for the control of the synthesis and release of oxytocin from the posterior pituitary gland (Cross, 1966). In later studies Tindal and Knaggs (1969) implanted chronic stimulating electrodes and assessed the effect of daily stimulation in various sites on the release of prolactin (measured by the extent of mammary growth on the pseudopregnant rabbit). The pathways were similar, but when the oxytocin pathway diverged, only the ventral pathway through the rostral central grey was found to elicit prolactin release.

Three main routes—the primitive substantia gelatinosa–Lissauer's tract system, the ancient spinothalamic system and the most recently developed and highly discriminating dorsal column–medial leminiscus system—serve to convey somaesthetic information to the forebrain. It would appear that in the rabbit, which is the only species for which we can combine data from spinal cord transection and midbrain stimulation, the spinothalamic system is necessary and sufficient for the suckling induced release of oxytocin. In the goat, however, in which the dorsal columns appear essential in the spinal cord, we might expect to find that electrical stimulation of the medial lemniscus would more readily provoke oxytocin release than stimulation of the spinothalamic system. Recording of activity in the various pathways has not been performed during suckling, but it seems likely that components of all three systems would be excited to some extent by the suckling stimulus. In the human, however, the skin of the nipple and areola has only limited powers of sensory discrimination (Wood-Jones and Turner, 1931); this might be taken as indirect evidence for a relatively small involvement of the lemniscal system in mammary sensory innervation.

Aulsebrook and Holland (1969a, b) have examined the effect of electrical stimulation in the brain stem on oxytocin release evoked by stimulation by suckling, or by electrical stimulation of a second site. The pathways excitatory to oxytocin were fairly similar to those described by Tindal and Knaggs (1970), but in addition they described areas in the brain stem inhibitory to oxytocin release. These areas were similar to, but more extensive than, the brain stem areas in which stimulation would elicit ADH release. These experiments provide some insight into possible mechanisms for the stress-induced inhibition of suckling-induced release of oxytocin.

Recording of hypothalamic unit activity in response to a suckling-like stimulation has been performed by Brooks et al. (1966). In the lightly chloralose-anaesthetised cat, they showed that neurones in the paraventricular region (which were not antidromically identified) were less sensitive to osmotic changes than cells in the supraoptic region, but more sensitive to excitation by such stimuli as gentle suction applied to the nipples, and vaginal and uterine stimulation. They did not correlate cell activity with the EEG, and some at least of the responses observed may have been nonspecific. The experiments reported in this paper were initially surprising in view of the finding of many workers from Gaines (1915) onwards that anaesthesia blocks the milk-ejection reflex. But recently Wakerley and Lincoln (1971) have demonstrated that milk-ejection can be elicited by suckling stimulation in the lightly urethane-anaesthetised rat. This apparent insensitivity of the reflex to light anaesthesia seems to open up great possibilities for a thorough examination of the details of mammary input mechanisms by electrical recording of single units at various parts of the pathway. Already we can say that it seems highly likely that some, at least, of the excitatory afferents to the paraventricular nuclei are cholinergic. Shute and Lewis (1966) found that some of the cells of the nuclei contain small or moderate amounts of acetylcholinesterase in their cell bodies, but none in their axons; this pattern was said to be characteristic of cholinoceptive neurones. Cross et al. (1971) have recently reported the effects of iontophoretic application of acetylcholine and noradrenaline to antidromically identified paraventricular neurones. Twenty-two out of 23 cells had their spontaneous discharge rate accelerated by acetylcholine; noradrenaline elicited a short latency depression of firing rate in 21 of the cells. Oba et al. (1971) have shown that atropine implanted into the paraventricular nucleus causes a blockade of the milk-ejection reflex in rats.

Finally, the behavioural significance of afferent nervous input from the mammary gland should not be overlooked. Rats find the medial forebrain bundle a rewarding structure to stimulate (Olds, 1956) and it is thought that certain kinds of goal-seeking behaviour might in part be organised by neurones in that area. We have recently found that rabbits will display nursing behaviour even when the state of the mammary glands is quite inappropriate; if the intensity of suckling stimulation is reduced, then they will display nursing behaviour for longer periods (Findlay and Tallal, 1971). Perhaps nursing behaviour is, via mammary inputs to the medial forebrain bundle, a form of peripheral self-stimulation.

The female genital tract

The effects of mechanical stimulation of the female genital tract on reproductive endocrine function fall into three main groups:

1. Effects on posterior pituitary gland function, and particularly oxytocin release, during labour and copulation.

2. Effects of the stimuli of copulation on anterior pituitary function, and particularly on ovulation and corpus luteum formation.

3. Effects of uterine foreign bodies and distension on corpus luteum lysis.

The first two of these effects are attained by neurally mediated hypothalamic input mechanisms, but the last may, in some species, be brought about by release directly from the uterus of a luteolytic factor, possibly prostaglandin F2α (Blatchley et al., 1971). The stimuli which cause oxytocin release are reviewed by Cross (1966). Cobo et al. (1964) found no significant milk-ejection activity during labour in women; but oxytocin was detected in appreciable quantities in goats during the second stage of labour (Folley and Knaggs, 1965), suggesting that its release is triggered by neural stimuli arising from the stretching of cervix and vagina. We must remember that stress is an important inhibitor of oxytocin release; the failure of investigators, particularly those working in obstetric clinics, to find evidence of oxytocin release after vaginal or cervical (Fisch et al., 1964) distension, or during labour, cannot be held to invalidate other results obtained in subjects more accustomed to, and less apprehensive about, their surroundings.

Vaginal distension caused the release of oxytocin in normal cycling ewes, and this release was inhibited after two weeks of progesterone treatment, but was enhanced after two weeks of oestradiol treatment (Roberts and Share, 1969). The stimulus of vaginal distension arises during parturition, but the same receptors are also likely to be stimulated during copulation; there is evidence for milk-ejection and raised blood oxytocin levels in women and in animals during copulation (Fox and Fox, 1971).

Very little is known about the properties of vaginal receptors, though a little information is available on the properties of the uterine mechanoreceptors in the rabbit (Bower, 1959). We know little about the afferent pathways employed in the spinal cord or brain stem, though it seems likely that, at least more rostrally, these are shared with afferent pathways from the mammary glands as the two converge upon hypothalamic neurosecretory nuclei (see previous section). Electrical stimulation of the cat uterus is followed after a long latency (30–50 msec) by evoked potentials in the preoptic and tuberal regions of the hypothalamus, and particularly in the supra-optic nucleus (Abrahams *et al.*, 1964). Distension of the uterus in post-partum cats anaesthetized with chloralose causes oxytocin release and an increase in the activity of neurones in the paraventricular region (Brooks *et al.*, 1966). I have recently been attempting to elicit specific activation of hypothalamic neurones in conscious rabbits by distension of the vagina with 10–20 ml of fluid in a balloon implanted in the vagina. On many occasions, vaginal distension caused arousal of the animal with associated changes in unit activity. But on only one occasion was I able to elicit a change in cell activity attributable to the stimulus (Fig. 5); curiously enough, the cell was determined by histological criteria to be lying in or close to the paraventricular nucleus. In the anaesthetized rat, Lincoln (1969a) found neurones in the anterior hypothalamus which would respond specifically during cervical stimulation.

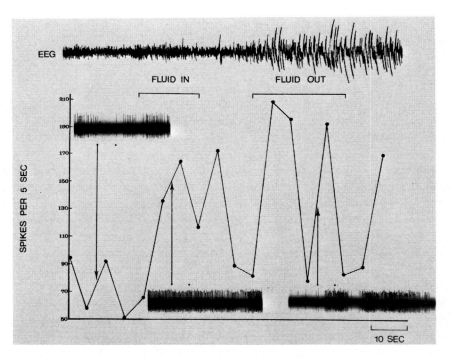

Fig. 5. The activity of a single neurone in the region of the paraventricular nucleus of a conscious unrestrained rabbit. During arousal (low-voltage EEG) the cell fired slowly until the distension (fluid in) of the vagina by injection of 20 ml fluid in a vaginal balloon. On removal of the fluid (fluid out) the animal passed into slow-wave sleep (high-voltage EEG) and the cell firing rate increased with a rather irregular pattern of firing. Photographs of cell activity at three different times are shown; the dots adjacent to the photographs are separated by a distance which represents one second of photographed record.

But in addition to the relatively brief responses to vaginal stimulation so far mentioned, there are phenomena of longer duration. Vincent *et al.* (1970), in a study of the effects of stimulation of the rabbit vagina with a vibrating lucite rod, reported that 15 out of 19 cells in the hypothalamus of the conscious animals showed clear responses lasting up to 30 min post-stimulation which were unrelated to non-specific EEG effects. Kawakami and his collaborators (Kawakami and Saito, 1967; Kawakami and Kubo, 1971) have also studied the events following vaginal stimulation in the cat and the rat. In the rat, they obtained significant responses only when the animal was in the oestrous state. They recorded from a variety of sites in midbrain, limbic system and hypothalamus concluding from these complex data that all these structures participate in the responses to vaginal stimulation.

The above are only a selection of the many studies which have attempted to correlate central events with vaginal stimulation. This subject has given rise to much attention, for as well as affecting the posterior pituitary, species-dependent effects on anterior pituitary function follow coitus. In rabbits, cats and some other species, vaginal stimulation causes ovulation, *i.e.* a surge in the production of luteinising hormone. In the rat and some other spontaneous ovulators, copulation causes the maintenance of corpus luteum life, and there is evidence that in many "spontaneous" ovulators, copulation hastens or facilitates ovulation (Zarrow *et al.*, 1968). The effect of vaginal stimulation on plasma gonadotrophin levels has been clearly demonstrated by Spies and Niswender (1971); they showed that pelvic nerve section did not affect the short-term (20 min) post-copulation rise of serum prolactin, LH and FSH levels, but abolished the long-term (8–24 h) rise in prolactin levels, which seemed crucial for corpus luteum activation. Furthermore, copulation is a stimulus which is probably, like the suckling stimulus, "pleasurable". This being so, it is possible that vaginal afferents project to and interact with neurones in areas positive for self-stimulation.

With so many important neural behavioural and endocrine consequences of such varying time course, we may expect that input mechanisms from the female genital tract to the hypothalamus will continue to attract much attention.

SUMMARY

Hypothalamic input mechanisms are listed and a variety of classification systems are suggested. Methods for the study of input mechanisms are discussed, with particular reference to the use of electrophysiological methods. Some suggestions for possible future tactics are put forward.

The effect of angiotensin on the hypothalamus is discussed. Evidence relating to the role of the kidney in the control of drinking via an action of angiotensin on hypothalamic neurones is given. Behavioural, endocrine and electrophysiological studies on olfactory input are described. Circadian and sleep–waking rhythms are shown to affect hypothalamic function; it is suggested that circadian activity cycles may act to influence many variables under hypothalamic control, in the absence of lighting cues.

References p. 184

Hypothalamic input from the mammary gland is discussed in some detail. Likely afferent pathways for the suckling stimulus are described, and the endocrine and behavioural implications of the suckling stimulus are mentioned. Finally, input from the female genital tract, which is activated both in labour and in copulation leads to hypothalamically mediated endocrine events. The neuronal activity which may underlie these endocrine reactions is discussed.

Note added in proof

Since this paper was written, much relevant work has been published of which the following must be mentioned. Komisaruk (1971) has surveyed possible experimental "strategies in neuroendocrine neurophysiology" in a review that contrasts with, but complements, some of the views that I have expressed. Nicoll and Barker (1971) have studied the responses of supraoptic neurosecretory cells to iontophoretically administered angiotensin. Intracarotid administration of angiotensin did not produce a measurable change in the activity of cells which had been responsive to the same drug administered by iontophoresis. The wide distribution of hypothalamic neurones sensitive to olfactory stimuli has been emphasized by the work of Komisaruk and Beyer (1972) in a paper which provides an extensive bibliography for those interested in olfactory input to the hypothalamus.

ACKNOWLEDGEMENTS

I am grateful to Dr. Paulette Setler for her helpful comments on the manuscript. Some of the work described was assisted by grants from the Agricultural Research Council, the Medical Research Council and the Lalor Foundation.

REFERENCES

ABRAHAMS, V. C., LANGWORTH, E. P. AND THEOBALD, G. W. (1964) Potentials evoked in the hypothalamus and cerebral cortex by electrical stimulation of the uterus. *Nature (Lond.)*, **203**, 654–656.

ANDERSSON, B. AND ERIKSSON, L. (1971) Conjoint action of sodium and angiotensin on brain mechanisms controlling water and salt balances. *Acta physiol. scand.*, **81**, 18–29.

ASCHOFF, J., FATRINSKA, M., GIEDKE, H., DOERR, P., STAMM, D. AND WISSER, H. (1971) Human circadian rhythms in continuous darkness: entrainment by social cues. *Science*, **171**, 213–215.

AULSEBROOK, L. H. AND HOLLAND, R. C. (1969a) Central regulation of oxytocin release with and without vasopressin release. *Amer. J. Physiol.*, **216**, 818–829.

AULSEBROOK, L. H. AND HOLLAND, R. C. (1969b) Central inhibition of oxytocin release. *Amer. J. Physiol.*, **216**, 830–842.

BACCELLI, G., GUAZZI, M., LIBRETTI, A. AND ZANCHETTI, A. (1965) Pressoceptive and chemoceptive aortic reflexes in decorticate and in decerebrate cats. *Amer. J. Physiol.*, **208**, 708–714.

BALLANTYNE, B. AND BUNCH, G. A. (1966) The neurohistology of quiescent mammary tissue in *Lepus albus. J. comp. Neurol.*, **127**, 471–487.

BEACH, F. A. (1970) Some effects of gonadal hormones on sexual behavior. In *The Hypothalamus*, L. MARTINI, M. MOTTA AND F. FRASCHINI (Eds.), Academic Press, New York, pp. 617–639.

BEYER, C. AND SAWYER, C. H. (1969) Hypothalamic unit activity related to control of the pituitary gland. In *Frontiers in Neuroendocrinology*, W. F. GANONG AND L. MARTINI (Eds.), Oxford Univ. Press, New York, pp. 255–287.

BLATCHLEY, F. R., DONOVAN, B. T., POYSER, N. L., HORTON, E. W., THOMPSON, C. J. AND LOS, M. (1971) Identification of Prostaglandin F2α in the utero-ovarian blood of guinea-pig after treatment with oestrogen. *Nature (Lond.)*, **230**, 243–244.

BLOCH, S. (1971) Enhancement of on-time nidations in suckling pregnant mice by the proximity of strange males. *J. Endocr.*, **49**, 431–436.

BLOOM, F. E., OLIVER, A. P. AND SALMOIRAGHI, G. C. (1963) The responsiveness of individual hypothalamic neurons to microelectrophoretically administered endogenous amines. *Int. J. Neuropharmacol.*, **2**, 181–193.

BOWER, E. A. (1959) Action potentials from uterine sensory nerves. *J. Physiol. (Lond.)*, **148**, 2–3P.

BRAIN, P. F. AND NOWELL, N. W. (1971) Isolation versus grouping effects on adrenal and gonadal function in albino mice. I. The Male. II. The Female. *Gen. comp. Endocr.*, **16**, 149–159.

BRINDLEY, G. S. (1970) *Physiology of the Retina and Visual Pathway*. Edward Arnold, London, p. 116.

BROOKS, C. M., ISHIKAWA, T., KOIZUMI, K. AND LU, H. (1966) Activity of neurones in the paraventricular nucleus of the hypothalamus and its control. *J. Physiol. (Lond.)*, **182**, 217–231.

BROWN, K. A. AND MELZACK, R. (1969) Effects of glucose on multi-unit activity in the hypothalamus. *Exp. Neurol.*, **24**, 363–373.

CATHCART, E. P., GAIRNS, F. W. AND GARVEN, H. S. D. (1948) The innervation of the human quiescent nipple, with notes on pigmentation, erection, and hyperneury. *Trans. roy. Soc. Edinb.*, **61**, 699–717.

CLEMENTE, C. D. AND STERMAN, M. B. (1963) Cortical synchronization and sleep patterns in acute restrained and chronic behaving cats induced by basal forebrain stimulations. *Electroenceph. clin. Neurophysiol.*, Suppl., **24**, 172–187.

COBO, E., DE BERNAL, M. M., QUINTERO, C. A. AND CUADRADO, E. (1964) Neuropophyseal hormone release in the human. III. Experimental study during labor. *Amer. J. Obstet. Gynec.*, **101**, 479–489.

COWLEY, J. J. AND WISE, D. R. (1970) Pheromones, growth and behavior. In *Chemical Influences on Behaviour, Ciba Foundation Study Group*. R. PORTER AND J. BIRCH (Eds.), No. 35, Churchill, London, pp. 144–166.

CREMER, J. E. AND BLIGH, J. (1969) Body-temperature and responses to drugs. *Brit. med. Bull.*, **25**, 299–306.

CROSS, B. A. (1966) Neural control of oxytocin secretion. In *Neuroendocrinology, Vol. I*, L. MARTINI AND W. F. GANONG (Eds.), Academic Press, New York, pp. 217–259.

CROSS, B. A. AND DYER, R. G. (1970) Characterization of unit activity in hypothalamic islands with special reference to hormonal effects. In *The Hypothalamus*, L. MARTINI, M. MOTTA AND F. FRASCHINI (Eds.), Academic Press, New York, pp. 115–122.

CROSS, B. A. AND FINDLAY, A. L. R. (1969) Comparative and sensory aspects of milk ejection. In *Lactogenesis*, M. REYNOLDS AND S. J. FOLLEY (Eds.), Univ. of Pennsylvania Press, Philadelphia, pp. 245–252.

CROSS, B. A., MOSS, R. L. AND URBAN, I. (1971) Effect of iontophoretic application of acetylcholine and noradrenaline to antidromically identified paraventricular neurones. *J. Physiol. (Lond.)*, **214**, 28–30P.

CROSS, B. A. AND SILVER, I. A. (1963) Unit activity in the hypothalamus and the sympathetic response to hypoxia and hypercapnia. *Exp. Neurol.*, **7**, 375–393.

CROSS, B. A. AND SILVER, I. A. (1966) Electrophysiological studies on the hypothalamus. *Brit. med. Bull.*, **22**, 254–260.

DAFNY, N., BENTAL, E. AND FELDMAN, S. (1965) Effect of sensory stimuli on single unit activity in the posterior hypothalamus. *Electroenceph. clin. Neurophysiol.*, **19**, 256–263.

DENAMUR, R. ET MARTINET, J. (1959) Le rôle du système nerveux de la glande mammaire dans l'entretien de la lactation. *Arch. Sci. physiol.*, **13**, 271–352.

DE WIED, D. AND WEIJNEN, J. A. W. M. (Eds.) (1970) Effects of ACTH and adrenocortical hormones on the nervous system. In *Progress in Brain Research, Vol. 32, Pituitary, Adrenal and the Brain*, D. DE WIED AND J. A. W. M. WEIJNEN (Eds.), Elsevier, Amsterdam, pp. 89–155.

DOMINIC, C. J. (1966) Observations on the reproductive pheromones of mice. *J. Reprod. Fertil.*, **11**, 415–421.

DONOVAN, B. T. (1970) *Mammalian Neuroendocrinology*, McGraw Hill, London.

DYBALL, R. E. J. (1971) Oxytocin and ADH secretion in relation to electrical activity in antidromically identified supraoptic and paraventricular units. *J. Physiol. (Lond.)*, **214**, 245–256.

TAMARI, I. (1970) Audiogenic stimulation and reproductive function. In *Physiological Effects of Noise*, B. L. WELCH AND A. S. WELSH (Eds.), Plenum Press, London, pp. 117–130.

TER HAAR, M. B. AND P. C. B. MACKINNON (1972) An investigation of cerebral protein synthesis in various states of neuroendocrine activity. *Progress in Brain Research, Vol. 38, Topics in Neuroendocrinology*, J. ARIËNS KAPPERS AND J. P. SCHADÉ (Eds.), Elsevier, Amsterdam, pp. 211–222.

TINDAL, J. S. AND KNAGGS, G. S. (1969) An ascending pathway for release of prolactin in the brain of the rabbit. *J. Endocr.*, **45**, 111–120.

spread to somatically evoked potentials in different areas of the hypothalamus. *Arch. ital. Biol.*, **103**, 119–135.

McCarley, R. W. and Hobson, J. A. (1971) Single neuron activity in cat gigantocellular tegmental field: selectivity of discharge in desynchronized sleep. *Science*, **174**, 1250–1252.

McClintock, M. K. (1971) Menstrual synchrony and suppression. *Nature (Lond.)*, **229**, 244–245.

McGinty, D. J. and Sterman, M. B. (1968) Sleep suppression after basal forebrain lesions in the cat. *Science*, **160**, 1253–1255.

Mena, F. and Beyer, C. (1968) Effect of spinal cord lesions on milk ejection in the rabbit. *Endocrinology*, **83**, 615–617.

~~Mena, F. and Grosvenor, C. E. (1971) Release of prolactin in rats by exteroceptive stimulation:~~

Tindal, J. S. and Knaggs, G. S. (1970) Environmental stimuli and the mammary gland. *Mem. Soc. Endocr.*, **18**, 239–258.

Tsaekhaev, G. A. (1955) Problem of reflex regulation of milk ejection. *Tr. Inst. Fiziol. (Mosk.)*, **4**, 5–16 (In Russian).

VanderLaan, W. P., Parker, D. C., Rossman, L. G. and VanderLaan, E. F. (1970) Implications of growth hormone release in sleep. *Metabolism*, **19**, 891–897.

Villamil, M. F., Nachev, P. and Kleeman, C. R. (1970) Effect of prolonged infusion of angiotensin II on ionic composition of the arterial wall. *Amer. J. Physiol.*, **218**, 1281–1286.

Vincent, J. D., Dufy, B. and Faure, J. M. A. (1970) Effects of vaginal stimulation on hypothalamic single units in unanesthetized rabbits. *Experientia (Basel)*, **26**, 1266–1267.

Von Euler, C. and Söderberg, U. (1957) The influence of hypothalamic thermoceptive structures on the electroencephalogram and gamma motor activity. *Electroenceph. clin. Neurophysiol.*, **9**, 391–408.

Wakerley, J. B. and Lincoln, D. W. (1971) Milk ejection in the rat: recordings of intramammary pressure during suckling. *J. Endocr.*, **51**, xiii–xiv.

Werner, G. and Mountcastle, V. B. (1963) The variability of central neural activity in a sensory system, and its implications for the central reflection of sensory events. *J. Neurophysiol.*, **26**, 958–977.

Whitten, W. K. (1966) Pheromones and mammalian reproduction. In *Advances in Reproductive Physiology, Vol. 1*, A. McLaren (Ed.), Logos and Academic Press, London and New York, pp. 155–177.

Wolstenholme, G. E. W. and Knight, J. (Eds.) (1971) *The Pineal Gland*, Churchill, Livingstone, Edinburgh and London.

Wood-Jones, F. and Turner, J. B. (1931) A note on the sensory characters of the nipple and areola. *Med. J. Austr.*, **1**, 778–779.

Wurtman, R. J. (1967) Effects of light and visual stimuli on endocrine function. In *Neuroendocrinology, Vol. II*, L. Martini and W. F. Ganong (Eds.), Academic Press, New York, pp. 19–59.

Yamada, M. (1971) A search for odour encoding in the olfactory lobe. *J. Physiol. (Lond.)*, **214**, 127–143.

Zanchetti, A. (1970) Control of the cardiovascular system. In *The Hypothalamus*, L. Martini, M. Motta and F. Fraschini (Eds.), Academic Press, New York, pp. 232–244.

Zarrow, M. X., Campbell, P. S. and Clark, J. H. (1968) Pregnancy following coital-induced ovulation in a spontaneous ovulator. *Science*, **159**, 329–330.

Zarrow, M. X., Estes, S. A., Denenberg, V. H. and Clark, J. H. (1970) Pheromonal facilitation of ovulation in the immature mouse. *J. Reprod. Fertil.*, **23**, 357–360.

DISCUSSION

Dreifuss: When you use angiotensin I or II how can you be sure that, once the substance has been ejected from the pipette it is still angiotensin I or II, but not glutamate or aspartate or one of the other amino acids that have excitatory action or γ-amino-butyrate that has an inhibitory action?

Findlay: No, of course you can't. There are ways of controlling that effect. I think, is it not right to say, that if you use strychnine you block amino-acid effects on neurons.

What you are supposed to do is to look at a particular effect. The problem with iontophoresis is that you can only test a limited number of drugs even with a five-barrelled pipette. You have one recording barrel, one isotonic saline barrel which you have to use to control the current effects, one barrel containing dye so you can mark the site of the neuron, and so you have only two barrels left to use for test substances of which one has to contain angiotensin. The first control we have to do is to put ammonium-acetate in one of the barrels because that also contaminates the available angiotensin solutions.

Moll: Do you think it is really of much importance for our understanding of the biological significance of what is going on, if there is one synapse, two synapses or no synapses at all in the retina?

Findlay: No, I don't.

gland. In *Frontiers in Neuroendocrinology*, W. F. GANONG AND L. MARTINI (Eds.), Oxford Univ. Press, New York, pp. 255–287.

BLATCHLEY, F. R., DONOVAN, B. T., POYSER, N. L., HORTON, E. W., THOMPSON, C. J. AND LOS, M. (1971) Identification of Prostaglandin F2α in the utero-ovarian blood of guinea-pig after treatment with oestrogen. *Nature (Lond.)*, **230**, 243–244.

BLOCH, S. (1971) Enhancement of on-time nidations in suckling pregnant mice by the proximity of strange males. *J. Endocr.*, **49**, 431–436.

BLOOM, F. E., OLIVER, A. P. AND SALMOIRAGHI, G. C. (1963) The responsiveness of individual hypothalamic neurons to microelectrophoretically administered endogenous amines. *Int. J. Neuropharmacol.*, **2**, 181–193.

BOWER, E. A. (1959) Action potentials from uterine sensory nerves. *J. Physiol. (Lond.)*, **148**, 2–3P.

BRAIN, P. F. AND NOWELL, N. W. (1971) Isolation versus grouping effects on adrenal and gonadal function in albino mice. I. The Male. II. The Female. *Gen. comp. Endocr.*, **16**, 149–159.

BRINDLEY, G. S. (1970) *Physiology of the Retina and Visual Pathway*. Edward Arnold, London, p. 116.

BROOKS, C. M., ISHIKAWA, T., KOIZUMI, K. AND LU, H. (1966) Activity of neurones in the paraventricular nucleus of the hypothalamus and its control. *J. Physiol. (Lond.)*, **182**, 217–231.

BROWN, K. A. AND MELZACK, R. (1969) Effects of glucose on multi-unit activity in the hypothalamus. *Exp. Neurol.*, **24**, 363–373.

CATHCART, E. P., GAIRNS, F. W. AND GARVEN, H. S. D. (1948) The innervation of the human quiescent nipple, with notes on pigmentation, erection, and hyperneury. *Trans. roy. Soc. Edinb.*, **61**, 699–717.

CLEMENTE, C. D. AND STERMAN, M. B. (1963) Cortical synchronization and sleep patterns in acute restrained and chronic behaving cats induced by basal forebrain stimulations. *Electroenceph. clin. Neurophysiol.*, Suppl., **24**, 172–187.

COBO, E., DE BERNAL, M. M., QUINTERO, C. A. AND CUADRADO, E. (1964) Neuropophyseal hormone release in the human. III. Experimental study during labor. *Amer. J. Obstet. Gynec.*, **101**, 479–489.

COWLEY, J. J. AND WISE, D. R. (1970) Pheromones, growth and behavior. In *Chemical Influences on Behaviour, Ciba Foundation Study Group*. R. PORTER AND J. BIRCH (Eds.), No. 35, Churchill, London, pp. 144–166.

CREMER, J. E. AND BLIGH, J. (1969) Body-temperature and responses to drugs. *Brit. med. Bull.*, **25**, 299–306.

CROSS, B. A. (1966) Neural control of oxytocin secretion. In *Neuroendocrinology, Vol. I*, L. MARTINI AND W. F. GANONG (Eds.), Academic Press, New York, pp. 217–259.

CROSS, B. A. AND DYER, R. G. (1970) Characterization of unit activity in hypothalamic islands with special reference to hormonal effects. In *The Hypothalamus*, L. MARTINI, M. MOTTA AND F. FRASCHINI (Eds.), Academic Press, New York, pp. 115–122.

CROSS, B. A. AND FINDLAY, A. L. R. (1969) Comparative and sensory aspects of milk ejection. In *Lactogenesis*, M. REYNOLDS AND S. J. FOLLEY (Eds.), Univ. of Pennsylvania Press, Philadelphia, pp. 245–252.

CROSS, B. A., MOSS, R. L. AND URBAN, I. (1971) Effect of iontophoretic application of acetylcholine and noradrenaline to antidromically identified paraventricular neurones. *J. Physiol. (Lond.)*, **214**, 28–30P.

CROSS, B. A. AND SILVER, I. A. (1963) Unit activity in the hypothalamus and the sympathetic response to hypoxia and hypercapnia. *Exp. Neurol.*, **7**, 375–393.

CROSS, B. A. AND SILVER, I. A. (1966) Electrophysiological studies on the hypothalamus. *Brit. med. Bull.*, **22**, 254–260.

DAFNY, N., BENTAL, E. AND FELDMAN, S. (1965) Effect of sensory stimuli on single unit activity in the posterior hypothalamus. *Electroenceph. clin. Neurophysiol.*, **19**, 256–263.

DENAMUR, R. ET MARTINET, J. (1959) Le rôle du système nerveux de la glande mammaire dans l'entretien de la lactation. *Arch. Sci. physiol.*, **13**, 271–352.

DE WIED, D. AND WEIJNEN, J. A. W. M. (Eds.) (1970) Effects of ACTH and adrenocortical hormones on the nervous system. In *Progress in Brain Research, Vol. 32, Pituitary, Adrenal and the Brain*, D. DE WIED AND J. A. W. M. WEIJNEN (Eds.), Elsevier, Amsterdam, pp. 89–155.

DOMINIC, C. J. (1966) Observations on the reproductive pheromones of mice. *J. Reprod. Fertil.*, **11**, 415–421.

DONOVAN, B. T. (1970) *Mammalian Neuroendocrinology*, McGraw Hill, London.

DYBALL, R. E. J. (1971) Oxytocin and ADH secretion in relation to electrical activity in antidromically identified supraoptic and paraventricular units. *J. Physiol. (Lond.)*, **214**, 245–256.

EAYRS, J. T. AND BADDELEY, R. M. (1956) Neural pathways in lactation. *J. Anat. (Lond.)*, **90**, 161–171.

ECCLES, J. C. (1964) *The Physiology of Synapses*, Springer, Berlin, p. 18.

EDWARDSON, J. A. AND EAYRS, J. T. (1967) Neural factors in the maintenance of lactation in the rat. *J. Endocr.*, **38**, 51–59.

EISENMAN, J. S. (1969) Pyrogen-induced changes in the thermosensitivity of septal and preoptic neurons. *Amer. J. Physiol.*, **216**, 330–334.

ELIE, R. AND PANISSET, J. (1970) Effect of angiotensin and atropine on the spontaneous release of acetylcholine from cat cerebral cortex. *Brain Research*, **17**, 297–305.

EPSTEIN, A. N., FITZSIMONS, J. T. AND ROLLS, B. J. (1970) Drinking induced by injection of angiotensin into the brain of the rat. *J. Physiol. (Lond.)*, **210**, 457–474.

EVERETT, J. W. AND SAWYER, C. H. (1950) A 24-hour periodicity in the "L-H-release apparatus" of female rats disclosed by barbitol sedation. *Endocrinology*, **47**, 198–218.

FEDER, H. H., BROWN-GRANT, K. AND CORKER, C. S. (1971) Pre-ovulatory progesterone, the adrenal cortex and the "critical period" for luteinizing hormone release in rats. *J. Endocr.*, **50**, 29–39.

FELDMAN, S. AND DAFNY, N. (1968) Acoustic responses in the hypothalamus. *Electroenceph. clin. Neurophysiol.*, **25**, 150–159.

FELDMAN, S. AND SARNE, Y. (1970) Effect of cortisol on single cell activity in hypothalamic islands. *Brain Research*, **23**, 67–75.

FINDLAY, A. L. R. (1966) Sensory discharges in lactating mammary glands. *Nature (Lond.)*, **212**, 1183–1184.

FINDLAY, A. L. R. (1968) The effect of teat anaesthesia on the milk-ejection reflex in the rabbit. *J. Endocr.* **40**, 127–128.

FINDLAY, A. L. R. (1971) Neural and behavioural interactions with lactation. In *Lactation*, I. R. FALCONER (Ed.), Butterworths, London, pp. 75–91.

FINDLAY, A. L. R. AND HAYWARD, J. N. (1969) Spontaneous activity of single neurones in the hypothalamus of rabbits during sleep and waking. *J. Physiol. (Lond.)*, **201**, 237–258.

FINDLAY, A. L. R. AND TALLAL, P. A. (1971) Effect of reduced suckling stimulation on the duration of nursing in the rabbit. *J. comp. physiol. Psychol.* **76**, 236–241.

FISCH, L., SALA, N. L. AND SCHWARCZ, R. L. (1964) Effect of cervical dilatation upon uterine contractility in pregnant women and its relation to oxytocin secretion. *Amer. J. Obstet. Gynec.*, **90**, 108–114.

FISCHER-FERRARO, C., NAHMOD, V. E., GOLDSTEIN, D. J. AND FINKIELMAN, S. (1971) Angiotensin and renin in rat and dog brain. *J. Exp. Med.*, **133**, 353–361.

FITZSIMONS, J. T. (1970) The renin–angiotensin system in the control of drinking. In *The Hypothalamus*, L. MARTINI, M. MOTTA AND F. FRASCHINI (Eds.), Academic Press, New York, pp. 195–212.

FITZSIMONS, J. T. (1971) The effect on drinking of peptide precursors and of shorter chain peptide fragments of angiotensin II injected into the rat's diencephalon. *J. Physiol. (Lond.)*, **214**, 295–303.

FITZSIMONS, J. T. (1972) Thirst. *Physiol. Rev.*, **52**, 468–561.

FITZSIMONS, J. T. AND SETLER, P. E. (1971) Catecholaminergic mechanisms in angiotensin-induced drinking. *J. Physiol. (Lond.)*, **218**, 43–44p.

FOLLEY, S. J. AND KNAGGS, G. S. (1965) Levels of oxytocin in the jugular vein blood of goats during parturition. *J. Endocr.*, **33**, 301–315.

FOX, C. A. AND FOX, B. (1971) A comparative study of coital physiology with special reference to the sexual climax. *J. Reprod. Fertil.*, **24**, 319–336.

FREDERICKSON, C. J. AND HOBSON, J. A. (1970) Electrical stimulation of the brain stem and subsequent sleep. *Arch. ital. Biol.*, **108**, 564–576.

FRIGYESI, T. L. AND MACHEK, J. (1971) Basal ganglia–diencephalon synaptic relations in the cat. II. Intracellular recordings from dorsal thalamic neurons during low frequency stimulation of the caudatothalamic projection systems and the nigrothalamic pathway. *Brain Research*, **27**, 59–78.

FUCHS, A. R. AND WAGNER, G. (1963) Quantitative aspects of release of oxytocin by suckling in unanaesthetised rabbits. *Acta endocr. (Kbh.)*, **44**, 593–605.

FUXE, K. AND HÖKFELT, T. (1969) Catecholamines in the hypothalamus and the pituitary gland. In *Frontiers in Neuroendocrinology, 1969*, W. F. GANONG AND L. MARTINI (Eds.), Oxford Univ. Press, New York, pp. 47–96.

GAINES, W. L. (1915) A contribution to the physiology of lactation. *Amer. J. Physiol.*, **38**, 285–312.

GANDELMAN, R., ZARROW, M. X., DENEBERG, V. H. AND MYERS, M. (1971) Olfactory bulb removal eliminates maternal behaviour in the mouse. *Science*, **171**, 210–211.

GANTEN, D., HAYDUK, K., BRECHT, H. M., BOUCHER, R., AND GENEST, J. (1970) Evidence of renin release or production in splanchnic territory. *Nature (Lond.)*, **226**, 551–552.

GANTEN, D., MINNICH, J. L., GRANGER, P., HAYDUK, K., BRECHT, H. M., BARBEAU, A., BOUCHER, R. AND GENEST, J., (1971) Angiotensin-forming enzyme in brain tissue. *Science*, **173**, 64–65.

GLICK, S. M. (1969) The regulation of growth hormone secretion. In *Frontiers in Neuroendocrinology, 1969*, W. F. GANONG AND L. MARTINI (Eds.), Oxford Univ. Press, New York, pp. 141–182.

GROSVENOR, C. E. (1965) Evidence that exteroceptive stimuli can release prolactin from the pituitary gland of the lactating rat. *Endocrinology*, **76**, 340–342.

GROSVENOR, C. E. AND MENA, F. (1971) Evidence for a refractory period in the neuroendocrine mechanism for the release of prolactin. *Endocrinology*, **88**, 355–358.

GROSVENOR, C. E. AND TURNER, C. W. (1957) Release and restoration of pituitary lactogen in response to nursing stimuli in lactating rats. *Proc. Soc. exp. biol. Med.*, **96**, 723–725.

GUALTIEROTTI, T. AND BAILEY, P. (1968) A neutral buoyancy micro-electrode for prolonged recording from single nerve units. *Electroenceph. clin. Neurophysiol.*, **25**, 77–81.

HAMMEL, H. T. (1968) Regulation of internal body temperature. *Ann. Rev. Physiol.*, **30**, 641–710.

HARRIS, M. C., MAKARA, G. B. AND SPYER, K. M. (1971) Electrophysiological identification of neurones of the tubero-infundibular system. *J. Physiol. (Lond.)* **218**, 86–87p.

HAYWARD, J. N. (1972) Hypothalamic input to supraoptic neurones. In *Progress in Brain Research, Vol. 38, Topics in Neuroendocrinology*, J. ARIËNS KAPPERS AND J. P. SCHADÉ (Eds.), Elsevier, Amsterdam, pp. 145–161.

HEIMER, L. (1971) Pathways in the brain. *Sci. Amer.*, **225**, 48–60.

HEIMER, L. AND NAUTA, W. J. H. (1969) The hypothalamic distribution of the stria terminalis in the rat. *Brain Research*, **13**, 284–297.

HELLON, R. F. (1967) Thermal stimulation of hypothalamic neurones in unanaesthetized rabbits. *J. Physiol. (Lond.)*, **193**, 381–395.

HORRIDGE, G. A. (1968) *Interneurons*, Freeman, London, San Francisco.

HUGHES, J. AND ROTH, R. H. (1971) Evidence that angiotensin enhances transmitter release during sympathetic nerve stimulation. *Brit. J. Pharmacol.*, **41**, 239–255.

JOUVET, M. (1967) Neurophysiology of the states of sleep. *Physiol. Rev.*, **47**, 117–177.

KAWAKAMI, M. AND KUBO, K. (1971) Neuro-correlate of limbic-hypothalamo-pituitary-gonadal axis in the rat: change in limbic-hypothalamic unit activity induced by vaginal and electrical stimulation. *Neuroendocrinology*, **7**, 65–89.

KAWAKAMI, M. AND SAITO, H. (1967) Unit activity in the hypothalamus of the cat: effect of genital stimuli, luteinizing hormone and oxytocin. *Jap. J. Physiol.*, **17**, 466–486.

KHAIRALLAH, P. A., DAVILA, D., PAPANICOLAOU, N., GLENDE, N. M. AND MEYER, P. (1971) Effects of angiotensin infusion on catecholamine uptake and reactivity in blood vessels. *Circulat. Res.*, **28**, II-96–II-104.

KOMISARUK, B. R. (1971) Strategies in neuroendocrine neurophysiology. *Am. Zoologist*, **11**, 741–754.

KOMISARUK, B. R. AND BEYER, C. (1972) Responses of diencephalic neurons to olfactory bulb stimulation, odor, and arousal. *Brain Research*, **36**, 153–170.

KNOWLES, F. G. W. (1972) Ependyma of the third ventricle in relation to pituitary function. In *Progress in Brain Research, Vol. 38, Topics in Neuroendocrinology*, J. ARIËNS KAPPERS AND J. P. SCHADÉ (Eds.), Elsevier, Amsterdam, pp. 255–270.

LINCOLN, D. W. (1969a) Response of hypothalamic units to stimulation of the vaginal cervix: specific versus non-specific effects, *J. Endocr.*, **43**, 683–684.

LINCOLN, D. W. (1969b) Correlation of unit activity in the hypothalamus with EEG patterns associated with the sleep cycle. *Exp. Neurol.*, **24**, 1–18.

LINCOLN, D. W. AND CROSS, B. A. (1967) Effect of oestrogen on the responsiveness of neurones in the hypothalamus, septum and preoptic area of rats with light-induced persistent oestrus. *J. Endocr.*, **37**, 191–203.

LINZELL, J. L. (1963) Some effects of denervating and transplanting mammary glands. *Quart. J. exp. Physiol.*, **48**, 34–60.

LOFTS, B., FOLLETT, B. K. AND MURTON, R. K. (1970) Temporal changes in the pituitary–gonadal axis. *Mem. Soc. Endocr.*, **18**, 545–572.

LOWE, R. D. AND SCROOP, G. C. (1969) The cardiovascular response to vertebral artery infusions of angiotensin in the dog. *Clin. Sci.*, **37**, 593–603.

MALLIANI, A., RUDOMIN, P. AND ZANCHETTI, A. (1965) Contribution of local activity and electric spread to somatically evoked potentials in different areas of the hypothalamus. *Arch. ital. Biol.*, **103**, 119–135.

McCARLEY, R. W. AND HOBSON, J. A. (1971) Single neuron activity in cat gigantocellular tegmental field: selectivity of discharge in desynchronized sleep. *Science*, **174**, 1250–1252.

McCLINTOCK, M. K. (1971) Menstrual synchrony and suppression. *Nature (Lond.)*, **229**, 244–245.

McGINTY, D. J. AND STERMAN, M. B. (1968) Sleep suppression after basal forebrain lesions in the cat. *Science*, **160**, 1253–1255.

MENA, F. AND BEYER, C. (1968) Effect of spinal cord lesions on milk ejection in the rabbit. *Endocrinology*, **83**, 615–617.

MENA, F. AND GROSVENOR, C. E. (1971) Release of prolactin in rats by exteroceptive stimulation; sensory stimuli involved. *Hormones and Behavior*, **2**, 107–116.

MICHAEL, R. P., KEVERNE, E. B. AND BONSALL, R. W. (1971) Pheromones: isolation of male sex attractants from a female primate. *Science*, **172**, 964–966.

MOSS, R. L. (1971) Modification of copulatory behavior in the female rat following olfactory bulb removal. *J. comp. physiol. Psychol.*, **74**, 374–382.

MOTTA, M., FRASCHINI, F. AND MARTINI, L. (1969) "Short" feedback mechanisms in the control of anterior pituitary function. In *Frontiers in Neuroendocrinology*, W. F. GANONG AND L. MARTINI. (Eds.), Oxford Univ. Press, New York, pp. 211–253.

MOUW, D., BONJOUR, J., MALVIN, R. L. AND VANDER, A. (1971) Central action of angiotensin in stimulating ADH release. *Amer. J. Physiol.*, **220**, 239–242.

MUGFORD, R. A. AND NOWELL, N. W. (1971) Endocrine control over production and activity of the anti-aggression pheromone from female mice. *J. Endocr.*, **49**, 225–232.

MURPHY, M. R. AND SCHNEIDER, G. A. (1970) Olfactory bulb removal eliminates mating behavior in the male golden hamster. *Science*, **167**, 302–304.

NAKAYAMA, T. AND HARDY, J. D. (1969) Unit responses in the rabbit's brain stem to changes in brain and cutaneous temperature. *J. appl. Physiol.*, **27**, 848–857.

NAUTA, W. J. H. (1946) Hypothalamic regulation of sleep in rats. An experimental study. *J. Neurophysiol.*, **9**, 285–314.

NAUTA, W. J. H. (1963) Central nervous organization and the endocrine motor system. In *Advances in Neuroendocrinology*, A. V. NALBANDOV (Ed.), Univ. of Illinois Press, Urbana, pp. 5–21.

NAUTA, W. J. H. AND MEHLER, W. R. (1966) Projections of the lentiform nucleus in the monkey. *Brain Research*, **1**, 3–42.

NICOLL, R. A. AND BARKER, J. L. (1971) Excitation of supraoptic neurosecretory cells by angiotensin II. *Nature New Biology*, **233**, 172–174.

NORGREN, R. (1970) Gustatory responses in the hypothalamus. *Brain Research*, **21**, 63–77.

OBA, T., OTA, K. AND YOKOYAMA, A. (1971) Inhibition of milk-ejection reflex in lactating rats by systemic administration and intracerebral implantation of atropine. *Neuroendocrinology*, **7**, 116–126.

OLDS, J. (1956) A preliminary mapping of electrical reinforcing effects in the rat brain. *J. comp. physiol. Psychol.*, **49**, 281–285.

OOMURA, Y., OOYAMA, H., YAMAMOTO, T., ONO, T. AND KOBAYASHI, N. (1969) Behavior of hypothalamic unit activity during electrophoretic application of drugs. *Ann. N.Y. Acad. Sci.*, **157**, 642–665.

OSBORNE, M. J., POOTERS, N., D'AURIAC, G. A., EPSTEIN, A. N., WORCEL, M. AND MEYER, P. (1971) Metabolism of tritiated angiotensin II in anaesthetized rats. *Pflügers Arch. ges. Physiol.*, **326**, 101–114.

O'STEEN, W. K. AND VAUGHAN, G. M. (1968) Radioactivity in the optic pathway and hypothalamus of the rat after intraocular injection of tritiated 5-hydroxytryptophan. *Brain Research*, **8**, 209–212.

PALAIC, D. AND KHAIRALLAH, P. A. (1968) Effect of angiotensin on uptake and release of norepinephrine by brain. *Biochem. Pharmacol.*, **16**, 2291–2298.

PERKEL, D. H., GERSTEIN, G. L. AND MOORE, G. P. (1967) Neuronal spike trains and stochastic point processes. I. The single spike train. II. Simultaneous spike trains. *Biophys. J.*, **7**, 391–440.

PFAFF, D. W. (1971a) Statistical effects of sensitivity differences among neurophysiological preparations. *J. theor. Biol.*, **31**, 159–160.

PFAFF, D. W. (1971b) Interactions of steroid sex hormones with brain tissue: studies of uptake and physiological effects. In *The Regulation of Mammalian Reproduction*, S. SEGAL (Ed.), Thomas, Springfield.

PFAFF, D. W. AND GREGORY, E. (1971) Olfactory coding in olfactory bulb and medial forebrain bundle of normal and castrated male rats. *J. Neurophysiol.*, **34**, 208–216.

PFAFF, D. W. AND PFAFFMANN, C. (1969) Olfactory and hormonal influences on the basal forebrain of the male rat. *Brain Research*, **15**, 137–156.

RAISMAN, G. (1966) Neural connexions of the hypothalamus. *Brit. med. Bull.*, **22**, 197–201.

RAISMAN, G. (1970) Some aspects of the neural connections of the hypothalamus. In *The Hypothalamus*, L. MARTINI, M. MOTTA AND F. FRASCHINI (Eds.), Academic Press, New York, pp. 1–15.

RAISMAN, G. AND FIELD, P. M. (1971a) Anatomical considerations relevant to the interpretation of neuroendocrine experiments. In *Frontiers in Neuroendocrinology, 1971*, W. F. GANONG AND L. MARTINI (Eds.), Oxford Univ. Press, New York, pp. 3–44.

RAISMAN, G. AND FIELD, P. M. (1971b) Sexual dimorphism in the preoptic area of the rat. *Science* **173**, 731–733.

REICHLIN, S. (1966) Control of thyrotropic hormone secretion. In *Neuroendocrinology, Vol. I*, L. MARTINI AND W. F. GANONG (Eds.), Academic Press, New York, pp. 445–536.

REITER, R. J. AND FRASCHINI, F. (1969). Endocrine aspects of the mammalian pineal gland: a review. *Neuroendocrinol.*, **5**, 219–255.

RETIENE, K. (1970) Control of circadian periodicities in pituitary function. In *The Hypothalamus*, L. MARTINI, M. MOTTA AND F. FRASCHINI (Eds.), Academic Press, New York, pp. 551–568.

ROBERTS, J. S. AND SHARE, L. (1969) Effects of progesterone and estrogen on blood levels of oxytocin during vaginal distension. *Endocrinology*, **84**, 1076–1081.

ROSENDORFF, C., LOWE, R. D., LAVERY, H. AND CRANSTON, W. I. (1970) Cardiovascular effects of angiotensin mediated by the central nervous system of the rabbit. *Cardiovasc. Res.*, **4**, 36–43.

SCOTT, J. W. AND PFAFF, D. W. (1970) Behavioral and electrophysiological responses of female mice to male urine odors. *Physiol. Behav.*, **5**, 407–411.

SCROOP, G. C., KATIC, F., JOY, M. D. AND LOWE, R. D. (1971) Importance of central vasomotor effects in angiotensin-induced hypertension. *Brit. Med. J.*, **71**, 324–326.

SETLER, P. E. (1971) Drinking induced by injection of angiotensin II into the hypothalamus of the rhesus monkey. *J. Physiol. (Lond.)*, **217**, 59–60p.

SHARE, L. (1969) Extracellular fluid volume and vasopressin secretion. In *Frontiers in Neuroendocrinology, 1969*, W. F. GANONG AND L. MARTINI (Eds.), Oxford Univ. Press, New York, pp. 183–210.

SHUTE, C. C. D. (1970) Distribution of cholinesterase and cholinergic pathways. In *The Hypothalamus*, L. MARTINI, M. MOTTA AND F. FRASCHINI (Eds.), Academic Press, New York, pp. 167–179.

SHUTE, C. C. D. AND LEWIS, P. R. (1966) Cholinergic and monaminergic pathways in the hypothalamus. *Brit. med. Bull.*, **22**, 221–226.

SMELIK, P. G. (1970) Integrated hypothalamic responses to stress. In *The Hypothalamus*, L. MARTINI, M. MOTTA AND F. FRASCHINI, Academic Press, New York, pp. 491–497.

SMITH, G. P. AND BROOKS, F. P. (1970) Brain, behavior and gastric secretion. In *Progress in Gastroenterology, Vol. II*, G. B. J. GLASS (Ed.), Grune and Stratton, New York, pp. 57–72.

SOUSA-PINTO, A. (1970) Electron microscopic observations on the possible retinohypothalamic projection in the rat. *Exp. Brain Res.*, **11**, 528–538.

SOUSA–PINTO, A. AND CASTRO–CORREIA, J. (1970) Light microscopic observations on the possible retinohypothalamic projection in the rat. *Exp. Brain Res.*, **11**, 515–527.

SPIES, H. G. AND NISWENDER, G. D. (1971) Levels of prolactin, LH and FSH in the serum of intact and pelvic-neurectomized rats. *Endocrinology*, **88**, 937–943.

STEINER, F. A., RUF, K. AND AKERT, K. (1969) Steroid-sensitive neurons in rat brain: anatomic localization and responses to neurohumours and ACTH. *Brain Research*, **12**, 74–85.

SUTIN, J. (1966) The periventricular stratum of the hypothalamus. *Int. Rev. Neurobiol.*, **9**, 263–300.

SZENTÁGOTHAI, J., FLERKÓ, B., MESS, B. AND HÁLASZ, B. (1968) *Hypothalamic Control of the Anterior Pituitary*, Akademiai Kiado, Budapest, p. 59.

TAKAORI, S., SASA, M. AND FUKUDA, N. (1968) Responses of posterior hypothalamic neurons to electrical stimulation of the inferior alveolar nerve and distension of stomach with cold and warm water. *Brain Research*, **11**, 225–237.

TAMARI, I. (1970) Audiogenic stimulation and reproductive function. In *Physiological Effects of Noise*, B. L. WELCH AND A. S. WELSH (Eds.), Plenum Press, London, pp. 117–130.

TER HAAR, M. B. AND P. C. B. MACKINNON (1972) An investigation of cerebral protein synthesis in various states of neuroendocrine activity. *Progress in Brain Research, Vol. 38, Topics in Neuroendocrinology*, J. ARIËNS KAPPERS AND J. P. SCHADÉ (Eds.), Elsevier, Amsterdam, pp. 211–222.

TINDAL, J. S. AND KNAGGS, G. S. (1969) An ascending pathway for release of prolactin in the brain of the rabbit. *J. Endocr.*, **45**, 111–120.

TINDAL, J. S. AND KNAGGS, G. S. (1970) Environmental stimuli and the mammary gland. *Mem. Soc. Endocr.*, **18**, 239–258.

TSAEKHAEV, G. A. (1955) Problem of reflex regulation of milk ejection. *Tr. Inst. Fiziol. (Mosk.)*, **4**, 5–16 (In Russian).

VANDERLAAN, W. P., PARKER, D. C., ROSSMAN, L. G. AND VANDERLAAN, E. F. (1970) Implications of growth hormone release in sleep. *Metabolism*, **19**, 891–897.

VILLAMIL, M. F., NACHEV, P. AND KLEEMAN, C. R. (1970) Effect of prolonged infusion of angiotensin II on ionic composition of the arterial wall. *Amer. J. Physiol.*, **218**, 1281–1286.

VINCENT, J. D., DUFY, B. AND FAURE, J. M. A. (1970) Effects of vaginal stimulation on hypothalamic single units in unanesthetized rabbits. *Experientia (Basel)*, **26**, 1266–1267.

VON EULER, C. AND SÖDERBERG, U. (1957) The influence of hypothalamic thermoceptive structures on the electroencephalogram and gamma motor activity. *Electroenceph. clin. Neurophysiol.*, **9**, 391–408.

WAKERLEY, J. B. AND LINCOLN, D. W. (1971) Milk ejection in the rat: recordings of intramammary pressure during suckling. *J. Endocr.*, **51**, xiii–xiv.

WERNER, G. AND MOUNTCASTLE, V. B. (1963) The variability of central neural activity in a sensory system, and its implications for the central reflection of sensory events. *J. Neurophysiol.*, **26**, 958–977.

WHITTEN, W. K. (1966) Pheromones and mammalian reproduction. In *Advances in Reproductive Physiology*, *Vol. 1*, A. MCLAREN (Ed.), Logos and Academic Press, London and New York, pp. 155–177.

WOLSTENHOLME, G. E. W. AND KNIGHT, J. (Eds.) (1971) *The Pineal Gland*, Churchill, Livingstone, Edinburgh and London.

WOOD-JONES, F. AND TURNER, J. B. (1931) A note on the sensory characters of the nipple and areola. *Med. J. Austr.*, **1**, 778–779.

WURTMAN, R. J. (1967) Effects of light and visual stimuli on endocrine function. In *Neuroendocrinology*, *Vol. II*, L. MARTINI AND W. F. GANONG (Eds.), Academic Press, New York, pp. 19–59.

YAMADA, M. (1971) A search for odour encoding in the olfactory lobe. *J. Physiol. (Lond.)*, **214**, 127–143.

ZANCHETTI, A. (1970) Control of the cardiovascular system. In *The Hypothalamus*, L. MARTINI, M. MOTTA AND F. FRASCHINI (Eds.), Academic Press, New York, pp. 232–244.

ZARROW, M. X., CAMPBELL, P. S. AND CLARK, J. H. (1968) Pregnancy following coital-induced ovulation in a spontaneous ovulator. *Science*, **159**, 329–330.

ZARROW, M. X., ESTES, S. A., DENENBERG, V. H. AND CLARK, J. H. (1970) Pheromonal facilitation of ovulation in the immature mouse. *J. Reprod. Fertil.*, **23**, 357–360.

DISCUSSION

DREIFUSS: When you use angiotensin I or II how can you be sure that, once the substance has been ejected from the pipette it is still angiotensin I or II, but not glutamate or aspartate or one of the other amino acids that have excitatory action or γ-amino-butyrate that has an inhibitory action?

FINDLAY: No, of course you can't. There are ways of controlling that effect. I think, is it not right to say, that if you use strychnine you block amino-acid effects on neurons.

What you are supposed to do is to look at a particular effect. The problem with iontophoresis is that you can only test a limited number of drugs even with a five-barrelled pipette. You have one recording barrel, one isotonic saline barrel which you have to use to control the current effects, one barrel containing dye so you can mark the site of the neuron, and so you have only two barrels left to use for test substances of which one has to contain angiotensin. The first control we have to do is to put ammonium-acetate in one of the barrels because that also contaminates the available angiotensin solutions.

MOLL: Do you think it is really of much importance for our understanding of the biological significance of what is going on, if there is one synapse, two synapses or no synapses at all in the retina?

FINDLAY: No, I don't.

SCHARRER: To follow along this line, you spoke of photic input as one of the very important extero-ceptive controlling phenomena. Should we also consider the difference between visual stimuli which exists for instance in the case when a pigeon has to see either his own image or another pigeon in order to proceed with its productive behavior or as contrasted to that, the simple photic stimuli which are responsible for photoperiodic mechanisms?

FINDLAY: I would have thought it most unlikely that the effect of the visual stimulus of a pigeon seeing another pigeon in causing it to ovulate, is mediated directly to the hypothalamus. It must surely involve a lot of information processing and recognition.

SCHARRER: There is evidence of light sensitivity of hypothalamic centers which do not require the presence of the retina.

FINDLAY: I think in the mammal light-sensitive structures other than the eye are somewhat unlikely.

VAN DE VEERDONK: I think there are some reports that pineal melatonin is secreted in response to light; could you comment on its function?

FINDLAY: I was talking to Dr. Donovan about this last night and there are obviously clear circadian variations in many pineal functions. By circadian I mean approximately 24 hours. We agreed that there was no clear evidence that pinealectomy caused any differences in hypothalamic outputs dependent on longer time periods, but there is no clear evidence of circadian variations in hypothalamic activity under control of the pineal. We thought that perhaps, although there have been observed variations in pineal activity and mechanisms under pineal control, that these were smoothed, perhaps by a sort of high frequency filter. Frequencies higher than one cycle per week are probably filtered out.

DONOVAN: One of the problems with the suggestion that sleep–wakefulness is important, is that you would imagine a synchronous release of pituitary hormones. But if you look at the output of the several pituitary hormones in the rat, you see for instance, that LH is released around 2 o'clock in the afternoon, ACTH at about 6 o'clock or later on, TSH is released at about 4 or 5 hours before that. We get a separation in the output of the pituitary hormones. How could you account for that?

FINDLAY: Well, I don't see any real difficulty in that, because what you say is that there are phase differences in rhythms. The point is that we have rhythmic rest activities and waking cycles; there may be a certain critical point in that cycle which is important in the case of TSH. As we mentioned in the case of growth hormone, release occurs early in sleep during stages 3 and 4, so that is obviously the critical event for growth hormone release. On the other hand, in the case of the adrenal, or in the case of body temperature, it may be that it is primarily motor activity and non-specific inputs which are the trigger points. So it depends exactly on what the critical event is and the critical event may well be different for each of these. There are different controlling mechanisms and each hormone has its own hypothalamic integrating neuron, which is driven by many things. The particular balance to give maximal activity of the various releasing factors is going to be different in the case probably of every individual hormone. There is no reason why it should be the same.

DONOVAN: There may be a changing sensitivity on the part of the hypothalamus and the discharge of the various pituitary hormones may be related to different levels of sensitivity.

What do you think might be the neural mechanism underlying the changes in sensitivity, what is the neural basis of the clock?

FINDLAY: In the case of the circadian release of luteinizing hormone I would say that the evidence from Brown–Grant showed that one of the important variations in that case is adrenal progesterone. That is one of the extra input mechanisms one has to consider, but they are clearly so diverse that I think it would be pointless to speculate that there are particularly critical ones in every case.

DONOVAN: What do you imagine progesterone is doing to the cells within the hypothalamus?

FINDLAY: It will possibly have an effect on the membrane potential or an effect on intracellular en-zymes as Dr. Schadé thinks happens in the case of cortisol. Changing the membrane potential and making it more susceptible to what had previously been subthreshold input from other areas may also occur.

Control of Ovulation by the Anterior Pituitary Gland

G. P. van REES*

Department of Pharmacology, University of Leiden, Leiden (The Netherlands)

It is generally accepted that, at least in the rat, the acute increase of secretion of gonadotrophins, which is responsible for ovulation, is ultimately dependent on a steering mechanism with a 24-h activity. The first indications of such a circadian mechanism were provided by Everett and Sawyer (1950), who showed that rats given pentobarbital at 2 p.m. on the day of vaginal pro-oestrus, did not ovulate the following night, but 24 h later, and that the next day it was again possible to postpone ovulation for 24 h by giving pentobarbital at a certain defined time. It is also generally accepted that the impulses associated with the induction of ovulation originate in or pass through the preoptic region and end in the mediobasal hypothalamus, where they bring about the discharge of the appropriate releasing factors.

In the experiments to be discussed, these concepts are illustrated. They are concerned with time factors involved in the pre-ovulatory discharge of gonadotrophins, with the dependence of the hypothalamus on afferent impulses, with the question as to whether such afferent impulses originate in the preoptic area or pass through this region, and with the induction of ovulation by progesterone and oestrogen.

These experiments were carried out with rats from the Wistar-derived colony kept at our laboratory at the usual lighting schedule of 14 h of light and 10 h of darkness, the period of light beginning at 5 a.m. In this colony the rats show ovarian cycles of both 4 and 5 days' duration, and although a certain amount of switching occurs from one type of the cycle to the other, it is possible to predict the duration of a forthcoming cycle on the basis of previous cycles. For instance, if one takes as criterion two successive cycles of the same duration, the chance that the next cycle lasts as long is about 90% in the case of 4-day cycles and 70% in the case of 5-day cycles.

In the first experiment we considered two questions. First we wanted to know whether there is a difference between animals with 4- or 5-day cycles with regard to the timing of pre-ovulatory gonadotrophin secretion, since there is only limited information to be found in the literature in this respect. Hoffmann and Schwartz (1965) mention that pentobarbital, administered at 2 p.m. on pro-oestrus, did not block ovulation in rats with 5-day cycles as opposed to rats running 4-day cycles. Also, Schwartz (1969) mentions that on the day of pro-oestrus a positive lordosis response can be evoked at an earlier time in rats with 5-day cycles than in animals with 4-day

---

* In collaboration with G. A. Schuiling and J. Wildschut.

References p. 209

cycles. This might be caused by a difference in the timing of pre-ovulatory gonado-trophin discharge, mating behaviour resulting from increased blood levels of steroid sex hormones.

To settle this point we made hypophysectomies on the day of pro-oestrus in animals with 4- and 5-day cycles at 2, 3, 4 or 5 p.m. and the next morning it was noted which animals had ovulated, judging from the presence of ova in the oviducts.

The second question was the following. As mentioned before, it is generally accepted that the nervous impulses responsible for the pre-ovulatory discharge of gonadotrophins enter the hypothalamus from anteriorly situated structures. When the connections between the preoptic area and the hypothalamus are severed, ovulation is blocked. We wanted to know how long, after cutting through the connections between these two structures, the hypothalamus is able to sustain its ovulatory activity. Thus, in the same experiment in which rats running 4- and 5-day cycles were subjected to hypophysectomies at different times in the afternoon of pro-oestrus, we made, using a modification of the knife devised by Halász, cuts just behind the anterior commissure and the optic chiasm. Fig. 1 gives an example of such a retrochiasmatic or "P"-cut. These cuts were also made at different times of pro-oestrus.

The results of this experiment are presented in Fig. 2. It shows the percentages of the animals belonging to each group, in which ova were detected the next morning. The total number of rats per point was 20. From the results of the hypophysectomy experiment it can be seen that the lines drawn through the points run at a distance which represents about $1\frac{1}{2}$ hours. This indicates that in 5-day cyclic animals an amount

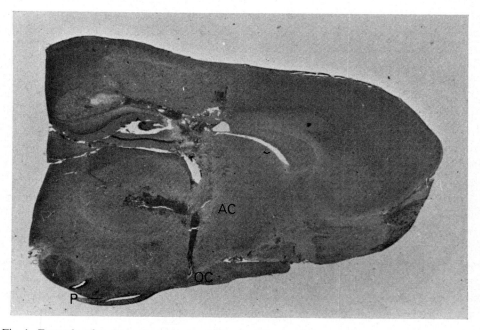

Fig. 1. Example of a retrochiasmatic or "P"-cut. AC, anterior commissure; OC, optic chiasm; P, pituitary stalk.

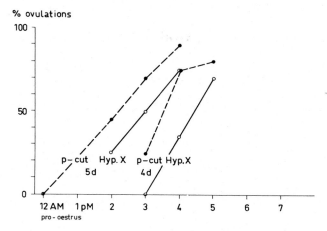

Fig. 2. Blocking effect of hypophysectomy and retrochiasmatic or "P"-cuts on ovulation when performed at various times on pro-oestrus in 4- and 5-day cyclic rats. The percentages of animals are shown in which ova were detected the next morning. Total number of animals per point: 20.

of gonadotrophins sufficient to cause ovulation has been discharged about $1\frac{1}{2}$ h earlier than in 4-day cyclic animals, which result confirms the afore-mentioned findings by Hoffmann and Schwartz (1965).

The effects of the retrochiasmatic cuts are comparable to those of the timed hypophysectomies: again the difference between rats with 4- and 5-day cycles is observed. Moreover, if we compare the effects of the cuts with those of the hypophysectomies, we see a difference in timing which is equivalent to about one hour. This may be interpreted as indicating that, after acute deafferentation, the hypothalamus can sustain its ovulatory activity for about this period and no longer. This then leads to the hypothesis that the cause of the fact that some animals run ovarian cycles with a duration of 4 days and others of 5 days must be sought in factors, possibly blood oestrogen levels, which have their site of action outside the hypothalamus.

Another question which may be posed is related to the origin of the impulses which trigger ovulation. One could think of the following possibilities: the preoptic area is the region in which these impulses are generated; fibre tracts along which these impulses are conducted may only pass through this region, and finally the preoptic area might be steered by impulses originating in other structures in the C.N.S. With regard to the latter possibility the experiments by Velasco and Taleisnik (1969) should be mentioned; they observed induction of ovulation by stimulation of the amygdaloid nuclei and inhibition by stimulation of hippocampal structures.

However, Köves and Halász (1970) made cuts around the preoptic area and part of the hypothalamus, which left the connections between preoptic area and hypothalamus intact. These animals showed an extremely high mortality rate, but the animals which survived ultimately showed spontaneous ovulations. We did nearly the same experiment, the results of which confirm the experiments of Köves and Halász.

Fig. 3 gives a summary of the cuts used in this and following experiments: the

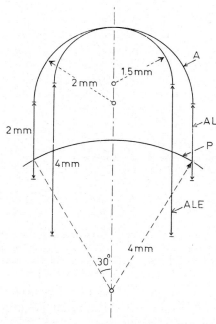

Fig. 3. Schematic presentation of the different cuts used, in a horizontal plane.

"ALE"-type cut resembles the one made by Köves and Halász. After a period of 3–4 weeks, the animals which survived the operation started to show ovarian cycles, although a large number of them were no more of the regular duration of 4 or 5 days. Still, in 6 out of 9 animals ova were found in the oviducts when they were in vaginal oestrus. When injected on pro-oestrus with pentobarbital at 2 p.m., ovulation was seen in only 1 out of 7 animals.

However, this does not necessarily apply to acute experiments, since it might be that some time after making these cuts some kind of reorganization takes place. From other experiments, especially those by Velasco and Taleisnik, mentioned before, it was supposed that fibre tracts in the immediate neighbourhood of the anterior commissure might be of importance.

Therefore, horizontal cuts (4 × 4 mm) were made at the level of the anterior commissure on the day of vaginal pro-oestrus in 4-day cyclic rats (see Fig. 4). Such cuts, made either at 1 or 2 p.m., blocked ovulation in all of the 20 animals. In a further experiment, conducted in 4-day cyclic rats at the same times on the day of pro-oestrus, two types of these so-called "roof-cuts" were made: either equal to the rostral half of the original roof-cut or to the posterior half. The results are summarized in Fig. 5. If the rostral half of the original cut was made, ovulation was still blocked in 11 out of 17 animals. The posterior half, however, did not inhibit ovulation in any of 10 rats.

Thus it appears that fibres entering the preoptic area just frontal to the anterior commissure are part of the mechanism involved in ovulation.

Finally, roof-sections were made in 4-day cyclic animals at different times on the

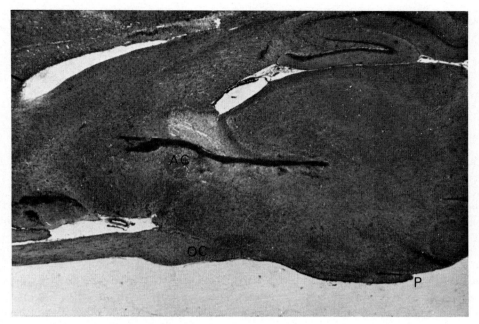

Fig. 4. Example of a preoptic "roof-cut". AC, anterior commissure; OC, optic chiasm; P, pituitary stalk.

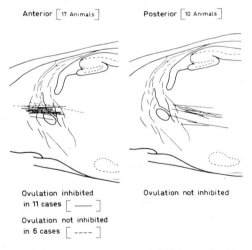

Fig. 5. Effect of ½-preoptic roof-cuts on spontaneous ovulation, when performed at 2 p.m. of pro-oestrus in 4-day cyclic rats.

day of pro-oestrus and their effects on ovulation were noted. The results are presented in Fig. 6. It can be seen that the effects of roof-cuts and those of retrochiasmatic cuts overlap completely. Since the roof-cuts do not affect the preoptic region, we must conclude that for spontaneous ovulation impulses are necessary originating in structures situated outside the preoptic area.

References p. 209

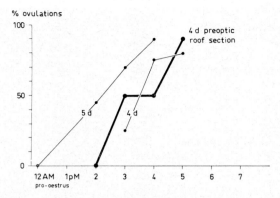

Fig. 6. Effect of timed preoptic roof-cuts on spontaneous ovulation in 4-day cyclic rats. For comparison, the results obtained with retrochiasmatic cuts in animals with 4- and 5-day cycles are also presented. See also Fig. 2.

Also, we must conclude that after making cuts between the preoptic area and the rest of the C.N.S., a considerable degree of reorganization can take place. This then should affect the preoptic area, since after making retrochiasmatic cuts, by which we sever the connections between preoptic area and hypothalamus, ovulation is blocked and remains blocked showing the development of the well-known persistent oestrus syndrome. The preoptic area, on the other hand, apparently becomes capable of inducing ovulation. It should be mentioned, however, that we do not know whether impulses from other areas in the C.N.S. now gain access to the preoptic area by fibre tracts which have not been severed and may be of little importance to the mechanism of ovulation in intact animals.

Since the original experiments of Everett (1948), it has been shown repeatedly that both oestrogen and progesterone, when administered at appropriate times during the ovarian cycle, can advance or induce ovulation. Apparently, oestrogen plays an important role in triggering ovulation. This has been demonstrated most clearly by the experiments of Ferin et al. (1969), who showed that antibodies to oestradiol, coupled to protein, administered to rats on the second day of dioestrus inhibit ovulation. This inhibition could be abolished by stilboestrol, a non-steroidal oestrogen. Also, it should be mentioned that Schwartz (1969) and Barnea et al. (1968) showed that on the day before pro-oestrus enough oestrogen is secreted to cause the development of a ballooning uterus or vaginal cornification. In this respect, it would be tempting to ascribe the occurrence of rats with ovarian cycles of 5 instead of 4 days' duration to a relative deficiency of oestrogen secretion at the early stages of the cycle; however, measurements of plasma levels of oestrogen at these times in both types of rats are not yet available.

Brown–Grant et al. (1970) measured plasma oestrogen on the second day of dioestrus of 4-day cyclic rats. They showed an increase of these levels which started at about 2 to 3 p.m. In our laboratory, the amount of oestradiol benzoate was estimated, which, injected at different times on the second day of dioestrus of the 5-day cycle, advanced ovulation for 24 h in 50% of the animals (ED 50). The result of this experiment is

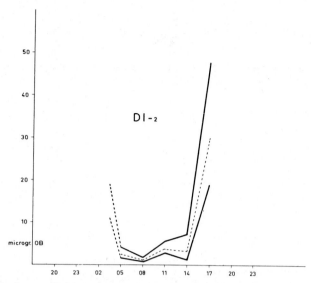

Fig. 7. The ED50 of oestradiol benzoate (OB), injected s.c. at different times on the second day of dioestrus of the 5-day cycle (DI-2) in order to advance ovulation. Area between lines represents the 95% confidence interval.

given in Fig. 7. During the afternoon of this day the effectiveness of oestradiol decreases rapidly. Thus, a relatively small delay in the increase of oestrogen secretion might result in a delay of ovulation of 24 h, leading to a cycle of 5 instead of 4 days' duration.

About the site of action of oestrogen, data are available which have been obtained essentially by two different approaches: either by implanting minute amounts of oestrogen at different sites of the C.N.S., or by studying the effect of injected oestrogen after making lesions in the C.N.S.

The results of the implantation experiments point to the mediobasal hypothalamus and the pituitary gland as sites of action as found by Weick and Davidson (1970) by implanting oestradiol on the second day of dioestrus in 5-day cyclic animals. However, implantation of substances at this time of the oestrous cycle inhibits ovulation. Weick and Davidson overcame this difficulty by a two-step procedure: first a permanent cannula was fixed in the brain, through which at a later time oestradiol could be implanted without stressing the animals.

We used a different procedure. The effect of oestradiol was studied in animals which had been pretreated with progesterone (1.5 mg, injected s.c. at 9 a.m.) daily for 10 days, starting on the first or second day of dioestrus. Injection of 50 μg of oestradiol benzoate at 9 a.m. of the 9th day of progesterone treatment resulted in ovulation in 20 out of 24 animals as judged from the presence of ova in the oviducts 48 hours later.

Implantation of 2 μg of oestradiol at 9 a.m. on the 9th day of progesterone pre-treatment induced ovulation when implanted in the ventromedial hypothalamic nucleus or anterior pituitary gland, which result is in agreement with that of Weick and Davidson mentioned above. A summary of the results of the implantation experiments is presented in Fig. 8. It can also be seen that implants in the dorsal hippocampus had some effect. The location of the implants in the mediobasal hypothalamus and dorsal hippocampus is given in Figs. 9 and 10.

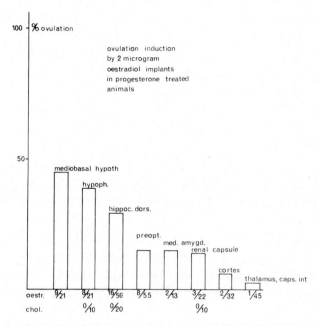

Fig. 8. Summary of the results of implantation of 2 μg oestradiol in progesterone-pretreated rats. Numbers of animals in which ovulation was induced, *vs.* total number of animals in each group are given under each column. Here also the results of cholesterol implants are presented. For details about progesterone-pretreatment, see text.

The effect of oestradiol at the level of the pituitary gland seems to coincide with an increased sensitivity to gonadotrophin releasing factors. This has been shown by Arimura and Schally (1971). Our preliminary results also indicate that pretreatment of 5-day cyclic animals with 7 μg of oestradiol benzoate on the first day of dioestrus enhances the effect of hypothalamic extracts, given 24 h later.

However, it is difficult to see how such an elevated sensitivity of the pituitary gland to releasing factors by itself could be responsible for oestrogen-induced ovulation. This conclusion is reached when we take into account the effect of cuts, performed with the Halász knife, on the effect of oestrogen.

In these experiments, retrochiasmatic cuts were made at different times of the afternoon prior to the expected ovulation, *i.e.*, on the day following the injection of oestradiol. This was done in animals which were given oestradiol benzoate (50 μg s.c. at 9 a.m.) on the second day of dioestrus of the 5-day cycle, or in progesterone-pretreated animals.

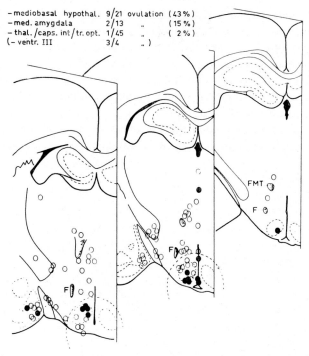

Fig. 9. Location of oestradiol implants in the mediobasal hypothalamus and some other brain areas of progesterone-pretreated rats. Closed circles, ovulation induced; open circles, no ovulation.

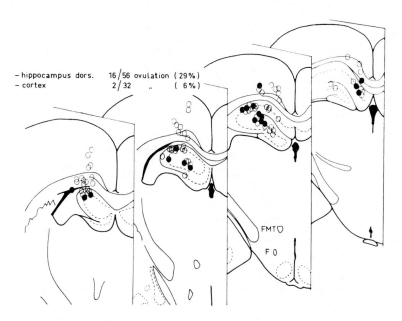

Fig. 10. Location of oestradiol implants in dorsal hippocampus and cerebral cortex of progesterone-pretreated rats. Closed circles, ovulation induced; open circles, no ovulation.

The effect of these cuts on ovulation in 5-day cyclic animals is summarized in Fig. 11. It can be seen that the cuts blocked oestrogen-induced ovulation as well as normal ovulation, although the "critical period" has shifted to later hours in the afternoon. The same result is observed in animals which were pretreated with progesterone (see Fig. 12). In this case the fact that the curve levels off at about 70% must await further explanation, although it can be explained, since by this method ovulation is not induced by oestradiol in all animals.

Moreover, in a following experiment the effect of cuts around the preoptic area was investigated in progesterone-pretreated animals. Cuts were made which were

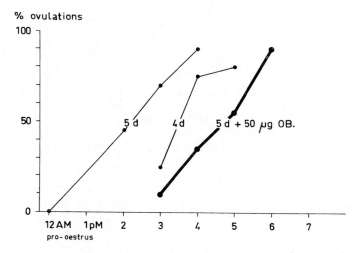

Fig. 11. Effect of timed retrochiasmatic cuts in 5-day cyclic rats given 50 μg oestradiol benzoate (OB) at 9 a.m. on the second day of dioestrus. Compare with Figure 2.

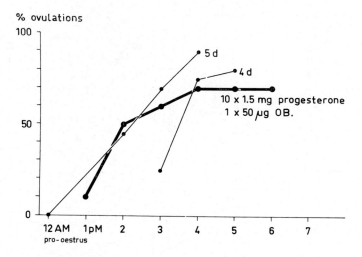

Fig. 12. Effect of timed retrochiasmatic cuts in progesterone-pretreated/oestradiol benzoate (50 μg at 9 a.m.) injected animals.

equal to the "AL"-type presented schematically in Fig. 3. Out of 25 animals with such cuts 16 ovulated after the injection of oestradiol immediately after the cut had been made. However, as shown in Fig. 13, histological control revealed that in 12 of these 16 animals the cut did not reach the anterior commissure. In other words, there appeared to be a "gap" between the distal end of the cut and the anterior border of the anterior commissure. Of the 9 animals which did not ovulate, only two showed the presence of such a "gap". Therefore, as was the case with spontaneous ovulation, fibre tracts in the immediate vicinity of the anterior commissure might be of importance with regard to ovulation induced by oestrogen.

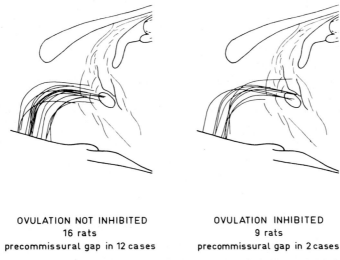

OVULATION NOT INHIBITED
16 rats
precommissural gap in 12 cases

OVULATION INHIBITED
9 rats
precommissural gap in 2 cases

Fig. 13. Effect of type "AL"-cuts on ovulation induced by 50 µg of oestradiol benzoate at 9 a.m. in progesterone-pretreated animals.

In a following experiment, roof-sections were made as described before. It may be recalled that such cuts sever in a horizontal plane all tracts at the level of the anterior commissure and block spontaneous ovulation. However, it was not possible to block the ovulations induced by oestradiol completely. In 8 out of 24 animals ovulation still occurred after injection of 50 µg of oestradiol, which is less than the 80% normally found in progesterone-pretreated rats, but certainly not zero. Thus, at least the large dose of 50 µg of oestradiol benzoate still seems to be able to induce ovulation in a minority of the animals after severing the dorsal connections of the preoptic area. It may be that in this instance such a strong stimulatory effect is produced, that in some animals centres situated in the preoptic area may be incited to act as an ovulatory stimulus. Severing the connections between the preoptic area and the hypothalamus completely blocked the effect of oestradiol.

With regard to the ovulation-inducing effect of progesterone, it is much more difficult to ascribe a physiologically important role to this substance than to oestrogen. Indeed, progesterone secretion does increase prior to ovulation, but all data available point to an increase which starts after, and not before the beginning of the pre-ovulatory discharge of gonadotrophins. Moreover, gonadotrophins, in particular LH, have been shown to promote progesterone secretion by pre-ovulatory ovaries.

Still, the effect of progesterone is clear-cut and easy to demonstrate, especially in the following two models: either advancement of ovulation by 24 h when given on the third day of the 5-day cycle, as demonstrated by Everett (1948), or induction of ovulation by progesterone given on the morning of pro-oestrus, followed by pento-barbital or hypophysectomy at 2 p.m. on the same day (Zeilmaker, 1966).

There are two striking differences between the effects of progesterone and oestrogen. The first is that progesterone induces ovulation in the night following its administra-tion, whereas it usually takes another 24 h in the case of oestrogen. The second difference is that progesterone induces ovulation combined with an advancement of the "critical period". This is best illustrated by the fact that after injection on the morning of pro-oestrus, at 2 p.m., enough gonadotrophins have been released in order to cause ovulation, as opposed to untreated animals. Oestrogen, on the other hand, does not change the timing of preovulatory gonadotrophin secretion in this sense, as has been shown before.

In studying the site of action of progesterone, lesion techniques and the implanta-tion method were also used. The results of both kinds of approaches, however, do not agree completely.

The first cut used was the type "A" cut (see Fig. 3). This cut around the preoptic area does not distally reach the anterior commissure. Thus it may be expected that this cut does not inhibit spontaneous ovulation. Such "A"-type cuts were made on the morning of the second dioestrous day in 4-day cyclic rats. The next morning (pro-oestrus) progesterone (15 mg) was injected subcutaneously at 11 a.m. followed by pentobarbital (30 mg/kg, i.p.) at 2 p.m. Table I shows that notwithstanding this cut spontaneous ovulation still occurred; the effect of progesterone was blocked, how-ever. It should be mentioned that using a different experimental design, the same result was obtained with regard to the effect of these cuts on progesterone-induced ovulation on the third day of dioestrus in the 5-day cycle (Kaasjager et al., 1971).

TABLE I

ACUTE EFFECTS OF CUTS AROUND THE PREOPTIC AREA (TYPE "A") ON SPONTANEOUS AND PROGESTERONE-INDUCED OVULATION

Cut*	Progesterone**	Pentobarbital[†]	Number of rats ovulating/total number of rats
A	none	none	6/8
Sham[††]	+	+	6/9
A	+	+	1/8

* Cuts made at 10 a.m. on the 2nd day of dioestrus in 4-day cyclic rats.
** 15 mg s.c. at 11.15 a.m. the next day (pro-oestrus).
[†] 30 mg/kg i.p. at 2 p.m. of pro-oestrus.
[††] knife lowered into the brain but removed without making a cutting movement to either side.

This indicates that the primary site of action of progesterone may be situated outside the complex formed by the preoptic area and the hypothalamus. Secondly, it must be concluded that this effect is apparently mediated by other fibre tracts than those involved in spontaneous ovulation. Finally, these results again point to the fact that the action of progesterone is not essential for spontaneous ovulation. This also fits in with the observations of Ferin *et al.* (1969), who could not inhibit spontaneous ovulation by the administration of antibodies against progesterone, as opposed to the blocking effect of antibodies against oestradiol.

In a following series, animals with cuts around the preoptic area were studied for a longer period. It has been mentioned above that such animals do show spontaneous ovulation after a certain interval following the operation. As shown in Table II,

TABLE II

CHRONIC EFFECTS OF CUTS AROUND THE PREOPTIC AREA ON SPONTANEOUS AND PROGESTERONE-INDUCED OVULATION

Type of cut	Progesterone*	Pentobarbital**	Number of rats ovulating/total number of rats
A	none	+	1/8
A	+	+	6/8
AL	none	+	3/9
AL	+	+	8/9
ALE	none	none	6/9
ALE	none	+	1/7
ALE	+	+	7/10

* 15 mg s.c. at 11.15 a.m. on pro-oestrus.
** 30 mg/kg i.p. at 2 p.m. on pro-oestrus.

animals with cuts of the types "A", "AL" and "ALE" usually ovulated when progesterone was injected on pro-oestrus, followed by pentobarbital at 2 p.m., as opposed to animals injected with pentobarbital only.

Therefore, the result of the "chronic" experiment is contrary to that of the "acute" one. Thus we have to reckon with the possibility that some time after making these cuts some kind of reorganization occurs, for instance resulting in an increased sensitivity of receptors to progesterone in the preoptic area of the hypothalamus.

When the effects of implants of progesterone were studied in rats with 4-day cycles by implanting 20 μg of progesterone between 10 and 10.30 a.m. on the day of pro-oestrus, followed by pentobarbital at 2 p.m., no effect was found of implants situated in the preoptic area. Bilateral implants in the mediobasal hypothalamus, however, readily caused ovulation. The results are summarized in Table III. In a second series the effect of unilateral implants in the mediobasal hypothalamus was studied. The sites of the implants are represented in Fig. 14. Although the unilateral implants were much less active than the bilateral ones, all implants except three which resulted in ovulation, were situated in the ventromedial nucleus.

References p. 209

TABLE III

EFFECTS OF PROGESTERONE IMPLANTS (20–25 μg) AT 10.15 A.M., FOLLOWED BY PENTOBARBITAL (30 mg/kg I.P.) AT 2 P.M. RATS WITH 4-DAY CYCLES, DAY OF PRO-OESTRUS

Site of implants	Number of rats ovulating/total number of rats
Preoptic area, unilaterally	0/8
Preoptic area, bilaterally	1/7
Mediobasal hypothalamus, bilaterally:*	
Both implants in N. ventromed./arc.	10/13
Both implants outside N. ventromed./arc.	1/9
(both cholesterol implants in N. ventromed./arc.)	1/6

* For the effects of unilateral implants of progesterone in the mediobasal hypothalamus, see Fig. 14.

OVULATION POSITIVE

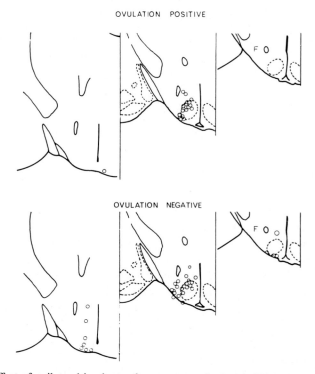

OVULATION NEGATIVE

Fig. 14. Effect of unilateral implants of progesterone in the mediobasal hypothalamus.

This result does not agree with that obtained by studying the effect of acute "A"-cuts on ovulation induced by progesterone. Then the conclusion was reached that the site of action of progesterone should be located outside the complex formed by the preoptic area and the hypothalamus. However, we must take into account that by implanting progesterone pellets very high concentrations are reached locally. Thus it is possible that there are receptors in the ventromedial hypothalamus, which have a limited sensitivity to progesterone, and are not stimulated when progesterone is injected systemically.

However, there are other arguments which point to a site of action situated within the hypothalamus. Döcke and Dörner (1969) observed that in animals, rendered persistently anovulatory by lesions situated in the anterior hypothalamus, progesterone did not induce ovulation. In such animals the effect of stimulation of the mediobasal hypothalamus was enhanced by previous administration of progesterone. This result may be interpreted as indicating that progesterone acts on the level of the medio-basal hypothalamus raising the sensitivity of structures present within this region to experimental stimulation. This then might also apply to the intact animal where progesterone could sensitize the hypothalamus for afferent ovulatory impulses. The result also explains why, in animals rendered anovulatory by large lesions in the anterior hypothalamus or in the preoptic area, progesterone has no effect in this

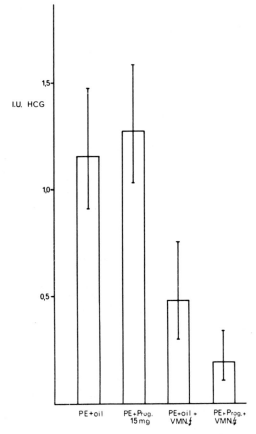

Fig. 15. Effect of progesterone and/or electrochemical stimulation of the mediobasal hypothalamus in animals with ovulation permanently blocked by retrochiasmatic cuts. Presented are estimations of the ED50 of HCG (with 95% confidence interval) in the 4 experimental groups. For details, see text.

respect since such afferent impulses may be expected to be absent in these animals.

In view of the importance of this hypothesis we performed a similar experiment in which the animals had been subjected to a retrochiasmatic cut. By this procedure all afferent fibres that enter the hypothalamus from frontally and dorsally situated regions are severed. Such animals were taken after 7 days of persistent vaginal oestrus and divided into the following 4 groups: (1) injection of oil at 11 a.m.; (2) injection of progesterone (15 mg s.c.) at 11 a.m.; (3) injection of oil at 11 a.m. followed by electrochemical stimulation (2 mA for 10 sec, unilaterally) of the mediobasal hypothalamus at 2 p.m., and (4) injection of 15 mg of progesterone followed by electrochemical stimulation of the hypothalamus at 2 p.m. All animals were also injected intravenously with Human Chorionic Gonadotrophin (H.C.G.) at 2 p.m. in order to estimate the dose of H.C.G. which would bring about ovulation in 50 % of the animals (the ED50 of H.C.G.). It was argued that an increase of gonadotrophin secretion by the anterior pituitary gland, by itself insufficient to cause ovulation, would be reflected in a decrease of the amount of H.C.G. which has to be given in order to cause ovulation.

The results of this experiment are summarized in Fig. 15. It can be seen that injection of progesterone exclusively had no effect. Stimulation of the mediobasal hypothalamus resulted in a lowering of the ED50, which indicates that this procedure caused a release of gonadotrophins by the anterior pituitary gland. However, after pretreatment with progesterone this decrease was significantly greater. Therefore, after progesterone, stimulation of the mediobasal hypothalamus resulted in a discharge of a greater amount of gonadotrophins than without this pretreatment, which is in agreement with the hypothesis discussed above. On the other hand, it still remains to be settled to what extent this also holds in intact animals. The rats used in the experiments discussed above had been operated on some time before and it still might be that this procedure changes the sensitivity of receptors to progesterone.

SUMMARY

First, arguments are brought forward pointing to the participation of structures situated outside the preoptic area and the hypothalamus in spontaneous ovulation. With regard to the ovulatory action of oestrogen, arguments are discussed which point to a site of action situated in the mediobasal hypothalamus and pituitary gland, although there are some indications that also other structures within the C.N.S. are involved. The same holds for the action of progesterone. In this respect a hypothesis is discussed which might explain its action within the hypothalamus.

Finally, the results presented indicate that the effects of cuts in the C.N.S. may vary according to the time elapsed between making these lesions and the experiment. It seems that we have to consider the possibility that after deafferentation a certain degree of reorganization can occur, although we have no idea as to the mechanisms involved.

REFERENCES

ARIMURA, A. AND SCHALLY, A. V. (1971) Augmentation of pituitary responsiveness to LH-releasing hormone (LH-RH) by estrogen. *Proc. Soc. exp. Biol. (N.Y.)*, **136**, 290–293.

BARNEA, A., GERSHONOWITZ, T. AND SHELESNYAK, M. C. (1968) Assessment of ovarian secretion of oestrogen during the oestrous cycle by the use of biological criteria. *J. Endocr.*, **41**, 281–288.

BROWN–GRANT, K., EXLEY, D. AND NAFTOLIN, F. (1970) Peripheral plasma oestradiol and luteinizing hormone concentrations during the oestrous cycle of the rat. *J. Endocr.*, **48**, 295–296.

DÖCKE, F. AND DÖRNER, G. (1969) A possible mechanism by which progesterone facilitates ovulation in the rat. *Neuroendocrinology*, **4**, 139–149.

EVERETT, J. W. (1948) Progesterone and estrogen in the experimental control of ovulation time and other features of the estrous cycle in the rat. *Endocrinology*, **43**, 389–403.

EVERETT, J. W. AND SAWYER, C. H. (1950) A 24-hours periodicity in the LH-release apparatus of the female rat, disclosed by barbiturate sedation. *Endocrinology*, **47**, 198–217.

FERIN, M., TEMPONE, A., ZIMMERING, P. E. AND VAN DE WIELE, R. L., (1969) Effect of antibodies to 17β-estradiol and progesterone on the estrous cycle of the rat. *Endocrinology*, **85**, 1070–1078.

HOFFMANN, J. C. AND SCHWARTZ, N. B. (1965) Timing of post-partum ovulation in the rat. *Endocrinology*, **76**, 620–625.

KAASJAGER, W. A., WOODBURY, D. M., VAN DIETEN, J. A. M. J. AND VAN REES, G. P. (1971) The role played by the preoptic region and the hypothalamus in spontaneous ovulation and ovulation induced by progesterone. *Neuroendocrinology*, **7**, 54–64.

KÖVES, K. AND HALÁSZ, B. (1970) Location of the neural structures triggering ovulation in the rat. *Neuroendocrinology*, **6**, 180–193.

SCHWARTZ, N. B. (1969) A model for the regulation of ovulation in the rat. *Recent Progress in Hormone Research, Vol. 25*, Academic Press, New York and London, p. 1.

VELASCO, M. E. AND TALEISNIK, S. (1969) Effect of hippocampal stimulation on the release of gonadotropins. *Endocrinology*, **85**, 1154–1159.

WEICK, R. F. AND DAVIDSON, J. M. (1970) Localization of the stimulatory feedback of estrogen on ovulation in the rat. *Endocrinology*, **87**, 693–700.

ZEILMAKER, G. H. (1966) The biphasic effect of progesterone on ovulation in the rat. *Acta Endocr. (Kbh.)*, **51**, 461–468.

DISCUSSION

FINDLAY: In terms of the extrahypothalamic sites of action of estrogen your evidence seems to suggest that the more important site is the hippocampus. This is surprising in terms of the information that we have on the uptake of radioactive estrogen, which seems not to be taken up in the hippocampus but rather in the amygdala. Do you have any comment on this?

VAN REES: No, it is difficult to give a reasonable answer to your question. We were surprised too when we found these effects, but we should regard these results with great caution, since we performed only one control experiment and many more experiments are needed before we would dare to draw conclusions about a possible site of action in the dorsal hippocampus.

SMELIK: I noticed that these implants were very close to the lateral ventricle.

VAN REES: Yes, and that is actually what makes me so cautious.

SWAAB: You implanted 2 micrograms of estradiolbenzoate. If I remember correctly, this drug has been used as a substitution therapy after ovariectomy, but it was then injected subcutaneously. Don't you think that you use a rather high dose?

VAN REES: We are aware of the fact that it is a high dose. We started with lower doses but they were not effective. When you implant such an amount of estrogen it is different from an injection. As further studies have shown in which radioactive estradiol has been implanted you may observe for at least one week a very slow decline of the radioactivity of the implant indicating that the release is very small.

An Investigation of Cerebral Protein Synthesis in Various States of Neuroendocrine Activity

M. B. ter HAAR* and P. C. B. MacKINNON

Department of Human Anatomy, University of Oxford, Oxford (Great Britain)

INTRODUCTION

Twenty years ago it was generally believed that cerebral proteins were metabolically inert and that little turnover occurred. This belief was engendered as a result of experiments in which the plasma levels of amino acids were grossly elevated and, although this led to an increased concentration of amino acids and protein in most organs of the body, little or no change was observed in the brain. (Friedberg and Greenberg, 1947; Borsook and Deasy, 1951; Kamin and Handler, 1951). However, with the introduction of radioactively labelled amino acids of high specific activity which could be injected into the systemic circulation in physiological dosages, measurement of uptake of radioactivity into brain proteins showed that new synthesis did in fact occur (Gaitonde and Richter, 1956; Piha *et al.*, 1962). Furthermore, introduction of these radiochemicals directly into the cerebrospinal fluid, either within or surrounding the brain, led to a rapid incorporation into cerebral proteins which then showed a relatively higher concentration of radioactivity than that of other tissues. It was clear therefore that the earlier ideas required revision, and the existence of a blood–brain barrier system was postulated to explain the impedance of flux of amino acids into the brain. In recent years much biochemical work has been undertaken and it is now accepted that under physiological conditions the adult brain exhibits a dynamic equilibrium with respect to protein metabolism, in that breakdown is largely balanced by synthesis. However, under certain conditions such as excitation or exhaustion, this state can be disturbed and a noncompensated breakdown or synthesis of protein may occur (see Waelsch and Lajtha, 1961; Krawczynski, 1961; Oja, 1967).

In a separate field of study it has been shown that many hormones exert their effects on extraneural target organs at the levels of transcription as well as translation, and evidence is beginning to accumulate which suggests that these effects may also obtain within the brain. In our laboratory interests lie in the neural control of reproductive activity and the effect of gonadal hormones not only in the regulation of gonadotrophic output but also in sexual differentiation and the onset of puberty.

---

* Berry Scholar of St. Andrew's University.

References p. 221

This paper presents the results of some investigations which are now in progress and which have as their objectives the correlation of protein synthetic activity with the physiological function of those areas of the brain which have been implicated in the control of reproductive activity.

MATERIALS AND METHODS

Animals

The animals used in these investigations were housed under regular lighting conditions (lights on 06.00–20.00 h BST) and fed on Dixon's 41B diet with water *ad libitum*. Wistar rats were used which showed regular 4-day cycles, as indicated by daily vaginal smears over at least two cycles, and a "critical period" which occurred between 15.00–17.00 h of pro-oestrus. Cyclic White Swiss mice (Tuck TO strain) were also used which were weaned and separated from the males at 15 days of age and which showed vaginal opening between 24–31 days of age with an average of 27 days. To ensure that the adult animals had attained maturity the ovaries, oviduct with uterus, and the vagina or the testes and seminal vesicles were removed from the carcasses and weighed; comparison with the weights of similar organs obtained from a control group of animals showed that they lay within the normal adult range. In addition the ovaries were examined for the presence of follicular and luteal tissue.

Methods

An hour before death [^{35}S]methionine (specific activity 40–500 mCi/mM, 0.4 μCi/g body weight) was injected subcutaneously into each animal. After decapitation and collection of blood from the neck, the pituitary gland and the brain were removed and placed on ice. The anterior pituitary and 2–5 mg samples of the brain (see MacKinnon *et al.*, 1972) were dissected out and homogenised in 1.0 ml 2.5% trichloroacetic acid (TCA). The protein was extracted by heating to 90°, washed with organic solvents at room temperature, and the precipitate finally dissolved in 0.45 N NaOH (0.5 ml) at 100°. Radioactivity was measured by liquid scintillation counting and protein by the method of Lowry *et al.* (1951) from which the protein specific activity (cpm/μg) protein) was estimated.

Levels of luteinising hormone in the plasma were measured by a micro-radioimmunoassay in a sheep system as described by Naftolin and Corker (1971).

RESULTS

Oestrus cycle changes

The incorporation of [^{35}S]methionine into protein (cpm/μg protein) in the anterior pituitary (AP) and selected areas of the brain, together with levels of serum LH, were measured in groups of 3-month-old Wistar rats at 6-hourly intervals throughout the oestrus cycle. Aspects of this work have already appeared in abstract form (Mac-Kinnon, 1970b; MacKinnon and ter Haar, 1971).

Serum LH. From Fig. 1 it can be seen that the preovulatory surge of LH in serum occurred in the evening of pre-oestrus; it extended from 15.00 h pro-oestrus to 03.00 h oestrus and reached a peak at 19.00 h pro-oestrus. This peak corresponds in level and timing with that observed by Brown Grant *et al.* (1970) in the same colony of rats, and provides a convenient time marker to which protein synthetic activity can be temporally related.

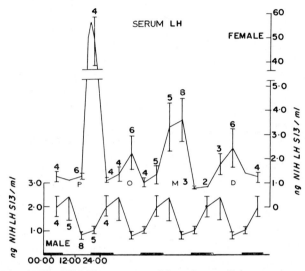

Fig. 1. Serum LH levels ($\pm$ S.E.M.) as measured by micro-radioimmunoassay in female Wistar rats at 6-h intervals over the 4-day oestrus cycle. LH levels in male Wistar rats over a 24-h period have been repeated for comparison with the female over 4 days. P, pro-oestrus; O, oestrus; M, metoestrus; D, dioestrus. The number of animals used at each point and the periods of light and darkness are indicated.

Protein synthesis. Incorporation of [^{35}S]methionine into protein in the AP (fig. 5) showed a peak of activity between 15.00 h pro-oestrus and 03.00 h oestrus, which was coincidental with the peak of serum LH. Statistical examination of the data by means of an analysis of variance and Duncan's multiple range test (Duncan, 1955) showed that the peak was significantly different ($P < 0.001$) from levels observed at any other time of the cycle. Values for the intact male were less than those obtained for the female at any stage of the oestrus cycle; however, values for males castrated 48 hours previously showed levels significantly higher ($P < 0.02$) than those of the intact male, and which were within the range of higher values shown by the female.

Data obtained for the area of the median eminence (ME) (Fig. 4), showed a peak of activity at pro-oestrus starting slightly earlier than that which occurred in the AP. An analysis of variance showed a smaller degree of significance ($P < 0.06$) for any single peak of activity in the ME. On the other hand, the application of Duncan's multiple range test showed that the pro-oestrus peak was significantly higher ($P <$

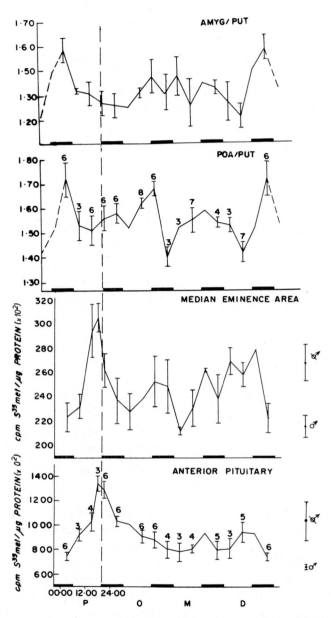

Figs. 2 and 3. Changes in incorporation of [³⁵S]methionine into protein (± S.E.M.) during a 4-day oestrus cycle in the amygdala (AMYG) and the preoptic area (POA) relative to the putamen (PUT), see text.

Figs. 4 and 5. Changes in incorporation of [³⁵S]methionine into protein (± S.E.M.) in the median eminence (ME) and the anterior pituitary (AP). Levels of male (♂) and castrated (♂̸) animals at 09.00 h are indicated. The time of the LH surge (19.00 h pro-oestrus) is indicated by a dotted line extending through all the figures. Note the temporal relationship of the peak values of incorporation for the AP and the brain to this line. Abbreviations as in Fig. 1.

0.01) than values obtained at the same time of day on any other day of the cycle. Again the values for the intact male were low, while the castrate levels were significantly higher ($P < 0.005$), falling within the upper limits shown by the female.

In Fig. 3 the values obtained for the preoptic area (POA) have been expressed as a ratio to those obtained for a control area (the putamen, PUT) at the same time. This treatment of the data was necessary in order to indicate those events which were related to the oestrus cycle and which were being masked by a well-defined circadian rhythm (Fig. 6). These curves for the POA and PUT were closely related ($r = 0.78$) and thus a ratio should indicate events which are not common to the two areas. The result of this treatment of the data, as shown in Fig. 3, is that the POA has a peak of activity at 03.00 h pro-oestrus, *i.e.*, about 16 hours earlier than the LH surge and the temporally related peaks in the AP and ME. A further peak of activity is apparent at 21.00 h oestrus. A statistical examination of the results, similar to that used for the data obtained in the AP and ME, showed that the pro-oestrus peak was significantly different ($P < 0.01$) from the rest of the cycle with the exception of the oestrus peak.

Similar statistical treatment of data obtained for the amygdala (AMYG) showed a peak of activity at pro-oestrus which was significantly different ($P < 0.05$) from all other values. This peak was coincidental with that observed in the POA at pro-oestrus.

Sex differences in circadian rhythms

In addition to the measurements on female rats, measurements of cerebral and pituitary protein synthesis as well as levels of serum LH were made on groups of 3-month-old intact male Wistar rats; the measurements were made at 6-hourly intervals over a 24-hour period.

Serum LH levels. Serum levels of LH measured at 6-hourly intervals throughout an

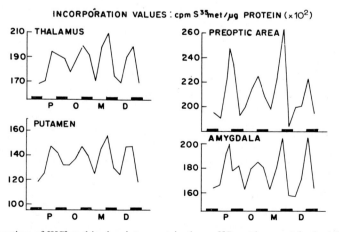

Fig. 6. Incorporation of [^{35}S]methionine into protein (cpm ^{35}S-met/µg protein ($\times 10^2$)) during the oestrus cycle of the rat in 2–5 mg samples of the thalamus, putamen, preoptic area and amygdala. Abbreviations as in Fig. 1.

References p. 221

oestrus cycle show that, in addition to the pre-ovulatory surge on the evening of pro-oestrus, there is an apparent circadian rhythm (Fig. 1). Moreover, this rhythm is more pronounced at metoestrus than at oestrus or dioestrus. An analysis of variance on this data showed that the levels around 15.00 h were significantly ($P < 0.05$) higher than around 03.00 h.

A circadian rhythm in male LH serum levels is also apparent (Fig. 1), though this rhythm is approximately 6 h ahead of that of the female. Values at 03.00 h and 15.00 h are significantly ($P < 0.01$) different as shown by Student's t-test.

Protein synthetic activity. Examination of the values which were obtained for the thalamus and which were combined for each time during the 4 days of the female cycle (Fig. 7) showed that protein synthetic activity is significantly higher ($P < 0.02$) at 21.00 h than at 09.00 h. However, in the male the reverse is seen with a maximal level at 09.00 h and a minimal level at 21.00 h. Hence, although levels of activity are similar in the male and female at 09.00 h, at 21.00 h the female levels are very significantly higher than those of the male ($P < 0.001$).

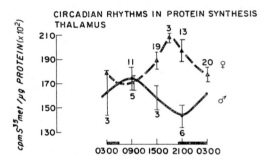

Fig. 7. Circadian rhythms in incorporation of [35S]methionine into protein ($\pm$ S.E.M.) in the thalamus over a 24-h period in female (– –▲– –) and intact male (—●—) Wistar rats.

Pubertal changes

Fig. 8 shows low resolution autoradiographs taken through the preoptic area (POA) of (a) an immature and (b) an adult mouse, both of which had been injected with [35S]methionine one hour prior to death. A marked increase in the concentration of silver grains in the POA of the adult animal can be seen. The density of silver grains in the POA (related to that in the putamen) in a group of adult (60–75 days) male and female litter mates, when compared with relative densities obtained from a similar group of immature (15 day) animals indicated that the relative rates of incorporation of amino acid into protein in the POA were significantly higher ($P < 0.001$) in the adult animals (MacKinnon, 1970a). These findings were confirmed in a further investigation where biochemical extraction of the protein in these areas indicated that the relative increase in incorporation of labelled amino acid into protein in the POA

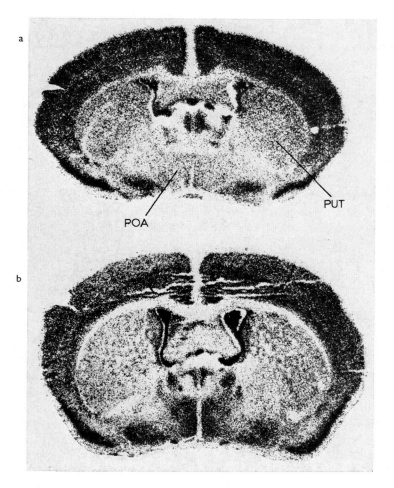

Fig. 8. Low resolution autoradiographs of 25 μm sections through the preoptic area of a, an immature White Swiss mouse (15 days) and b, an adult White Swiss mouse (60 days) injected with [^{35}S]methionine an hour before death. Abbreviations as in Figs. 2 and 3.

of adult animals occurred gradually between the fifteenth to the thirty-fifth day of age, during which time vaginal opening (an overt sign of puberty) occurred (see Fig. 9).

DISCUSSION

Many different techniques have been used in the study of brain metabolism. Autoradiographs of brain sections following intrathecal or systemic injection of radioactively labelled methionine (MacLean *et al.*, 1956; Richter *et al.*, 1960) have provided useful information as to the location and relative concentrations of the label in different areas of the brain, but they yield little information as to the metabolism of the amino acid or of the protein into which it is incorporated. Many *in vitro* methods

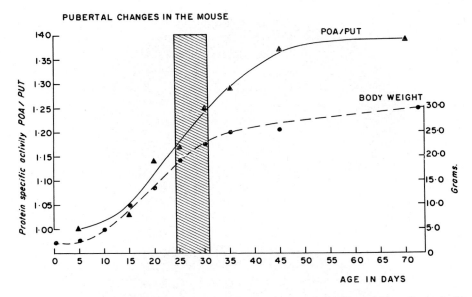

Fig. 9. Changes in White Swiss mice in body weight (– –●– –) and specific activities of protein (cpm ^{35}S-met/μg protein) in the preoptic area relative to the putamen (—▲—). Hatched area indicates average age of vaginal opening. For abbreviations see Figs. 2 and 3.

utilising cell-free systems, cell suspensions, tissue slices or blocks of hypothalamic tissue have also been used but it is often difficult to extrapolate the results obtained from such a system to those which might obtain *in vivo*. Although the estimation of nucleic acids or protein metabolism in single cells (Hyden, 1962) is perhaps the most elegant technique available, it too possesses inherent problems in the form of adequate sampling. In the present investigations, use has been made of both autoradiographic and biochemical *in vivo* methods to study, after the systemic injection of radioactive methionine, the specific activity of protein (cpm/μg protein) in discrete (2–5 mg) samples of the rodent brain and, in particular, in those areas which are concerned with the control of gonadotrophic output.

In an initial study of cerebral protein metabolism, autoradiographs were made of serial sections of brains taken from mice of various ages which had been previously injected with radioactively labelled amino acids (MacKinnon, 1970a). Measurement of silver grain densities showed that an increase in the concentration of label within the preoptic area relative to that in the putamen existed in post-pubertal compared with prepubertal animals. This finding was further investigated by the use of bio-chemical techniques which enabled measurements to be made of the amount of radioactivity which had incorporated into protein in the area. It was found that the specific activity of the protein in the preoptic area (relative to that in the putamen) increased gradually over the course of puberty, during which time vaginal opening occurred (MacKinnon *et al.*, 1972).

Since the preoptic area has been implicated in the control of the LH rise which precedes ovulation, a study of the preoptic area in different phases of the oestrus cycle was made using autoradiographic methods similar to those which were used in the original pubertal study. The concentration of labelled methionine was found to be higher in the afternoon of oestrus than at a similar time of day at dioestrus (MacKinnon, 1970b). Further studies of protein metabolism in the anterior pituitary and in several discrete areas of the brain at 6-hourly intervals throughout a 4-day oestrus cycle showed that peaks of protein synthetic activity occurred that were apparently associated with events of the oestrus cycle. A major peak of activity was seen in the preoptic area at 03.00 h pro-oestrus which preceded the surge of LH on the evening of pro-oestrus by about 16 hours. In the amygdala, which is considered to play a modulatory role in the output of gonadotrophins (Kawakami *et al.*, 1967; Velasco and Taleisnik, 1969), a similar peak of activity was observed which coincided with the preoptic 03.00 h pro-oestrus peak. Furthermore, on the evening of pro-oestrus (*ca.* 18.00 h) marked peaks of metabolic activity were also observed in the median eminence, from which gonadotrophin releasing factor (FRF/LRF) is released, and in the anterior pituitary from which LH is released. These latter peaks of activity were almost coincidental and occurred at the same time as the serum LH peak which rose from about 1 ng/ml to around 50 ng/ml as measured in terms of NIH LH S13 by radioimmunoassay. The important question which these findings pose is whether the biochemical events which occur during the oestrus cycle bear a *causal* relationship to changes in the output of gonadotrophins in addition to this *temporal* relationship.

A further point of interest that emerged from these studies was the observation that the incorporation of labelled amino acid into protein in the male rat 48 hours after castration was significantly higher than that of the normal male. This is in accordance with the autoradiographic study of Timiras and Litteria (1970) in which they reported that the incorporation of [^{14}C]lysine into the cerebellar cortex and various hypothalamic areas of ovariectomized rats was significantly decreased following treatment of the animals with large doses of oestrogen. Since the gonadal steroids appear to exert a feedback effect on protein metabolism in the brain, the possibility is worth considering whether feedback effects of either a positive or negative nature could influence the changes in cerebral metabolic activity which have been observed during the course of puberty and during the oestrus cycle in those areas which control the output of gonadotrophins.

During the investigations of protein metabolism over the course of the oestrus cycle, an additional and somewhat unexpected observation was made. In all the areas of the brain which were examined at 6-hourly intervals throughout a 24-hour period, a circadian rhythm in metabolic activity was observed. Similar observations of diurnal fluctuations in protein synthesis in the adult male rat have been reported in the pineal gland by Nir, Hirschmann, and Sulman (1971) and in the visual and motor cortices together with the geniculate nucleus by Richardson and Rose (1971). However, in the present studies adult females, though showing similar levels of activity to those of the male at 09.00 h, reached a zenith of activity 12 hours later when the male had reached its nadir. This divergence of the female rhythm from that of the male is interesting not only in relation to its possible effect on the regulation of the oestrus cycle (Strauss and Meyer, 1962; Schwartz, 1968; Zarrow and Dinius, 1971) but also as regards the concept of sexual differentiation of the brain which is currently regarded as affecting those regions which have been implicated in the cyclic control of ovulation (see Harris, 1970).

Furthermore, in spite of the fact that an apparent absence of a diurnal rhythm in serum and pituitary LH levels in intact male rats has been reported (Yamamoto *et al.*, 1970), in the present study, with the use of a micro-radioimmunoassay in which LH levels were measured in 50-μl volumes of serum (Naftolin and Corker, 1971), the sensitivity was such that circadian variations in the output of LH were detectable. LH serum levels were found to be higher in the morning than the evening (with the male peak preceding the female peak by 6 hours) which lends support to earlier reports of a diurnal fluctuation in the pituitary contents of LH and FSH which were lower in male rats in the morning than in the evening (Martini *et al.*, 1968). This raises a further pertinent question as to whether the variations in LH output are dependent upon circadian rhythms in protein metabolism within the anterior pituitary or, more indirectly, upon variations in cerebral protein metabolism.

SUMMARY

The incorporation of radioactivity into protein (cpm/μg protein) in the anterior pituitary (AP) and discrete areas of the brain has been measured in both mice and rats following systemic injection of [^{35}S]methionine. Serum levels of luteinising hormone (LH) were also measured by means of a micro-radioimmunoassay using a sheep system.

The incorporation of [^{35}S]methionine in the preoptic area (relative to that of the putamen) of groups of mice of different ages showed a gradual increase over the course of puberty, during which time vaginal opening occurred. Because the preoptic area controls the pre-ovulatory surge of LH, similar measurements were made on groups of rats every 6 hours over a 4-day oestrus cycle. On the morning of pro-oestrus, peaks of protein metabolism were observed in both the preoptic and amygdaloid areas which preceded, by 16 hours, similar peaks of activity in the median eminence and anterior pituitary, these latter being coincidental with the pre-ovulatory surge of LH.

The presence of a circadian rhythm in both LH serum levels and protein specific activity was also observed as in adult males. Adult females, however, showed a sexual difference in that their diurnal fluctuations were 12 hours out of phase with those of the other groups with respect to protein synthesis, and 6 hours with respect to serum LH levels.

ACKNOWLEDGEMENTS

We are grateful to the late Professor G. W. Harris, F.R.S., for his encouragement and support; to Miss Linda Palfrey for technical assistance; to the Population Council of the Ford Foundation for a grant (No. M70.039) to P. C. B. M. and St. Andrew's University for the Berry Scholarship awarded to M. B. ter H.

REFERENCES

Borsook, H. and Deasy, C. L. (1951) The metabolism of proteins and amino acids. *Ann. Rev. Biochem.*, **20**, 209–226.

Brown Grant, K., Exley, D. and Naftolin, F. (1970) Peripheral plasma oestradiol and luteinizing hormone concentrations during the oestrous cycle in the rat. *J. Endocr.*, **48**, 295–296.

Duncan, L. (1955) Multiple range and multiple S tests. *Biometrics*, **11**, 1–42.

Friedberg, F. and Greenberg, D. M. (1947) Partition of intravenously administered amino acids in blood and tissues. *J. biol. Chem.*, **168**, 411–413.

Gaitonde, M. K. and Richter, D. (1956) The metabolic activity of the proteins of the brain. *Proc. roy. Soc. B*, **145**, 83–99.

Harris, G. W. (1970) Hormonal differentiation of the developing central nervous system with respect to patterns of endocrine function. *Phil. Trans. B.*, **259**, 165–177.

Hyden, H. (1962) Cytophysiological aspects of the nucleic acids and proteins of nervous tissue. In *Neurochemistry*, K. A. C. Elliott, I. H. Page and J. H. Quastel (Eds.), 2nd ed., Thomas, Springfield, pp. 331–375.

Kamin, H. and Handler, P. (1951) The metabolism of parenterally administered amino acids. II. Urea synthesis. *J. biol. Chem.*, **188**, 193–205.

Kawakami, M., Seto, K., Terasawa, E. and Yoshida, K. (1967) Mechanisms in the limbic system controlling reproductive functions of the ovary with special reference to the positive feedback of progestin to the hippocampus. In *Progress in Brain Research, Vol. 27, Structure and Function of the Limbic System*, W. R. Adey and T. Tokizane (Eds.), Elsevier, Amsterdam, pp. 69–102.

Krawczynski, J. (1961) The effect of physical activity on the incorporation of radioactivity into proteins of the central nervous system, liver and kidney of the rat, after the intracranial injection of [^{35}S] methionine. *J. Neurochem.*, **8**, 50–54.

Lowry, O. H., Rosebrough, N. J., Farr, A. L. and Randall, R. J. (1951) Protein measurement with Folin phenol reagents. *J. biol. Chem.*, **193**, 265–275.

MacKinnon, P. C. B. (1970a) A comparison of protein synthesis in the brains of mice before and after puberty. *J. Physiol. (Lond.)*, **210**, 10–11P.

MacKinnon, P. C. B. (1970b) Some observations of protein synthesis in the medial preoptic area of mice before and after puberty and of female rats at different phases of the oestrous cycle. *J. Endocr.*, **48**, xliv.

MacKinnon, P. C. B. and ter Haar, M. B. (1971) Plasma LH levels and changes in protein synthesis in the median eminence and anterior pituitary during the oestrous cycle. *J. Physiol. (Lond.)*, **218**, 21–22P.

MacKinnon, P. C. B., ter Haar, M. B. and Burton, M. J. (1972) Preliminary observations of serum LH levels and of protein metabolism in the brain and anterior pituitary in the rodent around the time of puberty. *J. psychosom. Res.*, **16**, 271–278.

MacLean, P. D., Flanigan, S., Flynn, J. P., Kim, C. and Stevens, J. R. (1956) Hippocampal function: tentative correlation of conditioning, EEG, drug and radioautographic studies. *Yale J. Biol. Med.*, **28**, 380–395.

Martini, L., Fraschini, F. and Motta, M. (1968) Neural control of pituitary functions. *Recent Progr. Hormone Res.*, **24**, 439–485.

Naftolin, F. and Corker, C. S. (1971) An ultramicro method for the measurement of luteinising hormone by radio assay. In *Radioimmunoassay Methods*, K. E. Kirkham and W. M. Hunter (Eds.), Churchill, London, pp. 641–645.

Nir, I., Hirschmann, N. and Sulman, F. G. (1971) Diurnal rhythms of pineal nucleic acids and protein. *Neuroendocrinology*, **7**, 271–277.

Oja, S. S. (1967) Studies on protein metabolism in developing rat brain. *Ann. Acad. Sci. fenn. A*, **131**, 7–78.

Piha, R. S., Lehtovirta, E. O., Oja, S. S. and Uusitalo, A. J. (1962) The rate of incorporation of ^{14}C-labelled amino acids into the proteins of different organs and tissues. *Excerpta med. int. Congr. Ser.*, No. 48, 450.

RICHARDSON, K. AND ROSE, S. P. R. (1971) A diurnal rhythmicity in incorporation of lysine into rat brain regions. *Nature New Biology*, **233**, 182–184.

RICHTER, D., GAITONDE, M. K. AND COHN, P. (1960) The localisation of protein metabolism in the brain. In *Structure and Function of the Cerebral Cortex*, D. B. TOWER AND J. P. SCHADÉ (Eds.), Elsevier, London, p. 340.

SCHWARZ, N. B. (1968) New concepts of gonadotropin and steroid feedback control mechanisms. In *Textbook of Gynecologic Endocrinology*, J. J. GOLD (Ed.), New York, Hoeber, pp. 33–50.

STRAUSS, W. F. AND MEYER, R. K. (1962) Neural timing of ovulation in immature rats treated with gonadotrophin. *Science*, **137**, 860–861.

TIMIRAS, P. S. AND LITTERIA, M. (1970) *In vivo* inhibition of protein synthesis in specific hypothalamic nuclei by 17β-estradiol. *Proc. Soc. exp. Biol. (N.Y.)*, **134**, 256–261.

VELASCO, M. E. AND TALEISNIK, S. (1969) Release of gonadotropins induced by amygdaloid stimulation in the rat. *Endocrinology*, **84**, 132–139.

WAELSCH, H. AND LAJTHA, A. (1961) Protein metabolism in the nervous system, *Physiol. Rev.*, **41**, 709–736.

YAMAMOTO, M., DIEBEL, N. AND BOGDANOVE, E. M. (1970) Radioimmunoassay of serum and pituitary LH and FSH levels in intact male rats and of serum and pituitary LH in castrated rats of both sexes – apparent absence of diurnal rhythms, *Endocrinology*, **87**, 798–806.

ZARROW, M. X. AND DINIUS, J. (1971) Regulation of pituitary ovulating hormone concentration in the immature rat treated with pregnant mare serum. *J. Endocr.*, **49**, 387–392.

DISCUSSION

DONOVAN: You described a change in protein synthesis. Could you outline for us or could you make some suggestions as to what its significance may be, what is going up and what is going down?

TER HAAR: We have been looking at the synthesis of proteins over a period of one hour. This is an indication of activity. In experiments which we are just starting we are trying to find out whether any specific protein synthesis is occurring in any of these areas at any time.

DONOVAN: So you describe change in the rate of protein synthesis.

TER HAAR: This is really what it is.

BOUMA: You have shown that there is a change in protein synthesis around the time of puberty in the female mouse; did you try to manipulate the age of puberty occurrence in the species and look for consequent alterations in the protein synthesis process?

TER HAAR: It has been found in the rat that you can't start puberty before 25 to 26 days. We have not gone around to investigate the rat yet, but I think that there is a lot of interest for finding out the earliest moment one can push puberty back and correlating the curve of protein synthesis to these experiments.

SWAAB: You refer in your data to wet weight I saw.

TER HAAR: No, in fact we plot in absolute terms of incorporation to protein.

FINDLAY: When you say that protein synthesis is related to synthetic activity, would that be related to electrophysiological activity? It has been possible to show in experiments of different functional states that protein synthesis, *e.g.* in the visual cortex or the lateral geniculate body, is related to the amount of light input. A visually rich environment is different in that respect from a visually poor environment.

DE WIED: I would like to know how you came to use the methionine system. Is that because you just happened to make this choice or did you have experience with other radioactive amino acids before and then selected this?

TER HAAR: I have four answers to that, the major one being that methionine is the cheapest one can use. Methionine has a limited number of components which can be metabolized, the most obvious one being cysteine. About 10% will be formed in one hour. If you use C^{14}- or H^3- labelled material many other compounds are being labelled too. The previous work was done with autoradiographs and you will get some of your fastest pictures using S^{35} because it is quite a "hot label".

BATTA: I was just wondering whether you have any information on the effect of estrogen and androgen on the pregnant mothers and the activities seen later on in the babies?

TER HAAR: I have some information on the effect of androgen on neonatal females. We have animals growing up at the moment, which have been given estrogen neonatally. They should be ready by late September.

BATTA: You mentioned at one point that sexual differentiation occurs the day before pregnancy.

TER HAAR: My timing has been the day after birth, I did not mention pregnancy at all.

HALÁSZ: Just a very brief comment. You showed that these androgen-sterilized female rats show a male pattern as far as protein synthesis is concerned and at the same time the castrated males show also male patterns. That is interesting because you know that the castrated males, as far as gonadotropic hormone secretion is concerned, behave as females.

TER HAAR: Do they in fact produce estrogens?

HALÁSZ: Their brains show cyclic gonadotropin release.

TER HAAR: We are now preparing some chronic animals to study these effects.

The Hypothalamo-Neurohypophysial
System and Reproduction

D. F. SWAAB

Netherlands Central Institute for Brain Research, Amsterdam (The Netherlands)

INTRODUCTION

The hypothalamo-neurohypophysial system (HNS) consists of the magnocellular supraoptic and paraventricular nuclei (SON and PVN), the hypothalamo-neuro-hypophysial tract (HNT), and the posterior lobe of the pituitary. This system synthesizes, transports and releases the posterior lobe hormones and their carrier-proteins (see Chapter by Jongkind, in this volume).

The HNS is involved in the regulation of diuresis. Consequently, many studies on the HNS have concerned the activation of this system by means of osmotic stimuli such as thirsting (*e.g.*, Jongkind, 1967, 1969; Jongkind and Swaab, 1967; Swaab, 1970). In addition, a relationship seems to exist between this osmotically sensitive HNS and reproductive physiology. The present paper deals therefore with the HNS, its afferent pathways and peripheral effects during pregnancy, parturition, lactation, the oestrous cycle and mating.

Moreover, attention will be paid to the dual nature of stimuli that affect the HNS, and to some methodological problems in the study of this system.

A. PREGNANCY

The nature of the *afferent stimuli* activating the HNS during pregnancy is not known. Changes in gonadotropic hormone levels may however be concerned in this activation (see Swaab, 1970).

The HNS and peripheral effects

Enzymatic studies showed an undulating course in the synthesizing activity of posterior lobe hormones in the SON and PVN during the course of pregnancy. This activity rises in both of these neurosecretory nuclei to a peak at about mid-pregnancy, after which it gradually decreases again until parturition (Swaab and Jongkind, 1970a; Swaab, 1970). The neurosecretory material (NSM) increases in the HNS during the course of gestation (Malandra, 1956; Vazquez, 1970). During the second half of pregnancy the pituicytes and their nucleoli increase in size and show more mitoses (Malandra, 1956).

In spite of these signs of HNS-activation, no changes were observed in the vaso-pressin/oxytocin ratio nor in the content of these hormones in the rat's posterior lobe during pregnancy (Acher, 1956; Heller, 1959). Unfortunately, no reliable data are available on blood levels of posterior lobe hormones during the course of gesta-tion, while it is also unknown whether the HNS plays a role in the physiology of pregnancy.

B. PARTURITION

Maternal HNS

Mechanical stimulation of the female genital tract liberates oxytocin via a neuro-hormonal reflex (Ferguson, 1941). The neural component of this "Ferguson reflex" appears from its blockade by lesioning the neural afferent pathway (see below), while the humoral component is obvious both from cross-circulation experiments (Debackere et al., 1961) and from the long latency time (40–60 sec) between genital stimulation and peripheral effects (Richard, 1970).

Afferent pathways to the HNS

The major afferent fibers from the female genital tract run via the pelvic and pudendal nerves (Cross, 1966). Stimulation of mechanoreceptors in the uterus induces action potential discharge in its efferent nerves (Bower, 1959). The stimuli from the female genital tract are transmitted to the HNS via a spinal pathway that is mainly contra-lateral and diffusely distributed in the ventral and lateral fasciculi (Richard, 1970).

The HNS and peripheral effects

During parturition signs of increased production and release of posterior lobe hormones are observed. Enzymatic studies showed an increased synthesis of posterior lobe hormones in the SON and PVN (Swaab, 1970; Swaab and Jongkind, 1970a).

Stimulation of the female genital tract causes an increased firing rate of PVN cells (Brooks et al., 1966) and increased electrical activity in the HNT (Richard, 1970). These electrophysiological events are accompanied by a release of oxytocin (Roberts and Share, 1968, 1970) and of vasopressin (Kühn and Peeters, 1971), and by an in-crease of uterine pressure waves (Hindson et al., 1968, 1969).

That the Ferguson reflex is indeed an essential part of the mechanism of labor is a conclusion based partly on the signs of activation of this reflex arc that accompany parturition and partly on experiments which interfere with this arc and also influence parturition. Parturition is accompanied by a release of oxytocin and vasopressin as appears from their decreased posterior lobe levels (Fuchs and Saito, 1971) combined with the increased blood levels of oxytocin (Folley, 1969; Haldar, 1970) and of vasopressin (Cobo *et al.*, 1968; Coutinho, 1970) during the expulsive stage of labour. Moreover, expulsion of a litter is preceeded by strong oxytocin-like responses of the uterus (Fuchs and Poblete, 1970). Administration of oxytocin close to term advances the development of synchronous pressure waves that favour expulsion (Fuchs and Poblete, 1970) and induces labour (*e.g.*, Fuchs and Poblete, 1970; Fuchs and Saito, 1971). Direct evidence for a role of the Ferguson reflex in labour is obvious from the induction of labour by stimulation of the HNS (Cross, 1958; Lincoln, 1970) and from the occurrence of dystocia after blocking the reflex arc at the level of the spinal cord (Fitzpatrick, 1969; Beyer and Mena, 1970) or of the HNS (see Ginsburg, 1968). Moreover, labour is postponed by inhibition of oxytocin release (Fuchs, 1969; Fuchs *et al.*, 1967).

A role in the initiation of labour has been ascribed to many factors, *e.g.*, (1) the relative growth rates of uterus and conceptus or, (2) the release of a progesterone block on myometrial activity (Csapo, 1969), (3) the increased oestrogen production (Yoshinaga *et al.*, 1969) near term (*e.g.*, Csapo, 1969; Fuchs and Poblete, 1970), (4) the resistance of the cervix passage (Fuchs and Poblete, 1970), and (5) foetal factors (Liggins, 1969). Also (6) oxytocin has been mentioned frequently in this context (*e.g.*, Fuchs, 1966; Porter and Schofield, 1966; Schofield, 1969).

High spinal cord lesions induce dystocia, but the initiation of labour still occurs within the normal time (Beyer and Mena, 1970). This shows that the initiation of parturition is independent of neural stimuli from the genital tract. Oxytocin will therefore not trigger parturition via the Ferguson reflex, which must consequently be only concerned with acceleration of the expulsive stage. High oxytocin blood levels are in fact observed only in the second stage of labour (*e.g.*, Folley, 1969), which makes oxytocin release by whatever mechanism very improbable as the cause of the initiation of labour, although not impossible according to Fitzpatrick (1969).

Progesterone affects the uterus not only directly by inhibiting its spontaneous pressure waves (Csapo, 1969), but also indirectly by suppressing the Ferguson reflex. Oxytocin release (Roberts and Share, 1970) and uterine responses (Hindson *et al.*, 1969) induced by stimulation of the female genital tract are centrally (Fuchs, 1966; Hindson *et al.*, 1969) inhibited by progesterone. Withdrawal of the progesterone block will therefore not only influence labour via a direct action upon the myometrium, but also via disinhibition of the Ferguson reflex.

In contradistinction to oxytocin release, the liberation of vasopressin during parturition is probably only a consequence of labour pains (Cobo, 1968; Cobo *et al.*, 1968; Fuchs and Saito, 1971) or of emotional stress (Haldar, 1970). Teleologically, however, vasopressin release can be of importance because it would protect the mother from hypotension and excessive fluid loss (Coutinho, 1970).

Apart from its role in parturition, the Ferguson reflex has been applied since ancient times in cattle raising. The release of oxytocin in response to genital tract stimulation has been and is still being used in many parts of the world to assist the milking process (Folley, 1969).

References p. 237

Foetal HNS

Immediately after delivery, the vasopressin level is much higher in newborns' cord blood than in maternal blood during or after delivery (Hoppenstein *et al.*, 1968). High levels of oxytocin have recently been demonstrated in newborns' cord plasma (Chard *et al.*, 1970). Their finding that the arterial level was higher than the venous one suggests that oxytocin is produced by the foetus. Moreover, cord samples taken from forceps-delivered newborns were nearly all negative. These findings, combined with the observation that initiation of parturition failed to occur following lesion of the pituitary gland or stalk (Liggins *et al.*, 1967), suggests that the foetal HNS may play a role in delivery. Further work is needed to test this possibility.

C. LACTATION

Milk is liberated from the mammary gland partly by passive withdrawal, and partly by an active process. The HNS is involved in the latter as part of a neurohormonal reflex arc by which milk is forcibly ejected from the gland in response to oxytocin release (Bisset, 1968; Bisset *et al.*, 1970; Cleverley and Folley, 1970). The existence of a neural component of this milk ejection reflex arc is obvious from its blockade after lesioning the afferent pathway (see the next subchapter). The hormonal component is demonstrated by the finding that in rat, during suckling of the mammary glands cranial to the level of a spinal cord section, milk ejection also appears in the anaesthetic glands caudal to this section (Ingelbrecht, 1935). The long latency (40–50 sec) between suckling and milk ejection (Folley, 1969) is also to be expected for a humoral factor.

Afferent pathways to the HNS

Suckling activates the segmental mammary nerves via pressure and temperature sensitive nerve endings (Findlay, 1966, 1968).

The spinal tracts for the milk ejection reflex are mainly ipsilateral, but the exact localization differs appreciably in various species. In the ewe, the spinocervico-thalamic tract is probably involved. This is situated in the dorsal tract at thoracic levels and ventrally at cervical levels (Richard *et al.*, 1970). The spinal part of the reflex arc is situated in the dorsal tract in the goat (Popovici, 1963) and ventrolateral in the rabbit (Mena and Beyer, 1968). Tindal and co-workers (1967, 1968, 1969) showed by electrical stimulation studies that, in the mesencephalon, the milk ejection pathway is situated in the lateral tegmentum. In the diencephalon the pathway bifurcates into (1) a dorsal path situated close to the extreme rostral central grey, and (2) a ventral path ascending through the subthalamus. Both paths reunite in the posterior hypothalamus. This is a pathway for the preferential release of oxytocin, and not important for vasopressin release (Tindal *et al.*, 1968). The importance of these tracts for the milk ejection reflex needs, however, still to be confirmed by means of lesions made in them.

A release of oxytocin without activation of the HNS via the milk ejection reflex arc is possible in cows if the reflex becomes conditioned to stimuli associated with the milking routine (Cleverley, 1968; Cleverley and Folley, 1970) and in women by the sound of a baby crying (Newton, 1961, cited by Ginsburg, 1968).

In some species (*e.g.*, sheep and goats) milk ejection can still occur after complete denervation of the udder and without any oxytocin release, possibly through direct mechanical stimulation of the myoepithelium of the mammary gland (see Cleverley and Folley, 1970).

The HNS and peripheral effects

During lactation, the production and release of posterior lobe hormones and also the rate of axonal flow in the HNT are enhanced.

The increased production appears from the increased nucleolar size of the SON and PVN cells (Flament–Durand, 1967) and from enzymatic parameters for this production (Swaab and Jongkind, 1970a, b; Swaab, 1970; Swaab et al., 1971).

An enhancement of axonal transport appears from the observed quicker carriage of ^{35}S-cysteine along the HNT (Flament–Durand, 1967). According to Jones and Pickering (1970), however, vasopressin and oxytocin in rat are synthesized and transported to the posterior lobe within 2 h, whereas ^{35}S-cysteine appears in the posterior lobe only after 9 h (Flament–Durand, 1967). The latter method of labelling is, therefore, probably not specific for the posterior lobe hormones. Recent studies did not confirm an increased transport rate during lactation (Norström and Sjöstrand, 1971).

An activation of the pituicytes in the posterior lobe is obvious from their increased size and vacuolisation, and from their increased number of mitoses (Malandra, 1956).

Stimulation of the nipples induces a rise in firing rate of PVN cells (Brooks et al., 1966) and an increased release of posterior lobe hormones. This release is obvious from the decreasing amount of NSM-containing vesicles found in the posterior lobe during suckling (Monroe and Scott, 1966), combined with increased blood levels of oxytocin that appear in short bursts (Folley, 1969; Fox and Knaggs, 1969; Bisset et al., 1970; Cleverley and Folley, 1970). The amount of oxytocin released depends upon the number of pups suckling simultaneously (Fuchs and Wagner, 1963).

The controversy (see Ginsburg, 1968) whether oxytocin release during suckling is accompanied by a release of vasopressin or not (Cobo et al., 1967; Bisset et al., 1970) may be explained by a slight antidiuretic activity of oxytocin itself and by the vasopressin release caused by emotional stress (Bisset et al., 1970). Although such a possible vasopressin release would not be essential for milk ejection (Bisset et al., 1970), it could be considered as a physiological reaction to loss of fluid (Coutinho, 1970).

The released oxytocin gives rise to alveolar myoepithelium contraction (Linzell, 1955) resulting in milk ejection (see Bisset, 1968). Milk ejection in response to oxytocin in rat already occurs 12 h before parturition (Deis, 1968).

The reflex arc described has proved to be essential for milk ejection in most species by stimulation and destruction of its various parts. Milk ejection was observed after stimulation of the nipples (*e.g.* Folley, 1969; Brooks *et al.*, 1966; Richard *et al.*, 1970), stimulation of the afferent pathways in the brain (Tindal *et al.*, 1967, 1968, 1969), and direct stimulation of the SON and PVN (Aulsebrook and Holland, 1969; Cleverley *et al.*, 1968; Bisset *et al.*, 1969) or of the HNT (Brooks *et al.*, 1966; Bisset *et al.*, 1969). Suppression of the milk ejection reflex was found after anaesthesia of the teats or section of the mammary nerves (see Findlay, 1968), section of the spinal cord (Ingelbrecht, 1935; Mena and Beyer, 1968; Beyer and Mena, 1970), blocking (Oba *et al.*, 1971) of a cholinergic mechanism (Bisset, 1968) in the PVN, lesions made in the HNT (for reviews see Benson and Fitzpatrick, 1966; Cross, 1966), section of the stalk (Desclin, 1969), ablation of the posterior pituitary (see Benson and Fitzpatrick, 1966), and administration of oxytocin antibodies in the mother (Kumaresan *et al.*, 1971).

D. OESTROUS CYCLE

During the oestrus cycle, changes in posterior lobe hormone synthesizing activity were observed in the SON and PVN, both nuclei showing an increase during early oestrus (see below).

Afferent pathways to the HNS

In order to detect the possible hormonal stimuli inducing cyclic changes in the SON and PVN (Swaab, 1970), we studied the hormone synthesizing activity by means of enzymatic parameters in both of these neurosecretory nuclei during conditions that cause a change in gonadotropic or sex hormone levels. As appeared from the high activity in the SON and PVN during light-induced persistent oestrus, during early oestrus, and after gonadectomy, a parallelism exists between posterior lobe hormone synthesis in the HNS and blood levels of gonadotropic hormones (Swaab and Jongkind, 1970a, b; Swaab, 1970). The increase occurring in this synthetic activity after ovariectomy was inhibited by oestradiol benzoate. In ovariectomized oestrogen-primed rats, HCG (Pregnyl), HMG (Humegon), NIH–LH[1] and NIH–FSH[1] all caused an increase in posterior lobe hormone synthesizing activity. From these findings it could be concluded that the hormonal stimuli for the SON and PVN were LH and FSH (Swaab, 1970; Swaab and Jongkind, 1970a, b; 1971; Swaab *et al.*, 1971).

It was shown recently that gonadotropic hormones affect the neurosecretory nuclei directly (Swaab, unpublished observations). Cocoa butter pellets (approximately 300 μg) (Hirono *et al.*, 1970) containing 1 μg NIH-FSH-S8[1], placed within 50 μm of the SON, stimulated synthetic activity in the SON, as was indicated by the increased distribution of TPP-ase (Fig. 1) in this nucleus. No change was found in TPP-ase distribution after these implantations either in the same SON in sections

---

[1] NIH-LH and FSH were kindly provided by the Endocrinology Study Section, N.I.H., U.S.A.

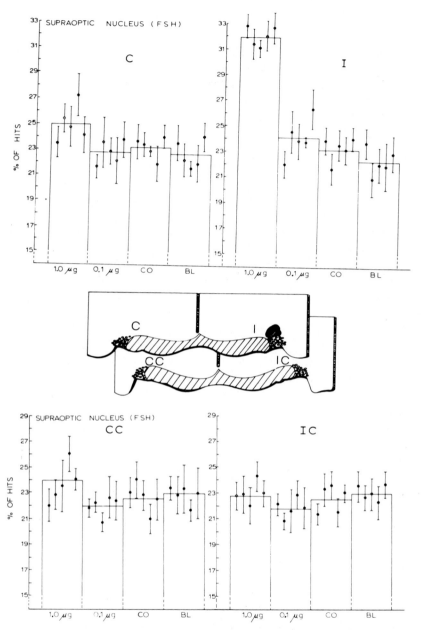

Fig. 1. Distribution of thiamine diphosphate-phosphohydrolase (TPP-ase) determined according to Swaab and Jongkind (1970, 1971) by a semi-quantitative histochemical method. The percentage of TPP-ase-produced lead sulphide hits was counted in the SON of individual male (200 g) rats 2 days after implantation of NIH-FSH-S8[1] adjacent to the SON. In these series 4 groups of 5 rats were used: (1) unilateral implantation of 1.0 μg FSH (1.0 μg), (2) implantation of 0.1 μg FSH (0.1 μg), (3) implantation of cocoa butter only (CO) and (4) animals that did not receive any treatment (BL). The distribution of TPP-ase was determined in each animal in 8 sections through the SON: at the site of implantation (I), at the corresponding place in the SON of the contralateral side (C), on the site of implantation but at least 160 μm remote from the implant (IC), and at the corresponding place on the contralateral side (CC). At these 4 localizations a significant difference ($P < 0.001$) between the 4 groups was observed only after implantation of 1 μg of FSH.

References p. 237

situated at least 160 μm from the implant, or in this nucleus after implants containing cocoa butter only, or in the contralateral SON during any of these conditions. These data show that the receptors for gonadotropic hormones must be situated within the SON.

HNS and peripheral effects

Using the same enzymatic parameters for neurosecretory activity, we found a high hormone synthetic activity in the SON and PVN during early oestrus, and a low activity during di- and metoestrus (Swaab, 1970; Swaab and Jongkind, 1970a; Swaab et al., 1971). Earlier studies using nuclear measurements (Smollich, 1969), changing amounts of NSM within cell bodies (Belajev et al., 1967) or autoradiographic observations (Belajev et al., 1967) also showed cyclic changes in activity of the neurosecretory nuclei.

These results could, however, not be interpreted as reflecting to hyperactivity of the HNS, since no correlation exists between these parameters and hormone production (see Swaab, 1970).

Parallel to the increased activity in the SON and PVN described in our work, the vasopressin and oxytocin content in the posterior lobe increases during pro-oestrus and oestrus (Heller, 1959; König and Böttcher, 1966). Blood levels of these hormones during the course of the oestrous cycle are not known.

According to the observations discussed above, the relation between the HNS and gonads (see, e.g., Zambrano and De Robertis, 1968; Stutinsky, 1970; Korfsmeier, 1970; Gabe et al., 1968) can be explained by the direct stimulating action of gonadotropic hormones upon the neurosecretory nuclei.

This mechanism thus provides an increased production of posterior lobe hormones during the fertile period of the oestrus cycle, a stage during which these hormones may play a role either in sperm or egg transport (see next subchapter).

E. MATING

Female HNS

G. W. Harris (1947) suggested that stimuli associated with coitus might result in a release of oxytocin that causes an increase in uterine activity and, in this way, influences sperm transport.

Afferent pathways to the HNS

As was shown in the subchapter on parturition, stimulation of the female genital tract induces posterior lobe hormone release. A similar mechanism was supposed to stimulate the HNS during mating (e.g., Cross, 1966). It was shown recently (McNeilly and Folley, 1970), however, that oxytocin is frequently released in the female goat, even before intromission. Consequently, it does not seem that mechanical stimulation of the female genital tract is necessary for oxytocin release during coitus. Although at present a mechanism similar to "conditioning" of the milk ejection reflex (see subchapter on lactation) cannot be excluded, the work of McNeilly and Folley (1970) points more to auditory, visual or olfactory stimuli as afferents for HNS stimulation.

HNS and peripheral effects

No data are available, either in female or in male individuals, on activity changes in the SON or PVN in connection with coitus.

Peripheral effects, *i.e.*, milk ejection, antidiuresis (Harris and Pickles, 1953) and pressure changes in the female genital tract (Michael and Reinke, 1970; Fox *et al.*, 1970), point to a release of posterior lobe hormones during mating. Moreover, increased oxytocin blood levels have been shown during this condition in human females (Fox and Knaggs, 1969) and in goats (McNeilly and Folley, 1970). Human blood values demonstrated a prolonged release in connection with mating (McNeilly and Folley, 1970), which is in contrast to the spurt-like release during milk ejection (see Lactation). In various species, spermatozoa ascend faster than can be accounted for by their flagellate activity (*e.g.* Fox *et al.*, 1970). The search for a physiological role of posterior lobe hormone release during mating has been concentrated, therefore, on the promotion of sperm transport by oxytocin (*e.g.* Mroueh, 1967; Morton, 1969). However, Coutinho (1970) showed that during the fertile period of the human menstrual cycle the uterus is refractory to oxytocin, whereas the fallopian tubes are very sensitive to this hormone during the entire menstrual cycle. This suggests that, at least in the human, oxytocin could not be of physiological importance in facilitation of sperm transport following uterine stimulation. Vasopressin, on the other hand, appeared to be a very potent myometrial stimulant. On the basis of sensitivity to posterior lobe hormones, therefore, vasopressin is more likely to stimulate the uterus and so facilitate the initial sperm ascent, whereas oxytocin might facilitate either sperm migration into the tubes or egg passage towards the uterus (Coutinho, 1970).

A sharp fall in uterine pressure, possibly causing sperm to be sucked inwards, has been reported following female orgasm (Fox *et al.*, 1970). It seems of interest to investigate whether this pressure fall is caused by a release of vasopressin, since administration of this hormone can produce a similar pressure drop (Coutinho, 1970).

Partly as a result of methodological problems (see below), it is not known whether destruction of the HNS impairs fertility. Until this kind of experiment has been carried out, no definite role in the physiology of reproduction can be attributed to the release of the posterior lobe hormones during mating.

Male HNS

On an average, similar posterior lobe contents of oxytocin and of vasopressin are found in female and male individuals (see Fuchs and Saito, 1971), despite the fact that no role can yet be assigned to oxytocin in the male. Certain data point, however, to a relationship between this hormone and sperm transport in the male.

Afferent pathways to the HNS

The increased blood levels of oxytocin found already prior to coitus (see below) indicate a release mechanism of posterior lobe hormones comparable to that in the female (see Female HNS).

The HNS and peripheral effects

A release of posterior lobe hormones in relation to coitus appears from demonstrations of changes in urine flow and electrolytes balance, increased oxytocin levels in jugular blood of a male donkey immediate before coitus (see Fitzpatrick, 1966), and high oxytocin levels in blood from bulls immediately before and after service (Bereznev, 1963; cited by Knight and Lindsay, 1970). Fox and Knaggs (1969) however, failed to find any oxytocin activity in human male blood taken either shortly before or just after coitus.

Administration of oxytocin immediately before ejaculation increases the volume of semen expelled and the number of spermatozoa per ejaculate (Fjellström *et al.*, 1968; Knight and Lindsay, 1970), but this effect declines during long-term administration and spermatogenesis becomes impaired (Knight and Lindsay, 1970). The influence of posterior lobe hormones on the contractive activity of the vas deferens, ductus epididymis (Melin, 1970) and seminiferous tubules (Neimie and Kormano, 1965) can explain the immediate stimulatory effects of oxytocin. Nevertheless, for the same reasons as were given for the female HNS, the physiological meaning of these findings remain doubtful. This also applies to the higher motivation reported in the male for copulation after oxytocin administration (Melin and Kihlström, 1963; Fjellström *et al.*, 1968).

F. DUAL QUALITY OF STIMULI AFFECTING THE HNS

The factors that activate the HNS can be grouped into neural and hormonal sources of stimulation.

Neural stimuli can reach the HNS via either short (Fig. 2b) or long (Fig. 2a) pathways. Osmoreceptors which are situated in the immediate perinuclear zone of the SON (Hayward and Vincent, 1970) activate the SON neurones via short neural pathways (Fig. 2b). Factors affecting the HNS via long neural pathways (Fig. 2a) are, *e.g.*, suckling (see Lactation), genital stimuli (see Parturition) stimuli from peripheral osmotic receptors (Haberich, 1968), and pain (Covey and Moran, 1966; Ginsburg, 1968).

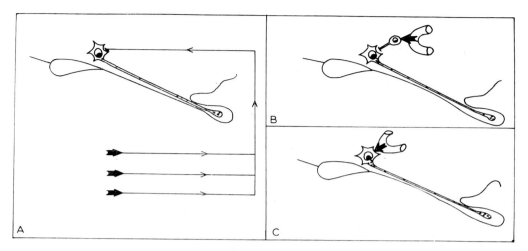

Fig. 2. The HNS is activated via long (a) and short (b) neural pathways and by hormonal (c) stimuli.

Hormonal stimuli (Fig. 2c) for the HNS are, *e.g.*, gonadectomy, early oestrus, light-induced persistent oestrus, and administration of gonadotropic hormones. These stimuli can all be explained by a direct stimulatory effect of gonadotropic hormones upon the hormone synthesizing activity of the neurosecretory cells (Swaab, 1970; Swaab and Jongkind, 1970a, b; 1971).

The activation of the magnocellular nuclei by these various kinds of stimuli does not involve activation of different cells within these nuclei. Rather the same cells become activated irrespective of the kind of stimulus (Swaab, 1970; Swaab and Jongkind, 1970b).

The subdivision into stimuli that affect the HNS by respectively neural and hormonal mechanisms reflects the dual quality of neurosecretory cells showing characteristics of neurones as well as of endocrine cells (*e.g.*, Scharrer, 1967; Stutinsky, 1970; Sawyer, 1970).

G. SOME METHODOLOGICAL PROBLEMS IN THE STUDY OF THE HNS

In the study of the physiological role of the HNS during the various reproductive stages it would be of great importance to be able to make observations following elimination of the HNS. *Lesion* studies involving the HNS are problematical however.

HNS function recovers soon after posterior lobectomy (Kawashima and Takasugi, 1968) or after stalk sectioning (Fendler *et al.*, 1970; Rodriguez and Dellmann, 1970), since the upper end of the stalk becomes reorganized into a "miniature neurohypophysis". Moreover, a large portion of PVN cells may not even innervate the neural lobe (Cross *et al.*, 1969). In addition, since islands of magnocellular elements are situated between the SON and PVN (Bodian and Maren, 1951) and even within the optic chiasm (Swaab, unpublished observations), elimination of all neurosecretory

analogues on the mammary gland. In *Handbook of Experimental Pharmacology*, *Vol. 23*, B. BERDE (Ed.), Springer, Berlin, Heidelberg, New York, pp. 475–544.

BISSET, G. W. AND CLARK, B. J. (1968) Synthetic 1-*N*-carbamylhemicystine-2-*O*-methyltyrosine-oxytocin (*N*-carbamyl-*O*-methyl-oxytocin): a specific antagonist to the actions of oxytocin and vasopressin on the uterus and mammary gland. *Nature (Lond.)*, **218**, 197–198.

BISSET, G. W., CLARK, B. J. AND ERRINGTON, M. (1969) The hypothalamic neurosecretory pathway for the release of oxytocin in the cat. *J. Physiol. (Lond.)*, **207**, 21P–22P.

BISSET, G. W., CLARK, B. J. AND HALDAR, J. (1970) Blood levels of oxytocin and vasopressin during suckling in the rabbit and the problem of their independent release. *J. Physiol. (Lond.)*, **206**, 711–722.

BODIAN, D. AND MAREN, TH. H. (1951) The effect of neuro- and adenohypophysectomy on retrograde degeneration in hypothalamic nuclei of the rat. *J. comp. Neurol.*, **94**, 485–511.

BOWER, E. A. (1959) Action potentials from uterine sensory nerves. *J. Physiol. (Lond.)*, **148**, 2P–3P.

BROOKS, C. McC., ISHIKAWA, T., KOIZUMI, K. AND LU, H. H. (1966) Activity of neurones in the paraventricular nucleus of the hypothalamus and its control. *J. Physiol. (Lond.)*, **182**, 217–231.

CHARD, T., BOYD, N. R. H., FORSLING, M. L., McNEILLY, A. S. AND LANDON, J. (1970) The development of a radioimmunoassay for oxytocin: the extraction of oxytocin from plasma, and its measurement during parturition in human and goat blood. *J. Endocr.*, **48**, 223–234.

CLEVERLEY, J. D. (1968) The detection of oxytocin release in response to conditioned stimuli associated with machine milking in the cow. *J. Endocr.*, **40**, 2P–3P.

CLEVERLEY, J. D. AND FOLLEY, S. J. (1970) The blood levels of oxytocin during machine milking in cows with some observations on its half-life in the circulation. *J. Endocr.*, **46**, 347–361.

CLEVERLEY, J. D., KNAGGS, G. S., TINDAL, J. S. AND TURVEY, A. (1968) Blood milk ejection activity after hypothalamic stimulation in the goat. *J. Endocr.*, **42**, 609–610.

COBO, E. (1968) Uterine and milk-ejecting activities during human labor. *J. appl. Physiol.*, **24**, 317–323.

COBO, E., DE BERNAL, M. M., QUINTERO, C. A. AND CUADRADO, E. (1968) Neurohypophyseal hormone release in the human. III. Experimental study during labor. *Amer. J. Obstet. Gynec.*, **101**, 479–489.

COBO, E., DE BERNAL, M. M., GAITAN, E. AND QUINTERO, C. A. (1967) Neurohypophyseal hormone release in the human. II. Experimental study during lactation. *Amer. J. Obstet. Gynec.*, **97**, 519–529.

COUTINHO, E. M. (1970) Effects of vasopressin and oxytocin on the genital tract of women. In *Proceedings of the Sixth World Congress on Fertility and Sterility, Tel Aviv, 1968.* The Israel Academy of Sciences and Humanities, Jerusalem, pp. 182–188.

COVEY, T. H. AND MORAN, W. H. (1966) Effect of cutaneous stimulation on blood antidiuretic hormone levels. *Surg. Forum*, **17**, 44–46.

CROSS, B. A. (1958) On the mechanism of labour in the rabbit. *J. Endocr.*, **16**, 261–271.

CROSS, B. A. (1966) Neural control of oxytocin secretion. In *Neuroendocrinology, Vol. 1*, L. MARTINI AND W. F. GANONG (Eds.), 217–259.

CROSS, B. A., NOVIN, D. AND SUNDSTEN, J. W. (1969) Antidromic activation of neurones in the paraventricular nucleus by stimulation in the neural lobe of the pituitary. *J. Physiol. (Lond.)*, **203**, 68–70.

CSAPO, A. (1969) The four direct regulatory factors of myometrial function. In *Progesterone: Its Regulatory Effect on the Myometrium*, G. E. W. WOLSTENHOLME AND J. KNIGHT (Eds.), Churchill, London, pp. 13–42.

DANIEL, A. R. AND LEDERIS, K. (1966) Effects of ether anaesthesia and haemorrhage on hormone storage and ultrastructure of the rat neurohypophysis. *J. Endocr.*, **34**, 91–104.

DATTA, H. AND CHAUDHURY, R. R. (1968) The antidiuretic hormone blocking effect of some oxytocin analogues. *J. Endocr.*, **42**, 345–346.

DEBACKERE, M., PEETERS, G. AND TUYTTENS, N. (1961) Reflex release of an oxytocic hormone by stimulation of genital organs in male and female sheep studied by a cross-circulation technique. *J. Endocr.*, **22**, 321–334.

DEIS, R. P. (1968) Oxytocin test to demonstrate the initiation and end of lactation in rats. *J. Endocr.*, **40**, 133–134.

DESCLIN, L. (1969) Hypothalamic control of lactation. In *The Hypothalamus*, W. HAYMAKER, E. ANDERSON AND W. J. H. NAUTA (Eds.), Thomas, Springfield, pp. 431–463.

FENDLER, K., VERMES, I., STARK, A., ENDRÖCZI, E. AND LISSÁK, K. (1970) Effect of cervical sympathectomy on the development of a "miniature posterior lobe" after pituitary stalk section. *Acta physiol. Acad. Sci. hung.*, **37**, 175–176.

FERGUSON, J. K. W. (1941) A study of the motility of intact uterus at term. *Surg. Gynec. Obstet.*, **73**, 359–366.

FINDLAY, A. L. R. (1966) Sensory discharges from lactating mammary glands. *Nature (Lond.)*, **211**, 1183–1184.

FINDLAY, A. L. R. (1968) The effect of teat anaesthesia on the milk-ejection reflex in the rabbit. *J. Endocr.*, **40**, 127–128.

FITZPATRICK, R. J. (1966) The posterior pituitary gland and the female reproductive tract. In *The Pituitary Gland, Vol. 3*, G. W. HARRIS AND B. T. DONOVAN (Eds.), Butterworths, London, pp. 453–504.

FITZPATRICK, R. J. (1969) In *Progesterone: Its Regulatory Effect on the Myometrium*, G. E. W. WOLSTENHOLME AND J. KNIGHT (Eds.), Churchill, London, p. 172 (discussion).

FJELLSTRÖM, D., KIHLSTRÖM, J. E. AND MELIN, P. (1968) The effect of synthetic oxytocin upon seminal characteristics and sexual behaviour in male rabbits. *J. Reprod. Fert.*, **17**, 207–209.

FLAMENT–DURAND, J. (1967) Contributions à l'étude de la neurosécrétion chez le rat par la méthode autoradiographique. In *Neurosecretion*, F. STUTINSKY (Ed.), Springer, Berlin, pp. 60–76.

FOLBERGROVÁ, J., LOWRY, O. H. AND PASSONNEAU, J. V. (1970) Changes in metabolites of the energy reserves in individual layers of mouse cerebral cortex and subjacent white matter during ischaemia and anaesthesia. *J. Neurochem.*, **17**, 1155–1162.

FOLLEY, S. J. (1969) The milk-ejection reflex: a neuroendocrine theme in biology, myth and art. *J. Endocr.*, ix–xx.

FOX, C. A. AND KNAGGS, G. S. (1969) Milk-ejection activity (oxytocin) in peripheral venous blood in man during lactation and in association with coitus. *J. Endocr.*, **45**, 145–146.

FOX, C. A., WOLFF, H. S. AND BAKER, J. A. (1970) Measurement of intra-vaginal and intra-uterine pressures during human coitus by radio-telemetry. *J. Reprod. Fert.*, **22**, 243–251.

FUCHS, A.–R. (1966) Studies on the control of oxytocin release at parturition in rabbits and rats. *J. Reprod. Fert.*, **12**, 418.

FUCHS, A.–R. AND WAGNER, G. (1963) Quantitative aspects of release of oxytocin by suckling in unanaesthetized rabbits. *Acta endocr. (Kbh.)*, **44**, 581–592.

FUCHS, A.–R. AND POBLETE, V. F. (1970) Oxytocin and uterine function in pregnant and parturient rats. *Biol. Reprod.*, **2**, 387–400.

FUCHS, A.–R. AND SAITO, S. (1971) Pituitary oxytocin and vasopressin content of pregnant rats before, during, and after parturition. *Endocrinology*, **88**, 574–578.

FUCHS, F. (1969) In *Foetal Autonomy*, G. E. W. WOLSTENHOLME AND M. O'CONNOR (Eds.), Churchill, London, pp. 233–234 (discussion).

FUCHS, F., FUCHS, A.–R., POBLETE, V. F. AND RISK, A. (1967) Effect of alcohol on threatened premature labor. *Amer. J. Obstet. Gynec.*, **99**, 627–637.

GABE, M., SCHRAMM, B. ET TUCHMANN–DUPLESSIS, H. (1968) Action d'un stéroide anticonceptionnel sur la voie neurosécrétrice hypothalamo-neurohypophysaire de la ratte albinos. *C.R. Soc. Biol. (Paris)*, **162**, 375.

GINSBURG, M. (1968) Production, release, transportation and elimination of the neurohypophysial hormones. In *Handbook of Experimental Pharmacology, Vol. 23*, B. BERDE (Ed.), Springer, Berlin, Heidelberg, New York, pp. 286–371.

HABERICH, F. J. (1968) Osmoreception in the portal circulation. *Fed. Proc.*, **27**, 1137–1141.

HALDAR, J. (1970) Independent release of oxytocin and vasopressin during parturition in the rabbit. *J. Physiol. (Lond.)*, **206**, 723–730.

HARRIS, G. W. (1947) The innervation and actions of the neurohypophysis; an investigation using the method of remote control stimulation. *Phil. Trans. B*, **232**, 385–441.

HARRIS, G. W. AND PICKLES, V. R. (1953) Reflex stimulation of the neurohypophysis (posterior pituitary gland) and the nature of posterior pituitary hormone(s). *Nature (Lond.)*, **172**, 1049.

HAYWARD, J. N. AND VINCENT, J. D. (1970) Osmosensitive single neurones in the hypothalamus of unanaesthetized monkeys. *J. Physiol. (Lond.)*, **210**, 947–972.

HELLER, H. (1959) The neurohypophysis during the estrous cycle, pregnancy and lactation. In *Recent Progress in the Endocrinology of Reproduction*, C. W. LLOYD (Ed.), Academic Press, New York, London, pp. 365–387.

HINDSON, J. C., SCHOFIELD, B. M. AND TURNER, C. B. (1968) Parturient pressures in the ovine uterus. *J. Physiol. (Lond.)*, **195**, 19–28.

HINDSON, J. C., SCHOFIELD, B. M. AND WARD, W. R. (1969) The effect of progesterone on recorded parturition and on oxytocin sensitivity in the sheep. *J. Endocr.*, **43**, 207–215.

HIRONO, M., IGARASHI, M. AND MATSUMOTO, S. (1970) Short- and auto-feedback control of pituitary FSH secretion. *Neuroendocrinology*, **6**, 274–282.

244

SLOPER: What other enzymes did you study by means of the cytochemical technique?

SWAAB: This work has been done by Dr. Jongkind. Perhaps he wants to comment on this point.

JONGKIND: By means of the microchemical procedure we found in the stimulated supraoptic nucleus a slight increase in glucose-6-phosphate dehydrogenase activity. Golgi apparatus enzymes increased about 40% already after 3 days of water deprivation.

SLOPER: What other Golgi-apparatus enzymes did you study?

JONGKIND: UDP-phosphohydrolase, GDP-phosphohydrolase and IDP-phosphohydrolase, which showed about the same increase as TPP-ase.

Neuroendocrine Adaptation

P. G. SMELIK

Department of Pharmacology, Free University, Amsterdam (The Netherlands)

Neuroendocrinology, the field which is covered by this conference, has been a rapidly expanding science during the last decades. This can be said, however, of many scientific areas; witness the enormous and terrifying hypertrophy of scientific literature. Neuroendocrinology is also an intriguing science, most of all because within this discipline endocrinology has become part of the neurosciences, which study the regulation and integration of the systems serving self-preservation and preservation of the species. In this field neuroanatomy, neurochemistry, neurophysiology, neuro-endocrinology, neuropharmacology and behavioural sciences come together, forming an interdisciplinary scientific activity of great interest.

It is in this context that the word "adaptation" receives its modern meaning. The concept of adaptation has been slowly accepted, and it still has different meanings. If adaptation is essentially an active change of the organism in response to stimuli from the environment, the word can be and has been used for the concept that evolution can best be explained by the existence of mechanisms which adapt the body to resist abnormal environmental conditions. In Darwinism this meant that successful adaptation resulted in survival, and failure resulted in death. In this sense, adaptation to the demands of the environment has become a guiding principle in evolutionary and Marxist philosophy. Evolutionary adaptation is a slow process, thought to be progressive and including changes in the genetic pool over many generations.

Adaptation nowadays is often associated with ecological adjustments of individuals or populations to a rather extreme and hostile environment, such as high or low temperatures, lack of oxygen, low atmospheric pressure, radiation, etc. Section 4 of the Handbook of Physiology is called "Adaptation to the Environment", but it is completely devoted to adaptation in this sense. To quote from the Preface: ". . . the scope will extend from bacteria to mammals, from the deep sea to the upper atmosphere, from dark caves to intense sunlight, from the arctic winter to the tropical rain forest".

In this lecture we will restrict ourselves to another type of adaptation: the rapid adjustment to stimuli from the normal environment, as they can occur in the everyday life of any organism.

The dynamic equilibrium of living cells presupposes the capacity for adjusting all physiological processes to the changing demands of the environment. This adjustment can be quickly made and is of a temporary nature: the organism is capable of following

medullary hormones do not play a crucial role in the activation of the pituitary-adrenal axis. The stimulating effect of adrenaline on this system is a puzzling phenomenon, since there are several indications that, in contrast, an adrenergic inhibition of ACTH release may exist.

There is one feature which may give us some valuable information in this respect: it appears that the posterior part of the hypothalamus is involved in the activation of the sympathetic-adrenomedullary pathway.

In contrast, there are several indications that the anterior part is involved in the regulation of ACTH secretion. In the rat, the placement of lesions or corticoid implants in the antero-basal area appears to be most effective.

Several workers (Ranson and Magoun, 1939; Hess, 1949; Gellhorn, 1957) have suggested a sort of balance between these two areas of the hypothalamus, which roughly corresponds with the division in an ergotropic or sympathetic and a trophotropic or parasympathetic side. The suggestion of a more or less antagonistic function of the two hypothalamic areas may be applicable to the regulation of the adaptive mechanism. Such an antagonism would render it unlikely that both areas are activated simultaneously, because a mutual inhibition would exist. However, if activation of one component would precede that of the other one, such an arrangement would be meaningful.

There are some arguments in favour of the idea. In the first place it is very likely that adrenomedullary secretion precedes ACTH secretion, because the adrenal medulla is activated by a purely neural reflex, whereas for ACTH release a neurohumoral link is involved. The reflex adrenaline discharge is a very fast phenomenon, as anybody can experience who is startled by a sudden frightening event. This reaction is identical to the so-called "alarm reaction" of Selye, and is followed by a counterphase which is marked by the subsequent adrenocortical secretion. Secondly, it would make sense (and this has been pointed out by several workers) that glucocorticoids act to prevent eventual damage, provoked by overactivity of the sympathetic system. This would also place the pituitary–adrenal system at the trophotropic side, as a system which would serve to restore the balance of the internal environment. Thirdly, there are some indications that the control of ACTH has a cholinergic component, since atropine implants in the anterior part of the hypothalamus rapidly block stress-induced ACTH secretion (Hedge and Smelik, 1968).

Moreover, a central adrenergic inhibition on ACTH release seems to be localized within the posterior hypothalamus (Smelik, 1959). Although we have not been able to find clear indications for an adrenergic character of such an inhibition (Fig. 1), others have collected several pieces of evidence in favour of this idea (see Marks *et al.*, 1970; Ganong, in this symposium).

If we would accept this idea of cholinergic stimulation and adrenergic inhibition of ACTH secretion, then this is certainly but a part of the story. However, it would imply that the alarm reaction starts off with activation of posterior hypothalamic centers, resulting in reflex adreno–medullary discharge of catecholamines. This would be followed by activation of the anterior hypothalamus causing the release of ACTH and adrenocortical secretion.

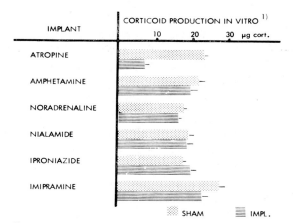

1) 1 hr after implantation under Nembutal anesthesia

Fig. 1.

Although stimulation of the adrenal glands certainly can be considered as the central event in neuroendocrine adaptive reflexes, it is probable that other hormones are also involved. Stressful stimuli have been reported to cause a rapid release of vasopressin from the posterior lobe, and of growth hormone and prolactin from the anterior lobe of the pituitary. It is possible that the adaptive reaction consists of a genetically fixed pattern of release of a number of pituitary hormones, and it would be interesting to know how a coupling between the secretion of different pituitary hormones is effectuated in the hypothalamus. In this respect, neurotransmitter systems may play an important role, and it is suggestive, that *e.g.* the control of ACTH seems to have a (muscarinic) cholinergic link, and vasopressin a (nicotinic) cholinergic control (Walker, 1957), and that dopamine recently has been reported to induce the concomitant release of LH-RF, FSH-RF and PIF (Kamberi *et al.*, 1971). It could be speculated, therefore, that neurotransmitters may translate the code for the release pattern of the hypophysiotropic factors.

Moreover, it should be realized that the neuroendocrine adaptation reflex is only the vegetative and metabolic coordinate which accompanies adaptive behaviour. The behavioural responses to imminent danger, like avoidance or flight, defense or attack, originate also from the hypothalamus, as the pioneer work of Hess has shown. Simple electrical stimulation of different areas of the hypothalamus can provoke affective behaviour, and these areas have been mapped out in several species, most extensively in the cat. From this work it became clear that the autonomic and endocrine reactions are part of behavioural patterns, and that the integration and coordination of this complex, innate adaptive response is situated in the hypothalamus. The correlation of neuroendocrine function with emotional behaviour is of great interest to current medicine, particularly in the field of psychosomatics.

In this connection the concepts of "emergency" and "stress" should be mentioned again. It can be asked whether the adrenal medulla only comes into play in cases of emergency as Cannon thought, and whether the adrenal cortex is activated only by noxious stimuli. The answer must be that minor stimuli which occur in everyday life, already stimulate this system. This has been recognized much later. It could happen some twenty years ago, that animals were transferred to the experimental room to undergo a stressful procedure, and that the experimenters were not aware of the fact that the simple opening of the cage and handling had already activated the adrenal system. It appeared that actually not only the harmful stimulus or the life-endangering situation elicits the adaptive reflex, but the *anticipation* of danger already triggers off the alarm reaction. This anticipation, which is of course of utmost importance for survival in wild animals, is called fear in humans. Fear, and its correlate in more chronic situations of potential danger, anxiety, appear to be the most potent elicitors of neuroendocrine adaptive reactions in man, and perhaps also in higher animals.

Now, here a complication arises, because anticipation is not always followed by the actual appearance of the danger or emergency situation. The organism can be mistaken in its expectancy, but the adaptive reflex has already occurred with its autonomic and metabolic consequences. We can be suddenly alarmed by a speeding car which comes very close to hitting us. The next moment we realize that there is no immediate danger, but our adrenals are already put to work. The body was ready for action, but no action was needed. Another situation seems to be even more frustrating: we would like to react behaviourally, be it attack or flight, but the socio-cultural pattern or our "Über-Ich" (super-ego) forbids the reaction. The repression of aggressive or defensive behaviour in our society is a well-known cause of psychosomatic diseases. Analogous situations have been found in animals.

It was one of the merits of Selye's stress concept that he paid attention to the consequences of overshoot of the adaptation mechanism. His "general adaptation syndrome" (G-A-S) was actually a pathological state, including symptoms like gastro-intestinal ulceration. It now seems that a frequent or continuous overactivity of the neuroendocrine adaptation mechanism can be harmful to the organism. In such cases the adaptive reflex should be dampened, and this is one of the main goals in psycho-pharmacology. It should be clear now that the attenuation of fear and anxiety, aggression and defense reactions by drugs must have its consequences for the neuro-endocrine corollaries; in other words, tranquillizing drugs can be expected to exert inhibiting actions also on the neuroendocrine system. Since most if not all of these drugs are known or suspected to act on central neurotransmission, it can be anticipated that the analysis of the interplay of the neuronal systems in the brain stem will be the central field of research for those disciplines which study the mechanisms for self-preservation and preservation of the species.

REFERENCES

GELLHORN, E. (1957) *Autonomic Imbalance and the Hypothalamus.* Univ. of Minnesota Press, Minneapolis.
GUILLEMIN, R. (1955) A re-evaluation of acetylcholine, adrenaline, noradrenaline and histamine as possible mediators of the pituitary-adrenal-corticotrophic activation by stress. *Endocrinology*, **65**, 248–255.

HEDGE, G. A. AND SMELIK, P. G. (1968) Corticotropin release: inhibition by intrahypothalamic implantation of atropine. *Science*, **159**, 891–892.

HESS, W. R. (1949) *Das Zwischenhirn: Syndrome, Lokalisationen, Funktionen*, Schwabe, Basel.

KAMBERI, I. A., MICAL, R. S. AND PORTER, J. C. (1971) Effect of anterior pituitary perfusion and intraventricular injection of catecholamines on prolactin release. *Endocrinology*, **88**, 1012–1020.

MARKS, B. H., HALL, M. M. AND BHATTACHARYA, A. N. (1970) Psychopharmacological effects and pituitary–adrenal activity. In *Progress in Brain Research, Vol. 32, Pituitary, Adrenal and The Brain*, D. DE WIED AND J. A. W. M. WEIJNEN (Eds.), pp. 57–70.

McDERMOTT, W. V., FRY, E. G., BROBECK, J. R. AND LONG, C. N. H. (1950) Mechanism of control of adrenocorticotrophic hormone. *Yale J. Biol. Med.*, **23**, 52–64.

RANSON, S. W. AND MAGOUN, H. W. (1939) The Hypothalamus. *Ergebn. Physiol.*, **41**, 56–163.

SMELIK, P. G. (1959) *Autonomic Nervous Involvement in Stress-Induced ACTH Secretion*. Thesis, Born, Assen.

SMELIK, P. G. (1960) Mechanism of hypophysial response to psychic stress. *Acta Endocr. (Kbh.)*, **33**, 437–443.

VOGT, M. (1951) The effect of emotion and of β-tetra-hydronaphthylamine on the adrenal cortex of the rat. *J. Physiol. (Lond.)*, **114**, 465–470.

WALKER, J. M. (1957) In The Neurohypophysis, H. HELLER (Ed.), Butterworths, London, pp. 221–229.

DISCUSSION

VAN DER SCHOOT: You spoke about experiments that were designed to determine the site of action of corticosteroids in the regulatory mechanism of the hypothalamus. Dr. Schadé has presented data in which he suggested that a fundamental pattern in the regulatory mechanism would be neurons which show a particular background activity which may be influenced by a number of factors. I see a minor discrepancy; there seem to be many sites of action on a particular neuron which are not primarily concerned with the regulation of a particular level of a circulating hormone, but which are regulated by a synaptic input from various neural pathways.

SMELIK: It cannot be denied that there is a very general action of steroids of different nature on neurons. There are well-known examples of this: the anaesthetic effect of the various steroids, effects on the conduction of nerve fibres in the spinal cord and so on. When you study such effects you are bound to find changes in the electrical activity of neurons. The case here is, that there must be some effect on top of this, such as a specific sensitivity of particular neurons to particular steroids. There are many indications in the literature about specific sites of actions and also of a specific influence on certain structures. It is very difficult to visualize what exactly the mechanism of such an influence is. You could think of a situation that either the steroids have a specific effect on the sensitivity of the cell body for incoming stimuli, or, according to the concept of Dr. Schadé, that there is first a penetration of the steroid into the cell body which results in a secondary effect on the neuronal membrane. There are indications in the literature for both concepts.

BERN: You could say that there is a problem distinguishing between the general effects that agents have and the specific effects which make certain centers really estrogen-sensitive or really corticoid-sensitive.

SMELIK: Yes, I think that is one of the main difficulties in experimentation in this field.

SCHADÉ: In the rat and snail brain there is only a very small percentage of cells that show a specific sensitivity to a particular corticosteroid. Our data did not exclude the presence of specific receptors in or on neuronal membranes.

GOLDFOOT: I would like to ask a question about the reserpine implantation. Is it not true that systemically administered reserpine results in a large ACTH release? Your interpretation seems to indicate a locus which responded in a positive fashion.

SMELIK: There are two things. If you give reserpine systemically it apparently turns on the system. The result is that one observes an activation of the pituitary–adrenal system. After a longer period of time, however, it is going to depress the system. It is a sort of biphasic response. The general idea behind the concept is that the first or single injection of such a drug would represent a sort of stressful stimulus. I believe that this is not very likely for several reasons. An injection of reserpine induces a rather sustained hypersecretion of ACTH. It was then assumed that reserpine would have a specific action on catecholamines in the brain stem and therefore would be able to induce the hypersecretion. If it would be true that reserpine depletes catecholamines resulting in a long-lasting hypersecretion of ACTH, then apparently some kind of an inhibition would have been removed. At the time this theory was proposed I thought that the dopaminergic system in the hypothalamus was responsible for this mechanism. My reasoning was that if you deplete the neurons locally with reserpine so that they cannot function anymore, then reserpine should not act anymore when given systemically. I took animals with a local implantation of reserpine and then injected reserpine systemically, and got exactly the same hypersecretion of ACTH.

FINDLAY: There is an effect of frontal lobectomy on anxiety. Have you any idea of the pathways or mechanisms by which that can be achieved?

SMELIK: No, that is too difficult a question for me.

STOECKART: I always have difficulties with the terminology about stress or stress response. Is a stress response the combination of corticosteroid release, and adrenal catecholamine release?

SMELIK: In talking about stress one should consider every aspect of the system that is activated. I think we have used the word stress very loosely during the years like we do with words like feedback and so on. Originally, the idea was that stress is the result of the pressure from outside and the resistance from inside. The resultant then is called stress. When you are going to talk about major stress and minor stress, one will experience that minor stressors are actually very normal emotional stimuli which can happen a few times per hour. In that case there is no use in talking about stress anymore. When you are considering the activity of a particular neuronal system, it would be wise to forget the whole concept of stress. It has done some harm to use the word stress or the concept of stress without sticking to the definition of Selye. The term has been applied to many situations which he would not have called stress.

SCHADÉ: I assume that in your conceptional model of hypothalamic regulatory mechanisms stress is one part of the balancing system. In order to test the negative sign in your model the animals must be made very happy. In order to answer the question of the previous speaker, one should attempt to design an experimental situation in which "negative stress" may be tested.

SMELIK: I do not think this is a crazy idea at all, I think it is a very good idea. There have been very few studies in this direction of which I like to mention self-stimulation. I don't know the details but certainly effects on the pituitary adrenal system were found which point to this direction.

BERN: It seems to me that the most valuable thing to do with this kind of diagram is to obliterate the term stress or stress response. If you start to talk about coordinated responses that involve the hypo-thalamo-pituitary system then I think we have a basis for a lot of physiological investigation and discussion. Please let me add just one more point. If the system is correct one is obliged to ask questions, such as: what profit will the animal have from more prolactin or more MSH. The comparative endocrinologist will tell you that prolactin is very important in fishes and birds in regard to mineral metabolism. Recently Ramsay investigated the relationship between prolactin and the internal water movement in laboratory rat. He showed a definite relationship. This is not just a coincidence that is of no use to the organism.

SMELIK: I think it is true what you said, although I don't believe that every hormone which is secreted should have a function. I am not inclined to say that prolactin must have a function because, otherwise, it would not have been secreted. I think we should not be ashamed if we have to say that MSH or prolactin is released but has no specific function at a particular moment. But the compounds are always secreted simultaneously because that is the genetically fixed pattern.

BERN: But one can always ask the question: why a genetically determined pattern?

recessus preoptici), though in respect of granule size there may be differences. Vigh *et al.* (1967) suggest that the posterior recess first described in selachian fishes by Dammerman (1910) should be considered as a part of the paraventricular organ and it is, therefore, relevant to note the structure of this region.

Van de Kamer (1955), in a careful optical microscope study, showed that in this organ many fine protuberances project into the ventricle and that capillaries are abundant close to the ventricular surface. He suggested that these features indicated some kind or resorption from the CSF.

Electron microscopy of the posterior recess of *Scylliorhinus* (Knowles, Meurling and Vollrath, in preparation) has demonstrated some dense-core-vesicle-containing cells which are innervated, others which are apparently not, and ependymal cells with large electron-dense inclusions. The types thus far observed seem to resemble the elements present in *Xenopus* (Peute, 1969).

The paraventricular organ and pituitary function

Thus far, the evidence linking the paraventricular organ with pituitary activity depends mainly on anatomical connections which have been described. In the amphibians, for example, Goos and Van Halewijn (1968) have shown that a pair of fluorescent (catecholamine-containing) nuclei may be observed situated along the third ventricle. The rostral tip of each nucleus was situated at both ends of the entrance to the infundibular lumen. Goos and Van Halewijn suggested that this rostral tip may correspond to the *organon vasculosum hypothalami* as described in *Lacerta* by Braak (1968).

In his monograph on the nervous system of fishes, Sterzi (1909) depicted a nerve tract running from a nucleus adjacent to the posterior recess to the pituitary neuro-intermediate lobe. Goos (1969) was unable to trace fibres from the nuclei he studied to the pituitary intermediate lobe but he showed by ablation of the nuclei combined with reserpine injections that there is reason to believe that these nuclei affect colour change. If this is so, we may suspect the paraventricular organ of implication in pars intermedia function. Goos (1969) has suggested also that a possible gonadotropin-releasing activity of the paraventricular nuclei cannot be discounted.

Evidence for a vascular link between the paraventricular organ and the pituitary in fishes and amphibians is well-documented. Meurling (1967) has shown that a vein, draining the region of the posterior recess, passes to the pituitary pars intermedia. Dierickx *et al.* (1970) have shown in *Rana* that a branch of the encephalo-posthypophysial portal vein drains the paraventricular organ and, moreover, that pericapillary accumulation of monoamines may be demonstrated at the origin.

There are, therefore, suggestive lines of morphological evidence which point to a possible involvement of the paraventricular organ in pituitary pars intermedia function.

THE FLOOR AND VENTROLATERAL WALLS OF THE INFUNDIBULAR RECESS

There are indications that the cells lying in the floor of the infundibular recess differ from those in a slightly more lateral position. Tanycytes are present in both areas (Kobayashi et al., 1970), but "glandular" ependymal cells which are PAS-positive and appear to secrete into the CSF are characteristic of the mid-line lying less frequent laterally (Knowles, 1967). In a combined histochemical and electron microscopic study Leveque et al. (1967) showed that, in the posterior third of the infundibular recess of the rat, special ependymal cells stainable by PAS could be clearly distinguished. Two types were seen, one type more or less oval and with abundant cytoplasm; the other type was more elongated and less cytoplasm enveloped the nucleus. The authors remarked that basal prolongations were in general difficult to follow in the rat, but that in the mouse prolongations were seen to extend towards pituitary portal vessels close by the pars tuberalis. The authors suggested that the form and disposition of these special ependymal elements indicated a possible implication in pituitary control. They could be the source of "releasing factors". Knowles and Kumar (1969) also distinguished two kinds of cells in the *floor* of the infundibular recess of the rhesus monkey. One of these (Type C) formed a many-layered epithelium of loosely-packed cells with few secretory inclusions; the other type (Type C′) was scattered among the C cells and clearly distinguished from these by a strong affinity not only for connective tissue stains but also for silver stains; in this respect they differed from the normal ependyma and tanycytes in the area studied. Type C′ cells were degranulated at menstruation compared to their condition at other times during the cycle. Current work on the dogfish *Scylliorhinus* (Knowles, Meurling and Vollrath, in preparation) shows that in this species liquor-contacting neurones are found in the ependymal layer of the mid-line above the median eminence and there are some indications that these neurones, which are innervated by synapses with dense-core granules in the pre-synaptic region, may release their products into the ventricle.

It would be interesting to know whether the C′ cells described by Knowles and Kumar (1969) in the monkey could also be liquor-contacting neurones; their strong reaction to silver stains indicates this possibility.

In the selachian median eminence the character of the ependyma differs in anterior and posterior regions. As early as 1909, Sterzi drew attention to the unusual nature of the floor of the infundibular recess lying directly above the pituitary neuro-intermediate lobe of the pituitary in elasmobranch fishes and termed this the "hypophysial area". It was characterized by two kinds of ependymal elements; those which resemble tanycytes, and those which have little or no basal processes. These latter cells are filled with secretory granules.

Electron microscope observations on *Scylliorhinus* have shown that the "Sterzi cells" are filled with large electron-lucent vacuoles and contain also electron dense granules, variable in size ranging from 1400 Å–2000 Å (Knowles, 1970). The vacuolated nature of the "Sterzi cells" was also remarked upon by Van de Kamer and Verhagen (1955). The morphology of the "Sterzi cells" indicates that they secrete into the CSF.

In the eel most of the ependymal cells lining the fingerlike protrusions of the infundibular recess extending into the intermedia tissue contained electron-dense vesicles. These appeared to be associated with a PAS-positive substance, which was released into the ventricle when eels were maintained on an illuminated white (but not a black) background (Knowles and Vollrath, 1966).

Concurrently synaptoid junctions between Type A or peptidergic neurosecretory fibres and these secretory ependymal cells were found in white background (but not black background) animals. Knowles and Vollrath (1966) suggested that the ependymal elements might be concerned in a feedback regulation of the preoptic nucleus–pituitary system.

The ependymal cells lining the extensions of the infundibular recess into the neuro-intermediate lobe of the eel constitute the only recognizable pituicytes of this organ, and it is therefore of interest that Wittkowski (1967a, 1968) has described tanycyte ependyma in the posterior pituitary of the guinea pig and rat which receives synaptic innervation by Type A neurosecretory fibres. A distinction was made in the rat between "protosplasmic" glia which contained large osmiophilic granules and was innervated, and fibrous glia, which was not.

Wittkowski (1968) remarked that the "neuroglial" synapses occurred in the terminal area of the tractus tuberohypophyseus (outer layer of the median eminence), and in the terminal region of the tractus supraoptico-hypophyseus (posterior lobe). Some of the ependymal tanycytes thus innervated were in contact with the primary plexus of the pituitary portal system in the median eminence and Wittkowski (1967b) suggested that these tanycytes might have a receptor function related to pituitary releasing factors.

A number of authors have described tanycytes which extend from the IIIrd ventricle lumen to the pituitary portal vessels in amphibians, reptiles and mammals (Rodriguez, 1972; Knowles and Kumar, 1969; for a review see Kobayashi et al., 1970). As Rodriguez (1972) has remarked, at present it is not possible to decide whether these cells are neurones, ependymal cells or special nervous elements representing an intermediate form. They are characterized by large microvilli, often bulbous in shape, projecting into the ventricle, and the presence of electron-dense inclusions in their perivascular end-feet (Knowles and Kumar, 1969; Scott et al., 1972). These morphological features have led investigators to postulate that these elements may absorb substances from the CSF and secrete into the pituitary portal vessels.

Recently, attention has been drawn to a somewhat different area of tanycytes which appear to be spatially related to the infundibular (arcuate) dorsomedial and centromedial nuclei. Bleier (1972) has described how processes of ependymal cells appear to form claws and networks which may encircle cells of these nuclei in rabbits, rats, mice and cats. One such element, which Bleier describes as a "spider cell", appears to be confined almost exclusively to the infundibular (arcuate) nucleus.

Halasz et al. (1962) depicted tanycytes in the ventrolateral wall of the IIIrd ventricle close to the arcuate and ventromedial nuclei and considered the possibility that they might in some way be related to control of pituitary gonadotropic function.

References p. 267

Ependyma in relation to pituitary gonadotropic function

Reference has already been made to the paper by Leveque (1972) in which he showed that cells in the preoptic recess of the female rat brain contains a PAS-positive material which increased greatly in young female rats injected with testosterone propionate on the fourth day. The increase continued until the twentieth day but thereafter the stainable substance became greatly reduced in amount and little or no stainable substance remained in these androgen-sterilized animals by an age equivalent to that of puberty.

Fluctuations in a PAS-positive substance in ependymal cells in relation to reproductive activity was also noted by Anand Kumar (1968). He found that in the rhesus monkey PAS-positive cells in the floor of the IIIrd ventricle showed considerable granular contents during the preovulatory phase of the menstrual cycle, but at menstruation the cells in question were degranulated. Ovariectomy led to a degranulation but this post-castration effect could be reversed by the administration of exogenous oestrogen.

Anand Kumar found that the PAS-positive cells he studied were also Gomori-positive; it is, therefore, of interest to note that a suggestion that Gomori-positive secretion by ependymal elements in the floor of the IIIrd ventricle appears in a paper by Vigh *et al.* (1963). It is not yet known whether the PAS-positive cells in the floor of the recess described by Anand Kumar (1968) secrete into the ventricle or blood capillaries, but Leveque (1972) indicated that those which were studied might secrete into a capillary network of the *organon vasculosum laminae terminalis*.

In contrast, certain ependymal elements which seem to bear some relation to reproductive function show clear morphological indications of secretion into vessels of the pituitary portal system. These, which penetrate the ventral and ventrolateral regions of the median eminence, have the form of tanycyte ependymal cells but some difficulty of nomenclature becomes evident when considering superficially similar elements which have been described by Knowles and Anand Kumar (1969), Kobayashi and Matsui (1969) and McArthur (1970) and shown to bear some relation to reproductive function. These authors have described the elements in question as tanycytes or ependymal cells, but the fact that Knowles and Anand Kumar, and Kobayashi and Matsui mention dence-core vesicles in the cells and, moreover, that Kobayashi and Matsui refer to a synaptic innervation of these cells might indicate that they have neuronal characteristics. Since, however, the name tanycyte ependymal cells has been used in the descriptions it will be retained here. The tanycytes suspected of possible control of pituitary GTH activity extend from the wall of the ventricle to the blood-vessels of the primary plexus of the pituitary portal system in close juxtaposition to the pars tuberalis. Occasionally some of the distal endings seemed to make direct synaptoid contacts with cells of the pars tuberalis (Knowles and Anand Kumar, 1969). Thus far, the elements described seem to have one important feature in common, namely that they respond to castration and/or fluctuations in the amounts of circulating sex hormones.

Knowles and Anand Kumar (1969) showed that bulbous ventricular protrusions of the tanycytes became especially large in female Rhesus monkeys at oestrous mid-cycle and regressed almost to extinction at or about menstruation. Ovariectomy led to the menstrual condition, but this could be prevented by oestradiol administration. Comparable results have been reported by Kobayashi and Matsui (1969) in the female rat. These authors found also that after ovariectomy cytoplasmic organelles and electron-dense bodies increased in size and amount in the tanycytes, an observation which is in contrast to the findings of Knowles and Anand Kumar (1969) who remarked that cytoplasmic inclusions were more abundant near mid-cycle in normal animals and more evident in oestradiol-injected animals than in castrates. As yet we have no information about the nature of the secretory material in the tanycytes and, therefore, any conclusions as to its significance would be premature.

In male monkeys the ependymal wall of the region studied was strikingly two-layered (single-layered in the females) with the tanycyte cell bodies at two levels separated by a space. After castration this arrangement was no longer evident. McArthur (1970), in a preliminary note, described changes in tanycyte ependymal cells in male rats, following castration. The changes observed (an increase in tubular formations and dilatations of smooth E.R., an increase in electron-dense vesicles, etc.) were interpreted as indicative of a considerable increase in synthesis and release of secretory products.

McArthur (1970), Kobayashi and Matsui (1969), and Kobayashi and Ishii (1969) describe axotanycytic synapses in the infundibulum though it is not entirely clear from their descriptions precisely where the tanycytes in question were located. Though Kobayashi and Ishii do refer to the "posterior region of the median eminence", Knowles and Kumar (1969) did not observe axotanycytic synapses, but clearly this question requires further study. Some difficulty in comparing results of different workers results from the often inadequate topographical descriptions. For example Hagedoorn (1965) reported that ependyma on the lateral walls of the IIIrd ventricle of the skunk showed seasonal changes in relation to the sexual activity of the animal, but the precise limits of the area she describes are not clearly defined. Jones (1967) reported some changes in tanycyte ependyma in relation to reproductive activity in the ferret and indicated an area close to the anterior opening of the infundibular recess, in the ventro-lateral wall. The area she depicted corresponds broadly to the circumscribed area described by Knowles and Kumar (1969) in the rhesus monkey. At present one can only remark that tanycytes which have shown alteration in relation to reproductive function lie in the hypophysiotropic area not far from the arcuate and ventromedial nuclei, but that there is a great need for a careful systematic morphological study of the floor and walls of the infundibular recess for, as Schiebler and Mitro (1968) have pointed out, a great many distinct areas may be recognized by appropriate histochemical methods.

It is interesting to compare Bleier's (1972) observation that specialized ependymal elements link the CSF and the arcuate nucleus with the experimental observation by Oksche et al. (1972) that 6 days after ovariectomy of the white-crowned sparrow (Zonotrichia leucophrys gambelii) an increase in nuclear volume occurs in the ependymal cells of the median eminence and arcuate nucleus regions, but that after 12 days only the ependymal nuclei of the median eminence return to their average size. The adjacent ependyma of the arcuate nucleus remains in its stimulated state. These results indicate that it is necessary to differentiate between the two ependymal regions, and point to a possibility that ependyma which link the CSF and the arcuate nucleus may play some part in the control of pituitary gonadotropic function.

DISCUSSION

Clearly, the ependymal wall of the hypothalamus is a mosaic of morphologically distinct elements. Some areas, it would seem, contain protrusions of cell bodies belonging to the magnocellular and parvocellular neurosecretory nuclei, which may be regarded as dendrites in contact with the CSF. There are indications also that part of the paraventricular organ, especially in lower vertebrates, consists of liquor-contacting neurones with dendritic (and possibly receptive) processes bathed by the CSF.

Many of the tanycyte ependyma which have terminal end-feet on pituitary portal vessels show bulbous protrusions into the CSF which might indicate absorption, and granules in their end-feet which might indicate secretion. Some cells of the paraventricular organ are similar in appearance.

There are, therefore, a number of elements in the hypothalamus which have a direct or indirect relationship with the pituitary, and are bathed by the CSF.

In 1959, Löfgren pointed out that the inflow of CSF into the IIIrd ventricle (from the lateral ventricles via the foramina of Monro) and the plexus chorioidei in its roof and its outflow via the aqueductus Sylvii are situated near the top of the ventricle and the currents must decrease towards the bottom. He suggested that the reduced flow of CSF in the recess would promote sedimentation of substances above its ventricular space and increased breadth of its floor just above the extension of the pars tuberalis. Löfgren noted, moreover, that capillary loops of the pituitary portal system are arranged in a wide meshwork just underneath the ependyma, an observation that has been greatly extended by Duvernoy and his colleagues (see Duvernoy et al., 1971). Based on these facts, a number of authors have inferred that the ependymal wall of the recess might play some part in an interchange of substances between the CSF, the pituitary, and its hypothalamic neurosecretory innervation. The presence of pituitary and gonadal hormones in the CSF has been demonstrated (Heller et al., 1968), and it has been shown that systemically ineffective amounts of a corticosteroid suppressed pituitary ACTH secretion when placed in the lateral ventricle, but not if placed adjacent to the ventricle (Kendall et al., 1969). There are, therefore, converging lines of evidence that indicate that hormones in the CSF may affect pituitary function and that modified ependymal elements may play some part in this process. Indeed, a possibility that the releasing factors, demonstrated by experimental means, might be present in ependymal elements cannot be discounted (Rodriguez, 1969; Knowles, 1970).

Certainly a number of neurosecretory and other elements which terminate in the pituitary or on blood vessels of the pituitary system are in intimate contact with the CSF. The possibility that these systems detect circulating hormones in the CSF and later secrete some factors regulating pituitary function merits serious attention (Knowles, 1972). In contrast to these elements there appears also to be some neurones or ependymal elements or forms intermediate between the two which, on morphological evidence, appear to discharge substances *into* the CSF. To this category belong the liquor-contacting neurones of the preoptic recess organ, the paraventricular organ and some cells in that portion of the infundibular recess adjacent to the pituitary pars nervosa. No satisfactory explanation of this possible secretion into the CSF has yet been forthcoming, though Knowles and Vollrath (1966) suggested that this activity might play some part in local feedback control of pituitary function. The number and the ubiquity of the liquor-contacting neurones and specialized ependymal elements in the ventral hypothalamus suggests that the composition of the CSF in the infundibular recess might differ greatly from that elsewhere in the brain, but unfortunately this question has not yet received attention. At present anatomical studies on ependyma have outpaced biochemical investigation.

The anatomical studies show the intimate relationships between specialized ependyma of the infundibular recess and the portal vessels supplying the pituitary. Moreover, correlations in structure of this ependyma and endocrine activity have been described. Nevertheless, the functional implications are far from clear. It has been suggested that ependymal cells might be involved in the production or transport of pituitary releasing factors and certainly this possibility must be borne in mind as the site of origin of releasing factors has not yet been identified. An alternative possibility is that the ependymal elements influence neurones which produce releasing factors. Until further investigations reveal the precise nature of the so-called secretory products which have been described in the specialized ependyma it is not possible to choose between these two alternatives. One can only meanwhile suspect the remarkable ependymal elements in the infundibular recess of an important role in the regulation of pituitary function.

REFERENCES

ANAND KUMAR, T. C. (1968) Modified ependymal cells in the ventral hypothalamus of the rhesus monkey and their possible role in the hypothalamic regulation of anterior pituitary function. *J. Endocr.*, **41**, 17–18 (Abstract).

ARIËNS KAPPERS, C. U. (1920) *Die vergleichende Anatomie des Nervensystems der Wirbeltiere und des Menschen, Vol. I.*, De Erven F. Bohn, Haarlem.

ARIËNS KAPPERS, C. U. (1921) *Die vergleichende Anatomie des Nervensystems der Wirbeltiere und des Menschen, Vol. II.* De Erven F. Bohn, Haarlem.

BERTLER, A., FALCK, B. AND VON MECKLENBERG, C. (1963) Monoaminergic mechanism in special ependymal areas in *Salmo irideus* L. *Gen. comp. Endocr.* **3**, 685–686.

BLEIER, R. (1972) Structural relationships of ependymal cells and their processes within the hypothalamus. In *Brain-Endocrine Interaction*, K. M. KNIGGE, D. E. SCOTT AND A. WEINDL (Eds.), Karger, Basel, pp. 306–318.

BRAAK, H. (1967) Elektronenmikroskopische Untersuchungen an Catecholaminkernen im Hypothalamus vom Goldfisch *(Carassius auratus)*. *Z. Zellforsch.*, **83**, 398–415.

BRAAK, H. (1968) Zur Ultrastruktur des Organon vasculosum hypothalami der Smaragdeidechse *(Lacerta viridis)*. *Z. Zellforsch.*, **84**, 285–303.

CAJAL, S. RAMÓN Y (1909) *Histologie du Système Nerveux de l'Homme et des Vertébrés. I. Généralités, Moelle, Ganglions Rhachidiens, Bulbe et Protubérance.* Maloine, Paris, 1909.

DAMMERMAN, K. W. (1910) Der Saccus vasculosus der Fische, ein Tiefeorgan. *Z. wiss. Zool.*, **96**, 654–726.

DIERICKX, K., GOOSSENS, M. AND DE WAELE, G. (1970) The vascularization of the Organon vasculosum Hypothalami of *Rana temporaria*. *Z. Zellforsch.*, **109**, 327–335.

DUVERNOY, H., KORITKE, J. G. ET MONNIER, G. (1971) Sur la vascularization du tuber postérieur chez l'homme et sur les rélations vasculaires tubéro-hypophysaires. *J. Neurovisc. Rel.*, **32**, 112–142.

FLEISCHHAUER, K. (1957) Untersuchungen am Ependym des Zwischen- und Mittelhirns der Land-schildkröte *(Testudo graeca)*. *Z. Zellforsch.*, **46**, 729–767.

FOX, C. A., DE SALVA, S., ZEIT, W. AND FISHER, R. (1948) Demonstration of supra-ependymal nerve endings in the third ventricle and synaptic terminals in the cerebral cortex. *Anat. Rec.*, **100**, 767.

FRONTERA, J. G. (1952) A study of the anuran diencephalon. *J. comp. Neurol.*, **96**, 1–69.

GOOS, H. J. TH. (1969) Hypothalamic control of the pars intermedia in *Xenopus laevis* tadpoles. *Z. Zellforsch.*, **97**, 118–124.

GOOS, H. J. TH. AND VAN HALEWIJN, R. (1968) Biogenic amines in the hypothalamus of *Xenopus laevis* tadpoles. *Naturwissenschaften*, **55**, 393–394.

HAGEDOORN, J. (1965) Seasonal changes in the ependyma of the third ventricle of the skunk, *Mephitis mephitis nigra*. *Anat. Rec.*, **151**, 453 (Abstract).

HALÁSZ, B., PUPP, L. AND UHLARIK, S. (1962) Hypophysiotropic area in the hypothalamus. *J. Endocr.*, **25**, 147–154.

HELLER, H., HASSAN, S. H. AND SAIFI, A. Q. (1968) Antidiuretic activity in the cerebrospinal fluid. *J. Endocr.*, **41**, 273–280.

HOFER, H. (1958) Zur Morphologie der circumventriculären Organe des Zwischenhirns der Säuge-tiere. *Verh. Dtsch. Zool. Ges. Frankfurt.* 202–251.

JONES, C. (1967) *Changes in Specialized Ependyma of the Ferret in Relation to the Oestrous Cycle.* Thesis presented for the degree of B.Sc. Birmingham University, Birmingham, England.

KAMBERI, I. A., MICAL, R. S. AND PORTER, S. C. (1969) Luteinizing hormone-releasing activity in hypophysial stalk blood and elevation by dopamine. *Science*, **166**, 388–390.

KENDALL, J. W., GRIMM, Y. AND SHIMSHAK, G. (1969) Relation of cerebrospinal fluid circulation to the ACTH-suppressing effects of corticosteroid implants in the rat brain. *Endocrinology*, **86**, 200–208.

KNIGGE, K. M. AND SCOTT, D. E. (1970) Structure and function of the median eminence. *Amer. J. Anat.*, **129**, 223–244.

KNOWLES, SIR F. (1967) Neuronal properties of neurosecretory cells. In *Neurosecretion*, F. STUTINSKY (Ed.), Springer, Berlin, pp. 8–19.

KNOWLES, SIR F. (1970) Ependymal secretion, especially in the hypothalamic region. *J. Neurovisc. Rel.* Suppl. 9, 97–110.

KNOWLES, SIR F. (1972) Concluding remarks. In *Internat. Symposium on Brain–Endocrine Interaction*, München, 1971, K. M. KNIGGE, D. E. SCOTT AND A. WEINDL (Eds.), Karger, Basel, 1971, p. 364–368.

KNOWLES, SIR F. AND ANAND KUMAR, T. C. (1969) Structural changes, related to reproduction, in the hypothalamus and the pars tuberalis of the Rhesus monkey. *Phil. Trans. B.*, **256**, 357–375.

KNOWLES, SIR F. AND VOLLRATH, L. (1966) Neurosecretory innervation of the pituitary of the eels *Anguilla* and *Conger*. *Phil. Trans. B*, **250**, 311–342.

KOBAYASHI, H. AND ISHII, S. (1969) The median eminence as storage site for releasing factors and other biologically active substances. In *Progress in Endocrinology*, *Proc. Third int. Congr. Endocrinol.*, *Mexico, 30 June–5 July, 1968*, pp. 548–554.

KOBAYASHI, H. AND MATSUI, T. (1969) Fine structure of the median eminence and its functional significance. In *Frontiers in Neuroendocrinology* W. F. GANONG AND L. MARTINI (Eds.), Oxford Univ. Press, London, pp. 3–46.

KOBAYASHI, H., MATSUI, K. AND ISHII, S. (1970) Functional electron microscopy of the hypothalamic median eminence. *Internat. Rev. Cytol.*, **29**, 281–381.

LEATHERLAND, J. F. AND DODD, J. M. (1969) Histology and fine structure of the pre-optic nucleus and hypothalamic tracts of the European Eel (*Anguilla anguilla.* L.). *Phil. Trans. B*, **256**, 135–145.

LEONHARDT, H. (1966) Über ependymale Tanycyten des III. Ventrikels beim Kaninchen in elektronen-mikroskopischer Betrachtung. *Z. Zellforsch.*, **74**, 1–11.

A more detailed investigation of the "contact" area yielded the following results:

A. After aldehyde fixation according to Karnovsky (1965) the membrane of the "presynaptic" element tends to show a few thickenings, which resemble dense projections of typical synapses. A "postsynaptic" thickening in the adjacent supporting cell cannot be observed (Fig. 3).

B. The Zn-I-OsO$_4$ method (Akert and Sandri, 1968; fixation as in A) brings about a heavy impregnation of the vesicles of the "presynaptic" element. A small number of the vesicles usually remains unstained (Fig. 4).

C. Bi-I impregnation (Pfenninger *et al.*, 1969; fixation as in A) reveals cone-shaped "presynaptic" dense projections (base about 400 Å, height about 500 Å) in the entire "presynaptic" area. A "postsynaptic" electron-opaque band is not observed. Instead, some paramembranous "postsynaptic" thickenings appear directly opposite the "presynaptic" dense projections. Sometimes they seem to attain the size of the latter, but their appearance is not uniform. In the synaptic cleft an electron-opaque line is seen, the double nature of which is most apparent below the "presynaptic" dense projections (Fig. 5a). In frontal sections the "presynaptic" dense projections occur in hexagonal patterns (Fig. 5b). The E-PTA method according to Bloom and Aghajanian (1966) yields the same results.

Compared to these synaptoid structures, the neuro-neuronal contacts at the CSF-contact neurones show a significant postsynaptic electron-opaque band in addition to presynaptic dense projections. Zn-I-OsO$_4$ impregnation stains the electron-lucent, but not the dense-core vesicles of these synapses.

DISCUSSION

CSF-contact neurones bearing similar contacts have been described in the ependyma of the ventricle and the central canal of numerous vertebrates, most recently by Peute (1971), Vigh *et al.* (1971) and Vigh–Teichmann *et al.* (1971). In fish, CSF-contact neurones have also been investigated electron-microscopically in the area of the nucleus recessus posterioris and lateralis hypothalami (Braak, 1967) and lateralis tuberis (Vigh–Teichmann *et al.*, 1970b). Their function is unknown. The significance of the "innervation" of glial cells in the CNS of vertebrates is not clear. It has to be ascertained, whether such morphological relationships may represent synapses in the sense of structures for the transmission of excitation.

A synaptoid type of innervation was found in studies of pituicytes of teleosts (for literature see Knowles, 1969). That this type of innervation occurs in vertebrates up to mammals was confirmed in more recent investigations (Wittkowski, 1967; Sterba and Brückner, 1969; Nakai, 1970; Zambrano, 1970; and others).

The innervation of the ependyma found by Rodríguez (1969) in the median eminence, and by Wittkowski (1969) in the infundibular recess, shows similar structural characteristics.

It should be noted that all these neuro-glial contacts show clear membrane thickenings only—if at all—in the presynaptic element. Similar contacts have also been

References p. 276

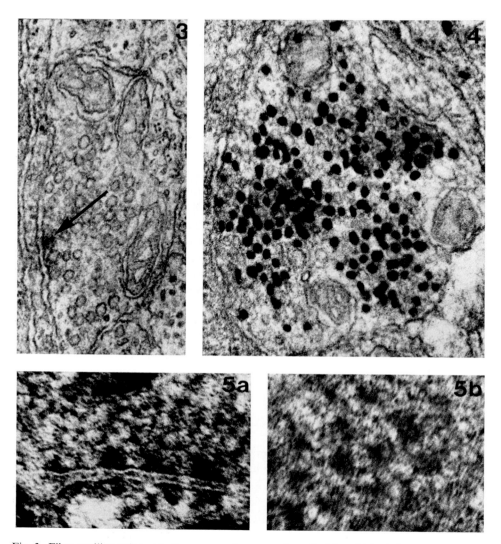

Fig. 3. Fibre swelling adjacent to the process of a supporting cell. After aldehyde fixation, membrane thickenings (↑) are scarcely observable. × 78 500.

Fig. 4. Vesicles in the fibre swellings are blackened after Zn-I-OsO₄ impregnation. × 78 500.

Fig. 5. Neuro-glial "contact" after Bi-I impregnation. a, In a transversal section, "presynaptic" dense projections, a line in the synaptic cleft, and small "postsynaptic" paramembranous thickenings are demonstrated. × 140 000. b, The hexagonal pattern of the "presynaptic" dense projections in a frontal section is shown. × 140 000.

reported on ependymal cells of the subcommissural organ (for literature see Diederen, 1970). Leonhardt and Backhus–Roth (1969) and Noack and Wolff (1970) observed synapse-like contacts between intraventricular axons and ependymal cells.

Even axon terminals, which do not border directly upon other cells (Leonhardt, 1970) or touch the basement membrane directly, as observed in the pulvinar of *Bombina* (Altner and Bayrhuber, 1969) or in the pituitary (Vollrath, 1967; and others), may show membrane thickenings like typical presynaptic knobs in addition to vesicles.

The interpretation of the relationship between neurones and glial cells in the saccus epithelium seems still more complicated: in contrast to the ependymal cells cited above, these ependymal cells contain only a small amount of cytoplasm seeming scarcely to possess the morphological precondition for an intense metabolic activity.

The innervation of the supporting cells present within the epithelium of the saccus vasculosus of the trout, according to Jansen and Flight (1969), which would be realized by conventional synapses could not be confirmed in the perch.

With the aid of the Zn-I-OsO_4 method, vesicles in the presynaptic elements of different tissues can be blackened. It is known, however, that this reaction occurs not only in synapses but also in other cytoplasmic structures like mitochondria, Golgi cisternae, smooth ER, MVB, etc. (Wienker, 1967; Niebauer *et al.*, 1969; Peute, 1971; Kolnberger, in press; Zimmermann, in preparation). Furthermore, this method does not supply direct evidence concerning the chemical nature of the material in the impregnated structures (Matus, 1970; and others). The vesicle impregnation in the terminal knobs in the saccus epithelium has to be considered also in the light of these limitations.

In all synapses, studied thus far, by means of the E-PTA or the Bi-I method (for literature see Bloom, 1970; Pfenninger, 1971) the postsynaptic band appears as a more or less uniform paramembranous thickening. This postsynaptic band is absent in the neuro-glial synaptoid contacts of the saccus vasculosus, although the axon terminal shows the typical arrangement of presynaptic dense projections. Therefore, the possibility of a particular relationship to the intercellular space giving access to the inner or outer cerebrospinal fluid spaces should be considered. On the other hand, the small thickenings of the "postsynaptic" membrane directly opposite to the "presynaptic" dense projections may be an indication of a functional relationship between the "pre-" and the "postsynaptic" element.

SUMMARY

The nerve fibre bundles in the epithelium of the saccus vasculosus in *Perca fluviatilis* contain three components.

1. Afferent fibres running to the hypothalamus proceed from the CSF-contact neurones which are situated between the coronet cells and the supporting cells of the saccus epithelium.

2. Efferent fibres terminate in synaptic contact with the perikaryon, the dendrite

or the axon of the CSF-contact neurones. The synapses show presynaptic dense projections and a postsynaptic band.

3. Other efferent fibres terminate along the surface of the bundles in large swellings which contact the surrounding supporting cells and are packed with electron-lucent vesicles. After aldehyde fixation, a few membrane thickenings are to be seen only in the "presynaptic" elements of these neuro-glial contacts. Bi-I and E-PTA impregnation reveal cone-shaped dense projections in a hexagonal pattern in the "presynaptic" element, but no "postsynaptic" band. The Zn-I-OsO$_4$ method brings about a heavy impregnation of the vesicles in the "presynaptic" element.

The possibility of a functional relationship of the latter fibre endings with the intercellular space, which is in open connection with the inner or outer cerebrospinal fluid spaces, is discussed.

REFERENCES

AKERT, K. AND SANDRI, C. (1968) An electron-microscopic study of zinc–iodide–osmium impregnation of neurons. I. Staining of synaptic vesicles at cholinergic junctions. *Brain Research*, 7, 286–295.

ALTNER, H. UND BAYRHUBER, H. (1969) Über den Charakter synaptoider Endstructuren markloser Fasern im Epiphysenpolster (Pulvinar corporis pinealis) der Gelbbauchunke (*Bombina variegata* L.). *Z. Zellforsch.*, **96**, 600–608.

ALTNER, H. UND ZIMMERMANN, H. (in press) The saccus vasculosus. In *The Structure and Function of Nervous Tissue*, G. H. BOURNE (Ed.), Academic Press, New York.

BLOOM, F. E. (1970) Correlating structure and function of synaptic ultrastructure, In *The Neurosciences, Second Study Program*, F. O. SCHMITT (Ed.), Rockefeller Univ. Press, New York, pp. 729–747.

BLOOM, F. E. AND AGHAJANIAN, G. K. (1966) Cytochemistry of synapses: selective staining for electron microscopy. *Science*, **154**, 1575–1577.

BRAAK, H. (1967) Elektronenmikroskopische Untersuchungen an Catecholaminkernen im Hypothalamus vom Goldfisch *(Carassius auratus)*. *Z. Zellforsch.*, **83**, 398–415.

DIEDEREN, J. H. B. (1970) The subcommissural organ of *Rana temporaria* L. A cytological, cytochemical and electronmicroscopical study. *Z. Zellforsch.*, **111**, 379–403.

JANSEN, W. F. AND FLIGHT, W. F. (1969) Light- and electronmicroscopical observations on the saccus vasculosus of the rainbow trout *(Salmo irideus)*. *Z. Zellforsch.*, **100**, 439–465.

KARNOVSKY, M. J. (1965) A formaldehyde–glutaraldehyde fixative of high osmolality for use in electron microscopy. *J. Cell Biol.*, **27**, 137A–138A.

KNOWLES, F. (1969) Ependymal secretion, especially in the hypothalamic region, *J. Neuro-Visc. Rel.*, Supp. IX, 97–110.

KOLNBERGER, I. (in press) Über die Zugänglichkeit des Intercellularraums und Zellkontakte im Riechepithel des Jacobsonschen Organs. *Z. Zellforsch.*

LEONHARDT, H. (1970) Über Plasmazellen im Nervengewebe (Eminentia mediana des Kaninchens). *Acta neuropath. (Berl.)*, **16**, 148–153.

LEONHARDT, H. UND BACKHUS-ROTH, A. (1969) Synapsenartige Kontakte zwischen intraventrikulären Axonendigungen und freien Oberflächen von Ependymzellen des Kaninchengehirns. *Z. Zellforsch.*, **97**, 369–376.

MATUS, A. J. (1970) Ultrastructure of the superior cervical ganglion fixed with zinc iodide and osmium tetroxide. *Brain Research*, **17**, 195–203.

NAKAI, Y. (1970) Electron microscopic observations on synapse-like contacts between pituicytes and different types of nerve fibres in the anuran pars nervosa. *Z. Zellforsch.*, **110**, 27–39.

NIEBAUER, G., KRAWCZYK, W. S., KIDD, R. AND WILGRAM, G. F. (1969) Osmium zinc iodide reactive sites in the epidermal Langerhans cells. *J. Cell. Biol.*, **43**, 80–89.

NOACK, W. UND WOLFF, J. R. (1970) Über neuritenähnliche intraventriculäre Fortsätze und ihre Kontakte mit dem Ependym der Seitenventrikel der Katze. Corpus callosum und Nucleus caudatus. *Z. Zellforsch.* **111**, 572–585.

PEUTE, J. (1971) Somato-dendritic synapses in the paraventricular organ of two anuran species. *Z. Zellforsch.*, **112**, 31–41.

PFENNINGER, K. H. (1971) The cytochemistry of synaptic densities. I. An analysis of the bismuth iodide impregnation method, *J. Ultrastruct. Res.*, **34**, 103–122.

PFENNINGER, K. H., SANDRI, C., AKERT, K. AND EUGSTER, C. H. (1969) Contribution to the problem of structural organization of the presynaptic area. *Brain Research*, **12**, 10–18.

RODRÍGUEZ, E. M. (1969) Ependymal specializations. I. Fine structure of the neural (internal) region of the toad median eminence, with particular reference to the connection between the ependymal cells and the subependymal capillary loops. *Z. Zellforsch.*, **102**, 153–171.

STERBA, J. UND BRÜCKNER, G. (1969) Elektronenmikroskopische Untersuchungen über die Reaktion der Pituicyten nach Hypophysenstieldurchtrennung bei *Rana esculenta. Z. Zellforsch.*, **93**, 74–83.

VIGH, B., VIGH–TEICHMANN, J. UND AROS, B. (1971) Ultrastruktur der spinalen Liquorkontaktneurone beim Krallenfrosch *(Xenopus laevis). Z. Zellforsch.*, **112**, 201–211.

VIGH–TEICHMANN, J., VIGH, B. UND AROS, B. (1970a) Enzymhistochemische Studien am Nervensystem IV. Acetylcholinesteraseaktivität im Liquorkontaktneuronensystem verschiedener Vertebraten. *Histochemie*, **21**, 322–337.

VIGH–TEICHMANN, J., VIGH, B. UND AROS, B. (1971) Liquorkontaktneurone im Nucleus infundibularis des Kükens. *Z. Zellforsch.*, **112**, 188–200.

VIGH–TEICHMANN, J., VIGH, B., UND KORITSÁNSZKY, S. (1970b) Liquorkontaktneurone im Nucleus lateralis tuberis von Fischen. *Z. Zellforsch.*, **105**, 325–338.

VOLLRATH, L. (1967) Über die neurosekretorische Innervation der Adenohypophyse von Teleostiern, insbesondere von *Hippocampus cuda* und *Tinca tinca. Z. Zellforsch.*, **78**, 234–260.

WIENKER, H. G. (1967) Elektronenmikroskopische Untersuchungen zur Spezifität der Osmium-Zink-Jodid-Methode. *Z. mikr.-anat. Forsch.* **76**, 70–102.

WITTKOWSKI, W. (1967) Synaptische Strukturen und Elementargranula in der Neurohypophyse des Meerschweinchens. *Z. Zellforsch.*, **82**, 434–458.

WITTKOWSKI, W. (1969) Ependymokrinie und Rezeptoren in der Wand des Recessus infundibularis der Maus und ihre Beziehung zum kleinzelligen Hypothalamus. *Z. Zellforsch.*, **93**, 530–546.

ZAMBRANO, D. (1970) The nucleus lateralis tuberis system of the gobiid fish *Gillichthys mirabilis*. II. Innervation of the pituitary. *Z. Zellforsch.*, **110**, 496–516.

ZIMMERMANN, H. UND ALTNER, H. (1970) Zur Charakterisierung neuronaler und gliöser Elemente im Epithel des Saccus vasculosus von Knochenfischen. *Z. Zellforsch.*, **111**, 106–126.

DISCUSSION

HAYWARD: I would like to know two things: What does the saccus vasculosus do and where do those nerve fibres go?

ZIMMERMANN: Both questions are very difficult to answer. The function of the organ is still unknown. There have been several attempts to draw up a concept, *e.g.* by Dr. Jansen from Utrecht who has spent several years studying the function of the saccus vasculosus, especially of the coronet cells. Dr. Jansen thinks that these elements could have some function in the ion exchange between the inner and outer cerebrospinal fluid. As far as your second question is concerned, I don't know where the axons of the liquor-contacting neurones end.

STOECKART: You showed in the axonal terminals, fixed with the conventional glutaraldehyde–osmium technique, small lucid vesicles and large granular vesicles. Do you think that this is in accordance with the Dale principle that means that a neurone can only synthetize one transmitter.

ZIMMERMANN: My personal experience is, that one should not put a specific functional label on neurones on the basis of a fixation method.

---

† Present address: Department of Pharmacology, Free University of Amsterdam, Amsterdam, The Netherlands.

region of the subcommissural area reduced aldosterone production, experimental nephrosis induced by puromycin administration in lesioned and sham-operated rats alike produced similar increases in aldosterone production, indicating that the zona glomerulosa responds in a normal fashion in rats bearing lesions in the subcommissural area.

After 1960, attention was focussed on the renin-angiotensin system as a major control mechanism for aldosterone secretion. Various groups at the same time showed that the octapeptide angiotensin II stimulates the secretion of aldosterone by a direct action on the zona glomerulosa (Carpenter *et al.*, 1961; Davis *et al.*, 1961a; Davis *et al.*, 1961b; Davis *et al.*, 1962; Ganong and Mulrow, 1961, 1962; Blair–West *et al.*, 1962; Ganong *et al.*, 1962; Kaplan and Bartter, 1962; Mulrow and Ganong, 1961, 1962; Mulrow *et al.*, 1962; Mulrow *et al.*, 1963). However, whereas most of these studies were done in dogs, sheep and man, attempts to demonstrate a similar effect of angiotensin II in rats were met with dubious success. Chronic administration (Gláz and Sugár, 1962) or high doses (van der Wal *et al.*, 1965) were required to induce a moderate stimulation of aldosterone secretion. Single doses of pressor quantities of angiotensin II failed to increase aldosterone secretion (Marieb and Mulrow, 1965) and infusions either produced an occasional elevation (Dufau and Kliman, 1966) or variable and non-dose dependent alterations in the secretion of this mineralocorticosteroid (Singer *et al.*, 1964; Marieb and Mulrow, 1965).

These results suggested that the zona glomerulosa of the sodium-replete rat is not very sensitive to angiotensin II. In fact, more recent studies showed that high sodium intake reduces (Dufau and Kliman, 1968; Dufau *et al.*, 1969) while low sodium intake enhances (Kinson and Singer, 1968) the sensitivity of the zona glomerulosa of the rat to angiotensin II. Similar effects of alterations in sodium intake have also been observed in dogs (Ganong, 1968). Our demonstration that cross-circulation between sodium-deficient rats with high aldosterone production rates and rats on a standard sodium-replete diet failed to affect the aldosterone production rates of the latter (Lee and de Wied, 1967) provided additional evidence suggestive of the relative refractoriness of the zona glomerulosa in the sodium-replete rat. This demonstration may be of particular significance because studies in animals with transplanted adrenals (Carpenter *et al.*, 1961) and cross-circulation experiments in sheep (Denton *et al.*, 1959) and dogs (Yankopoulos *et al.*, 1959) have clearly indicated the humoral nature of the mechanism(s) responsible for the control of aldosterone secretion.

Hypophysectomy in the dog (Davis *et al.*, 1960; Binnion *et al.*, 1965) and pituitary insufficiency in man (Lieberman and Luetscher, 1960; Dingman *et al.*, 1960) are known to reduce the normal rise in aldosterone secretion which occurs in response to dietary sodium restriction. This reduction is presumably the consequence of corticotropin (ACTH) deficiency since ACTH is known to stimulate aldosterone secretion in dogs (Ganong *et al.*, 1966), sheep (Blair–West *et al.*, 1962) and man (Tucci *et al.*, 1967), particularly during conditions of sodium deprivation in which the sensitivity of the zona glomerulosa is enhanced (Blair–West *et al.*, 1963; Ganong *et al.*, 1966). However, whether ACTH plays a definitive role in the control of aldosterone secretion is still a subject of intensive investigation. In the rat, at least, the possibility that ACTH may play an important role was first suggested by the work of Singer and Stack–Dunne (1954) who showed that ACTH administration effectively prevented the fall in aldosterone secretion which follows hypophysectomy in sodium-replete rats. In our studies in rats, maintained on a standard sodium-replete diet, aldosterone production *in vitro* was found to be slightly reduced by hypophysectomy, but not affected by procedures which mobilize endogenous ACTH (*e.g.*, exposure to ether) nor by nephrectomy (Csánky *et al.*, 1968). Administration of high doses of ACTH to acutely hypophysectomized rats similarly failed to affect the rate of aldosterone production. Only hypophysectomy and nephrectomy in the same animal induced a significant reduction in the production of aldosterone when studied 6 h after the operation. Similar findings were reported by others (Eilers and Peterson, 1964; Marieb and Mulrow, 1964, 1965; Cade and Perenich, 1965).

In view of the fact that sodium restriction in dogs (Blair–West *et al.*, 1963; Ganong *et al.*, 1965), man (Venning *et al.*, 1962) and rats (Müller, 1965) sensitizes the zona glomerulosa to ACTH, our subsequent experiments were performed in sodium-deficient rats (Csánky *et al.*, 1968). Acute hypophysectomy or nephrectomy caused no decrease in the elevated aldosterone production of sodium-deficient rats. However, 6 h after hypophysectomy and nephrectomy in the same animal a marked decrease in aldosterone production was observed, which was comparable to the decrease observed in rats on the standard sodium-replete diet. The intravenous administration of small amounts of ACTH in intact as well as hypophysectomized, sodium-deficient rats consistently induced a marked increase in the rate of aldosterone production (Fig. 1). Stress also caused an increase in the aldosterone production of sodium-deficient rats, and a correlation was found between the production of corticosteroids and aldosterone production *in vitro* suggesting that the increase in aldosterone secretion was due to an increase in circulating ACTH.

Further studies showed that the aldosterone- and glucocorticosteroid-stimulating

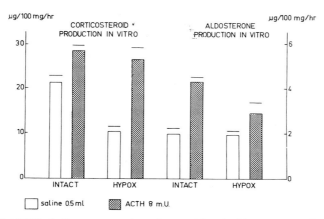

Fig. 1. Effect of ACTH challenge on total corticosteroid and aldosterone production *in vitro* by adrenals of sodium-deficient hypophysectomized rats. Animals were fed a low sodium diet for 2 weeks. Hypophysectomy was performed 24 h before the end of the experiment. ACTH was administered i.v. 15 min before decapitation. The data represent mean ± S.E.M. of 4–5 determinations.

activities of ACTH are apparently the inherent properties of the same part of the ACTH molecule (van der Wal and de Wied, 1968). Purified ACTH and synthetic β^{1-24} ACTH stimulated aldosterone as well as glucocorticosteroid production in sodium-deficient rats, but neither of the smaller synthetic ACTH-analogues studied, β^{1-16} ACTH and β^{1-10} ACTH, had any detectable steroidogenic effect.

Systemically administered angiotensin II also stimulated the production of aldosterone in sodium-deficient rats (van der Wal and de Wied, 1968). This effect, however, was most likely to have been mediated by pituitary ACTH-release, since prior hypophysectomy (24 h) or pretreatment with dexamethasone (16 h) prevented the aldosterone-stimulating effect of angiotensin II.

The significance of ACTH in the mechanism of aldosterone secretion in the sodium-deficient animal was further explored in "chronically" hypophysectomized rats. Hypophysectomy was performed on the 7th day of dietary sodium restriction and the animals were maintained postoperatively on the same low-sodium diet for an additional 7 days prior to study. Hypophysectomy not only prevented the increase in aldosterone production normally found in intact sodium-deficient rats, but also depressed the level of aldosterone production to below that of intact rats on a standard sodium-replete diet. Rats hypophysectomized for the same period but maintained on the standard diet showed a similar decrease in the rate of aldosterone production *in vitro* (Lee *et al.*, 1968). These findings are in accord with those of others who found that chronically hypophysectomized rats maintained on either a sodium-replete (Singer and Stack-Dunne, 1954, 1955; Venning and Lucis, 1962; Singer *et al.*, 1964) or sodium-restricted diet (Singer and Stack–Dunne, 1955) produced aldosterone *in vitro* and *in vivo* at rates lower than those of intact rats kept on a sodium-replete diet.

Experiments in adeno- and neurohypophysectomized rats indicated that the pituitary factor(s) required for a normal mineralocorticoid response to sodium restriction resided in the anterior pituitary (Lee *et al.*, 1968). Treatment of hypophysectomized sodium-deficient rats with long acting ACTH (β^{1-24} ACTH-Zn) in amounts which prevented adrenal atrophy did not restore aldosterone production to the levels of intact sodium-deficient rats. Moreover, whereas a challenging dose of 16 mU of ACTH given 15 min prior to decapitation elicited a normal glucocorticoid response, it failed to stimulate aldosterone production. On the other hand, treatment with anterior pituitary powder in quantities sufficient to prevent adrenal atrophy in the hypophysectomized sodium-deficient rat restored normal adrenal responsiveness, as evidenced by a normal aldosterone secretory response to the same challenging dose of ACTH. On the basis of these findings we then postulated the existence of a non-ACTH pituitary factor which, in addition to ACTH, plays a role in the control of aldosterone secretion. Studies in the rat by Palmore and Mulrow (1967) and in the dog by Ganong *et al.* (1966) also provided evidence for the existence of this factor.

Growth hormones (STH) of various species have been shown to prevent the reduction in the *in vitro* aldosterone production of chronically hypophysectomized sodium-replete rats when administered *in vivo* (Lucis and Venning, 1960; Venning and Lucis, 1962). It was possible, therefore, that STH might be the non-ACTH factor from the anterior pituitary whose presence is essential for the changes which enhance the sensitivity of the zona glomerulosa in response to sodium restriction (Lee and de Wied, 1968; Palkovits et al., 1970). Long term treatment with either an adrenal maintenance dose of ACTH or with growth promoting amounts of STH did neither restore adrenal responsiveness nor affect the low rate of aldosterone production of chronically hypophysectomized, sodium-deficient rats. However, when given simultaneously, ACTH and STH effectively restored the enhanced aldosterone secretory responsiveness which is characteristic of intact sodium-deficient rats (Fig. 2). These

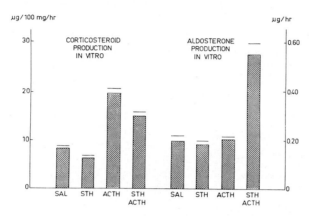

Fig. 2. Effect of treatment with ACTH (long acting β^{1-24} ACTH 2 i.u. injected s.c. every 48 h at 0, 2, 4 and 6 days after hypophysectomy), with STH (purified bovine somatotropin, 250 μg in 0.2 ml 7% gelatine injected s.c. twice daily for 7 days after hypophysectomy) and with ACTH plus STH on total corticosteroid and aldosterone production *in vitro* by adrenals of hypophysectomized rats subjected to a sodium-deficient diet for 14 days. Hypophysectomy was performed on the 7th day after starting diet. All animals received a challenge dose of 16 mU ACTH i.v. 15 min before decapitation. The data represent the mean ± S.E.M. of 8–13 animals.

results are at variance with the initial observations of Palmore and Mulrow (1967), but subsequent studies by these investigators (Palmore et al., 1968, 1970), using higher doses of STH more comparable to that used in our experiments, also showed that combined treatment with STH and ACTH restored the high rate of aldosterone secretion *in vivo* in hypophysectomized, sodium-deficient rats. These authors did not use the challenge with ACTH prior to the determination of the production of aldosterone, indicating that the secretion rates of aldosterone by adrenals of sodium-deficient rats can, in principle, be restored without the challenge. It is of interest to note that in rats after intravenous administration of ^{125}I-labeled human growth hormone a high concentration of radioactivity was noted in the kidney, liver and adrenal cortex with a slightly higher level in the zona glomerulosa than in the zona fasciculata (Mayberry et al., 1971). Still higher concentrations of ^{125}I-human growth hormone in the adrenal cortex were observed after pretreatment with ACTH.

Since the hypothalamus exerts control over pituitary secretions, subsequent experiments were designed to study the effects of elimination of this control by hypothalamic lesions on aldosterone secretion in sodium-deficient rats. For example, if it

were possible to selectively block the release of STH by specific lesions in the hypothalamus, the importance of STH for the regulation of aldosterone secretion might
then be demonstrated in the absence of other perturbations in pituitary function. In
these studies, female rats were first fed a sodium-deficient diet (9 μ-equiv. Na$^+$/g)
and one week later small electrolytic lesions were placed bilaterally in a variety of
locations within the hypothalamus. The animals received no treatment while continuing on the sodium-deficient diet and were studied one week after the operation.
The specificity of the lesions and their effects on the pattern of adrenal responsiveness
to elevated circulating levels of endogenous ACTH were assessed by subjecting the
animals to the stress of handling and transfer to a strange environment before sacrifice.
Lesions in a number of different locations reduced the high rate of aldosterone production which is characteristic for sodium-deficient rats subjected to the stress
procedure used (Fig. 3). Significant reductions in aldosterone production were found

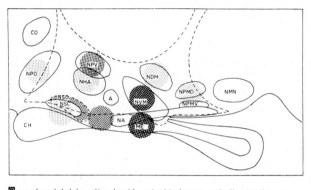

      reduced total corticosteroid and aldosterone poduction in vitro
      reduced aldosterone production in vitro
      no effect on steroid production in vitro

Fig. 3. Schematic representation of the lesions in the hypothalamus. Lesions in the median eminence
(ME) and in the nucleus ventromedialis (NVM) caused a reduced response to stress as indicated by a
significant reduction in the rate of corticosteroids as well as aldosterone production *in vitro*. Lesions in
the nucleus supraopticus (NSO), tractus supraoptico-neurohypophyseos (Tr.S.) and nucleus para-
ventricularis (NPV) caused a significant reduction in the rate of aldosterone production *in vitro* only.
CO, commissura anterior; NPO, nucleus preopticus; NSC, nucleus suprachiasmatis; CH, chiasma
opticum; NHA, nucleus hypothalamus anterior; A, nucleus ventromedialis anterior; NA, nucleus
arcuatus; NDM, nucleus dorsomedialis; NVM, nucleus ventromedialis; NPMD, nucleus premamillaris dorsalis; NPMV, nucleus premamillaris ventralis and NMN, nucleus mamillaris.

in rats bearing lesions in the median eminence (ME) and the ventromedial nucleus
(NVM). However, similar reductions in total corticosteroid production indicated
that these lesions had inhibited the release of ACTH. Similar findings have been
reported in dogs with median eminence or medial basal hypothalamic lesions (Ganong
et al., 1959; Ganong *et al.*, 1961). In contrast, while lesions in the nucleus para-
ventricularis (NPV) resulted in marked reductions in aldosterone production, total
corticosteroid production remained unaffected. Lesions in the nucleus supraopticus
(NSO) and in the tractus supraoptico-neurohypophyseos (Tr.S.) substantially reduced
the rate of aldosterone production, but these lesions also caused slight reductions in

total corticosteroid production. Lesions in the preoptic nucleus (NPO), premamillary nucleus (NPM), nucleus suprachiasmatis (NSC), nucleus hypothalamicus anterior
(NHA) and nucleus dorsomedialis (NDM), as well as lesions in various parts of the
thalamus, affected neither aldosterone nor total corticosteroid productions.

The reductions in aldosterone production observed in rats bearing lesions in the
NSO and in the Tr.S. might have been the consequence of disruptions in the release
of vasopressin. On the other hand, the effects of lesions in the NPV could have resulted
from growth hormone deficiency as suggested by the stunted growth rate of these
animals. The effects of vasopressin and growth hormone were, therefore, studied in
sodium-deficient rats with bilateral lesions in the Tr.S. and in the NPV. In rats
with lesions in the Tr.S., vasopressin, but not STH, restored aldosterone production
to the high levels found in sham-operated sodium-deficient rats. On the other hand,
whereas STH treatment in rats bearing lesions in the NPV restored normal aldosterone
secretory responsiveness, vasopressin was ineffective (Fig. 4).

The selective nature by which lesions in the paraventricular nucleus (NPV) reduced
the aldosterone secretory responsiveness in the sodium deficient rat and its reversal
by treatment with STH alone suggest that the NPV is involved in the control of
growth hormone secretion. This is supported by the data of O'Brien *et al.* (1964)
who showed that administration of STH restored the growth rate of kittens with

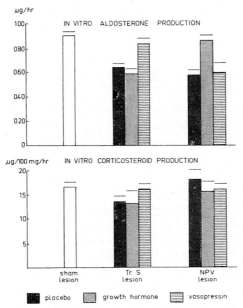

Fig. 4. Effect of treatment with STH and a crude vasopressin preparation on corticosteroid and
aldosterone production *in vitro* by adrenals of rats on a sodium-restricted diet and with bilateral
lesions in the tractus supraoptico-neurohypophyseos (Tr.S.) or in the area of the paraventricular
nuclei (NPV). Both preparations were given s.c. on the 5th and 6th postoperative day. Purified
bovine somatotropin (STH) 100 μg in 0.2 ml 7% gelatine twice daily; 0.25 mg posterior pituitary
powder (0.675 I.U. of vasopressin) in 0.2 ml 15% gelatine twice daily. The data represent mean
$\pm$ S.E.M. of 6–7 animals.

lesions in the NPV, and of Endröczi *et al.* (1957) who demonstrated the same in puppies. In addition, Sawano *et al.* (1968) reported decreased amounts of growth hormone releasing factor in the hypothalami of kittens with lesions in the NPV. However, Bernardis and Frohman (1971) failed to induce growth hormone release by electrical stimulation of the NPV in the rat.

The supraoptic nucleus (NSO) and vasopressin have been implicated in the release of growth hormone (Del Vecchio *et al.*, 1958; Bernardis *et al.*, 1963; Bernardis and Skelton, 1964; Arimura *et al.*, 1968). Rats with a lesion in the Tr.S. and in the NSO drank more, the rate of aldosterone production *in vitro* by adrenals of these animals was markedly reduced, and it was found that the neurosecretory material disappeared from the posterior pituitary. The deficient aldosterone response seen in these animals was not affected by growth hormone treatment but by the administration of vasopressin (Fig. 4). Vasopressin is capable of stimulating the discharge of ACTH from the anterior pituitary (de Wied *et al.*, 1967) and increases aldosterone production in sodium-deficient rats via its stimulation of ACTH release (van der Wal and de Wied, 1968). In addition, removal of the posterior pituitary interferes with the release of ACTH in response to emotional or neurogenic stress (de Wied *et al.*, 1964). Therefore, it might well be that the lesions in the supraopticoneurohypophysial tract reduced the release of ACTH and thereby the production of aldosterone. In fact, the total corticosteroid production *in vitro* of lesioned rats was slightly lower than that of sham-operated animals and treatment with vasopressin restored the corticosteroid response to normal (Fig. 4). Accordingly, the failure of animals with lesions in the supraopticoneurohypophysial tract might have been caused by a reduction in the release of ACTH or by the absence of a specific effect of vasopressin or a related peptide* on aldosterone secretion. Further experiments are needed to clarify this point.

The foregoing studies revealed the importance of the hypothalamo–pituitary complex in the regulation of aldosterone secretion in the rat. This control became obvious after subjecting rats to a sodium-deficient diet. Under these conditions the rat resembled sheep, dog and man much more than rats on a "regular" sodium intake. The difference with other species might be attributed to the fact that the sodium intake of rats in their laboratory habitat is generally higher than that of sheep, dog and man. Apart from this, other factors might be involved, for example, the method employed to determine aldosterone secretion. The production of this steroid by excised adrenal glands *in vitro* has been fruitfully used by us as a method to explore the mechanisms in the regulation of aldosterone secretion, assuming that its production *in vitro* reflects the trophic influences exerted on the zona glomerulosa *in vivo* prior to excision of the gland (de Wied *et al.*, 1965). The determination of aldosterone in blood has for many years been a time consuming procedure, associated with anaesthesia, traumatization and blood loss, because it had to be measured in adrenal venous blood. Recently, radioimmunological methods have been developed which will enable the determination of aldosterone in small quantities of blood. It is possible,

---

* A crude preparation of vasopressin was used in the present studies.

therefore, that the direct measurement of aldosterone *in vivo* in the non-anaesthetized rat with a highly sensitive method may reveal that the same pituitary factors which operate in the sodium-deficient rat also play a role in the secretion of this steroid under non-restricted sodium intake conditions.

Evidence is accumulating that the aforementioned pituitary factors operate in the regulation of aldosterone secretion in other species as well. Ganong recently found that STH has a similar action in the dog as we reported in the rat (Ganong, personal communication). Recent data from Williams *et al.* (1971) indicate that pituitary factors, in particular STH, are also involved in the regulation of aldosterone secretion in man. In contrast to normal subjects, hypopituitary patients failed to show a significant increase in aldosterone secretion during ACTH infusion, although the 17-hydroxycorticosteroid response to ACTH was not impaired. An abnormally low aldosterone response to sodium restriction was also an apparent characteristic seen in most of the hypopituitary patients. Moreover, practically all subjects who showed low basal growth hormone levels and an absent growth hormone response to arginine or insulin failed to respond to ACTH stimulation and to sodium restriction normally. While confirmatory evidence is still forthcoming, it is possible that further studies along these lines may eventually substantiate the hypothesis that the hypothalamus, the anterior and possibly the posterior pituitary exert a hitherto unrecognized role in the even more complex regulation of aldosterone secretion, not alone in the rat but in man and in other species as well.

REFERENCES

ARIMURA, A., SAWANO, S., REDDING, T. W. AND SCHALLY, A. V. (1968) Studies on retarded growth of rats with hereditary hypothalamic diabetes insipidus. *Neuroendocrinology*, **3**, 187–192.

BERNARDIS, L. L., BOX, B. M. AND STEVENSON, J. A. F. (1963) Growth following hypothalamic lesions in the weanling rat. *Endocrinology*, **72**, 684–692.

BERNARDIS, L. L. AND SKELTON, F. R. (1964) Contribution to the problem of growth hormone releasing effect of antidiuretic hormone. *Growth*, **28**, 263–272.

BERNARDIS, L. L. AND FROHMAN, L. A. (1971) Plasma growth hormone responses to electrical stimulation of the hypothalamus in the rat. *Neuroendocrinology*, **7**, 193–201.

BINNION, P. F., DAVIS, J. O., BROWN, T. C. AND OLICKNEY, M. J. (1965) Mechanisms regulating aldosterone secretion during sodium depletion. *Amer. J. Physiol.*, **208**, 655–661.

BLAIR–WEST, J. R., COGHLAN, J. P., DENTON, D. A., GODING, J. R., MUNRO, J. A., PETERSON, R. E. AND WINTOUR, M. (1962) Humoral stimulation of adrenal cortical secretion. *J. clin. Invest.*, **41**, 1606–1627.

BLAIR–WEST, J. R., COGHLAN, J. P., DENTON, J. R., WINTOUR, M. AND WRIGHT, R. D. (1963) The control of aldosterone secretion. *Recent Progr. Hormone Res.*, **19**, 311–363.

CADE, R. AND PERENICH, T (1965) Secretion of aldosterone by rats. *Amer. J. Physiol.*, **208**, 1026–1030.

CARPENTER, C. C. J., DAVIS, J. O. AND AYERS, C. R. (1961) Relation of renin, angiotensin II and experimental renal hypertension to aldosterone secretion. *J. clin. Invest.*, **40**, 2026–2042.

CARPENTER, C. C. J., DAVIS, J. O., HOLMAN, J. E., AYERS, C. R. AND BAHN, R. C. (1961) Studies on the response of the transplant of kidneys and the transplant of adrenal gland to thoracic inferior vena cava constriction. *J. clin. Invest.*, **40**, 196.

CSÁNKY, M. F. D., WAL, B. VAN DER, AND WIED, D. DE (1968) The regulation of aldosterone production in normal and sodium deficient rats. *J. Endocr.*, **41**, 179–188.

DAVIS, J. O., AYERS, C. R. AND CARPENTER, C. C. J. (1961a) Renal origin of an aldosterone-stimulating hormone in dogs with thoracic caval constriction and in sodium depleted dogs. *J. clin. Invest.*, **40**, 1466–1474.

DAVIS, J. O., CARPENTER, C. C. J., AYERS, C. R., HOLMAN, J. E. AND BAHN, R. C. (1961b) Evidence for secretion of an aldosterone-stimulating hormone by kidney. *J. clin. Invest.*, **40**, 684–696.

DAVIS, J. O., HARTROFT, P. M., TITUS, E., CARPENTER, C. C. J., AYERS, C. R. AND SPIEGEL, H. E. (1962) Role of the renin-angiotensin system in the control of aldosterone secretion. *J. clin. Invest.* **41**, 378–389.

DAVIS, J. O., YANKOPOULOS, N. A., LIEBERMAN, F., HOLMAN, J. E. AND BAHN, R. C. (1960) The role of the anterior pituitary in the control of aldosterone secretion in experimental secondary hyperaldosteronism. *J. clin. Invest.*, **39**, 765–775.

DEL VECCHIO, A., GENOVESE, E. AND MARTINI, L. (1958) Hypothalamus and somatotrophic hormone release. *Proc. Soc. exp. biol. (N.Y.)*, **98**, 641–644.

DENTON, D. A., GODING, J. R. AND WRIGHT, R. D. (1959) Control of adrenal secretion of electrolyte-active steroids. *Brit. med. J.*, **2**, 447 and 522.

DINGMAN, J. F., GAITON, E., STAUB, M. C., ARIMURA, A. AND PETERSON, R. E. (1960) Hypoaldosteronism in panhypopituitarism. *J. clin. Invest.*, **39**, 981.

DUFAU, M. L. AND KLIMAN, B. (1966) Acute effects of angiotensin and ACTH on aldosterone and corticosterone secretion in the intact rat. *Program of the Forty-eighth Meeting of the Endocrine Society*, Chicago, p. 103.

DUFAU, M. L. AND KLIMAN, B. (1968) Acute effects of angiotensin-II-amide on aldosterone and corticosterone secretion by morphine–pentobarbital treated rats. *Endocrinology*, **83**, 180–183.

DUFAU, M. L., CRAWFORD, J. D. AND KLIMAN, B. (1969) Effect of high sodium intake on the response of the rat adrenal to angiotensin II. *Endocrinology*, **84**, 462–463.

EILERS, E. A. AND PETERSON, R. E. (1964) Aldosterone secretion in the rat. In *Aldosterone*, E. E. BAULIEU AND P. ROBEL (Eds.), Blackwell Scientific Publications, Oxford, pp. 251–264.

ENDRÖCZI, E., KOVÁCS, S. UND SZALAY, G. (1957) Einfluss von Hypothalamusläsionen auf die Entwicklung des Körpers und verschiedener Organe bei neugeborenen Tieren. *Endokrinologie*, **34**, 168–175.

FARRELL, G. (1960) Adrenoglomerulotropin. *Circulation*, **21**, 1009–1015.

FARRELL, G. AND TAYLOR, N. A. (1962) Neuroendocrine aspects of blood volume regulation. *Ann. Rev. Physiol.*, **24**, 471–490.

GANONG, W. F. (1968) Variations in the aldosterone-stimulating activity of angiotensin: causes and physiological significance. In *Pharmacology of Hormonal Polypeptides and Proteins*, N. BLACK, L. MARTINI AND R. PAOLETTI (Eds.), Plenum Press, New York, pp. 517–526.

GANONG, W. F., BIGLIERI, E. K. AND MULROW, P. J. (1966) Mechanisms regulating adrenocortical secretion of aldosterone and glucocorticoids. *Recent Progr. Hormone Res.*, **22**, 381–429.

GANONG, W. F., BORYCZKA, A. T., SHACKLEFORD, R., CLARK, R. M. AND CONVERSE, R. P. (1965) Effect of dietary sodium restriction on adrenal cortical response to ACTH. *Proc. Soc. exp. Biol. (N.Y.)*, **118**, 792–795.

GANONG, W. F., LIEBERMAN, A. H., DAILY, W. J. R., YUEN, V. S., MULROW, P. J., LUETSCHER, J. A. AND BAILEY, R. E. (1959) Aldosterone secretion in dogs with hypothalamic lesions. *Endocrinology*, **65**, 18–28.

GANONG, W. F. AND MULROW, P. J. (1961) Evidence for secretion of an aldosterone stimulating substance by the kidney. *Nature (Lond.)*, **190**, 1115–1116.

GANONG, W. F. AND MULROW, P. J. (1962) Role of the kidney in adrenocortical response to hemorrhage in hypophysectomized dogs. *Endocrinology*, **70**, 182–188.

GANONG, W. F., MULROW, P. J., BORYCZKA, A. T. AND CERA, G. (1962) Evidence for a direct effect of angiotensin II on adrenal cortex of the dog. *Proc. Soc. exptl. Biol. (N.Y.)*, **109**, 381–384.

GANONG, W. F., NOLAN, A. M., DOWOY, A. AND LUETSCHER, J. A. (1961) The effect of hypothalamic lesions on adrenal secretion of cortisol, corticosterone, 11-desoxycortisol and aldosterone. *Endocrinology*, **68**, 169–171.

GLÁZ, E. AND SUGÁR, K. (1962) The effect of synthetic angiotensin II on synthesis of aldosterone by the adrenals. *J. Endocr.*, **24**, 299–302.

HUNGERFORD, G. F. AND PANAGIOTIS, N. M. (1962) Response of pineal lipid to hormone imbalances. *Endocrinology*, **71**, 936–942.

KAPLAN, N. M. AND BARTTER, F. C. (1962) The effect of ACTH, renin, angiotensin and various precursors on biosynthesis of aldosterone by adrenal slices. *J. clin. Invest.*, **41**, 715–724.

KINSON, G. A. AND SINGER, B. (1968) Sensitivity to angiotensin and adrenocorticotrophic hormone in the sodium deficient rat. *Endocrinology*, **83**, 1108–1116.

LEE, T. C. AND WIED, D. DE (1967) *In vitro* aldosterone production by adrenals of normal recipient rats cross-circulated with rats with secondary hyperaldosteronism of dietary sodium restriction. *Endocrinology*, **80**, 221–224.

LEE, T. C., WAL, B. VAN DER, AND WIED, D. DE (1968) Influence of the anterior pituitary on the aldosterone secretory response to dietary sodium restriction in the rat. *J. Endocr.*, **42**, 465–475.

LEE, T. C. AND WIED, D. DE (1968) Somatotropin as the non-ACTH factor of anterior pituitary origin for the maintenance of enhanced aldosterone secretory responsiveness of dietary sodium restriction in chronically hypophysectomized rats. *Life Sci.*, **7**, 35–45.

LIEBERMAN, A. H. AND LUETSCHER, J. A. (1960) Some effects of abnormalities of pituitary, adrenal or thyroid function on excretion of aldosterone and the response to corticotrophin or sodium deprivation. *J. clin. Endocrin.*, **20**, 1004–1016.

LUCIS, O. J. AND VENNING, E. H. (1960) *In vitro* and *in vivo* effect of growth hormone on aldosterone secretion. *Canad. J. Biochem. Physiol.*, **38**, 1069–1075.

MACHADO, A. B. M. AND DA SILVA, C. R. (1963) Pineal body and urinary sodium excretion in the rat. *Experientia (Basel)*, **19**, 264–265.

MARIEB, N. J. AND MULROW, P. J. (1964) The response of aldosterone secretion to angiotensin in the rat. *Fed. Proc.*, **23**, 300.

MARIEB, N. J. AND MULROW, P. J. (1965) Role of the renin-angiotensin system in the regulation of aldosterone secretion in the rat. *Endocrinology*, **76**, 657–664.

MAYBERRY, H. E., BRANDE, J. L. VAN DEN, WYK, J. J. VAN, AND WADDELL, W. J. (1971) Early localization of ^{125}I-labeled human growth hormone in adrenals and other organs of immature hypophysectomized rats. *Endocrinology*, **88**, 1309–1317.

MÜLLER, J. (1965) Aldosterone stimulation *in vitro*. I. Evaluation of assay procedure and determination of aldosterone-stimulating activity in a human urine extract. *Acta Endocr. (Kbh.)*, **48**, 283–296.

MULROW, P. J. AND GANONG, W. F. (1961) Stimulation of aldosterone secretion by angiotensin II. *Yale J. Biol. Med.*, **33**, 386–395.

MULROW, P. J. AND GANONG, W. F. (1962) Role of the kidney and the renin-angiotensin system in the response of aldosterone secretion to hemorrhage. *Circulation*, **25**, 213–220.

MULROW, P. J., GANONG, W. F. AND BORYCZKA, A. (1963) Further evidence for a role of the renin-angiotensin system in regulation of aldosterone secretion. *Proc. Soc. exp. Biol. (N.Y.)*, **112**, 7–10.

MULROW, P. J., GANONG, W. F., CERA, G. AND KULJIAN, A. (1962) The nature of the aldosterone-stimulating factor in dog kidney. *J. clin. Invest.*, **41**, 505–518.

NEWMAN, A. E., REDGATE, E. S. AND FARRELL, G. (1958) The effect of diencephalic-mesencephalic lesions on aldosterone and hydrocortisone secretion. *Endocrinology*, **63**, 723–736.

O'BRIEN, C. P., HAPPEL, L. AND BACH, L. M. N. (1964) Some hypothalamic effects on STH-influences, growth and insulin sensitivity in kittens. *Fed. Proc.*, **23**, 205.

PALKOVITS, M. (1965) Participation of the epithalamo-epiphyseal system in the regulation of water and electrolytes metabolism. In *Progress in Brain Research, Vol. 10, The Structure and Function of the Epiphysis Cerebri*, J. ARIËNS KAPPERS AND J. P. SCHADÉ (Eds.), Elsevier, Amsterdam, pp. 627–634.

PALKOVITS, M., JONG, W. DE, WAL, B. VAN DER, AND WIED, D. DE (1970) Effect of adrenocorticotrophic and growth hormones on aldosterone production and plasma renin activity in chronically hypophysectomized sodium-deficient rats. *J. Endocr.*, **47**, 243–250.

PALKOVITS, M. AND FÖLDVÁRI, P. J. (1963) Effect of the subcommissural organ and the pineal body on the adrenal cortex. *Endocrinology*, **72**, 28–32.

PALKOVITS, M., MONOS, E. AND FACHET, J. (1965) The effect of subcommissural-organ lesions on aldosterone production in the rat. *Acta Endocr. (Kbh.)*, **48**, 169–176.

PALMORE, W. P., ANDERSON, R. C. AND MULROW, P. J. (1968) Control of aldosterone secretion by the pituitary gland. *Proc. Third Intern. Congr. Endocrinology, Mexico D.F., July, 1968, Excerpta med. int. Congr. Ser.*, No. 157, 169–170.

PALMORE, W. P., ANDERSON, R. AND MULROW, P. J. (1970) Role of the pituitary in controlling aldosterone production in sodium-depleted rats. *Endocrinology*, **86**, 728–734.

PALMORE, W. P. AND MULROW, P. J. (1967) Control of aldosterone secretion by the pituitary gland. *Science*, **158**, 1482–1484.

PANAGIOTIS, N. M. AND HUNGERFORD, G. F. (1961) Response of the pineal and adrenal glands to sodium restriction. *Endocrinology*, **69**, 217–224.

RENNELS, E. G. AND DILL, R. E. (1961) Effect of pinealectomy on the histology and lipid content of the rat adrenal gland. *Texas Rep. Biol. Med.*, **19**, 843–850.

SLOPER: You have not really answered Dr. Hayward's question, have you? Can you make any speculations on the anatomical route by which your paraventricular lesion is working?

DE WIED: We think that the paraventricular nucleus may be involved in the production of the growth hormone releasing factor. By damaging the nucleus we may have diminished or reduced the amount of growth hormone releasing factor and therefore decreased the released of growth hormone.

SLOPER: I don't understand what you think of the role of vasopressin in this respect. What happens when you induce diabetes insipidus, and then give vasopressin? You restore the waterbalance, which you have disturbed. So I think you should conclude that the waterbalance has some effect, a rather specific effect of vasopressin.

DE WIED: We found, years ago, that the posterior lobectomized animal showed a reduced release of ACTH. We did not check in these animals the responsiveness after an injection of ACTH because we used an emotional stress to arouse the pituitary–adrenal system. I think these studies are not yet finished. To check whether there is a diminished release of ACTH, because this will explain why there is a reduced aldosterone production, one has to be able to measure the ACTH concentration.

SMELIK: What is known about the salt regulation in the normal rat, or is the sodium-restricted rat a normal animal?

DE WIED: I think the rat takes in general more salt. This animal has a larger salt intake than other species. So if we would lower slightly the salt intake of rats you would get a much more sensitive adrenal cortex.

SMELIK: Is this due to the diet we give them or is this true for every rat?

DE WIED: One can make the adrenal system more sensitive by restricting salt. The method we used to determine aldosterone secretion is too crude for registering small changes in the secretion. Recently, a new method has been developed for measuring aldosterone by way of a radioimmunoassay technique, which will enable us in the future to measure the variations in aldosterone secretion directly.

A Cybernetic Approach to the Hypothalamo-Pituitary/Adrenal System

E. PAPAIKONOMOU

Department of Pharmacology, Free University, Medical Faculty, Amsterdam (The Netherlands)

INTRODUCTION

"Let no man say that I have said nothing new—the arrangement of the materials is new. In playing tennis, we both use the same ball, but one of us plays it better. I would just as soon be told that I have used old terms. Just as the same thoughts differently arranged form a different discourse, so the same words differently arranged form different thoughts." (Pascal)

In his delightful book, "The Stress of Life", Dr. Hans Selye has occasionally remarked: "My advice to any young man at the beginning of his career is to try to look for the mere outlines of big things with his fresh, unstrained and unprejudiced mind". In forming the views we are going to present, we have tried to follow the advice of Dr. Selye; however, although these views might look fresh and unstrained, they are not unprejudiced: our preoccupation with biocybernetics has led us to look at the world of physiology—so also at the adrenal system—through a special kind of glasses.

It is widely known that Norbert Wiener (1961) christened in 1948 the new science of "Cybernetics", a name also used by Plato and Ampère; he defined it as "the science of control and communication in the animal and the machine". In modern terms, cybernetics can be defined as "the science of complex organized systems where information flows into, through, and out of the systems" (Papaikonomou, unpublished). This science introduced a new way of looking at old things (an information theoretic approach) and a new methodology (systems analysis). Consequently, a cybernetic approach to a biological system will, essentially, consist of making a systems analysis of it, using information-theoretical considerations in describing the phenomena inside the system and the system's behaviour. The ultimate aim of such an approach is to arrive at a synthesis—in general simulation on a computer—of the system's function, on the ground of systematically collected experimental information.

In the field of endocrinological research, the existence of automatically operating regulating systems was early recognized. However, biologists were not taken by surprise since this remarkable fact fits well in the line of thinking originated by Hippocrates with his belief in the "natural healing forces and rediscovered and further pursued by Claude Bernard with his notion of the constancy of the internal environment of any living organism, as well as by Walter Cannon with his theory of "homeo-stasis", the regulation phenomena in living systems (Papaikonomou, unpublished). So it happened that many terms, borrowed from cybernetics and control theory jargon, began to be used in endocrinological literature, although the underlying concepts were not always well understood. Some other colourful terms were created by these researchers themselves such as, *e.g.*, "internal" and "external feedback", "short" and "ultra-short feedback", etc. In the meantime these investigators did not always realize how important it is to investigate the dynamic properties of a biological functioning whole or system, *i.e.*, not only the system's function in the steady-state, but also the system's transient responses to external and/or internal influences.

Using a cybernetic approach, we have analyzed the published experimental evidence on the function of the adrenal system (Papaikonomou, 1970). The result of this analysis has been a three-level model of the communication and control hierarchy in the adrenal system. Since our ultimate aim is to make a synthesis (*i.e.*, computer simulation) of this system, we need special information about the system's dynamics, which, unfortunately, has not yet been fully documented. To get this information we have to design special cybernetic experiments which can provide the only right questions to ask in order to get the answers required by computer modeling. In designing these experiments, we have used as a starting point a simplified model of the communication network among the adrenal system components, developed by using certain theoretical cybernetic considerations. This model, the questions we want to ask, and our general strategy will be discussed in the sequel.

A STRATEGY FOR A SYSTEMS ANALYSIS OF COMPLEX BIOLOGICAL SYSTEMS

As a first attempt towards formalizing a general strategy for a system's analysis, we have assembled an algorithm or program as a systematic guide in such an endeavour; although it has not previously been explicitly formulated in this way, it is implicit in modern physiological work. This algorithm looks as follows:

step one: choose the resolution level;
step two: identify the organs or elements of the system under investigation;
step three: trace the pathways of interaction of the system with other systems and the environment;
step four: discover the signals which transfer information between the communicating components of the system;
step five: trace the exact communication network in the system and the polarity (excitation or inhibition) of the different interactions;
step six: discover a quantitative description of the static and dynamic characteristics of the system's components;
step seven: identify the "purpose" of the system or the criterion according to which the system functions.

This algorithm is a natural outgrowth from our definition of a (biocybernetic) system, which sounds as follows:

Definition: at a certain resolution level we conceive of a system as a collection of systems at a lower resolution level, also variably called subsystems, components, or elements, which are the nodal points in a network of pathways, or channels, through which information flows with mass and energy as carriers.

It is evident that the behaviour of a system is determined by the dynamic properties of the system's elements together with the dynamics of the organizing communication network inside the system, in other words, the system's dynamics. Therefore, whenever the system's dynamics have been discovered by means of a systems analysis, the system's behaviour can be predicted.

Naturally, in biological research we are dealing with an existing system, a "black-box" which we wish to "open", *i.e.* to analyze it, using, for example, the heuristic algorithm described above. Actually, we might achieve this by measuring, *i.e.*, by experimentation on real hardware examples, namely animals of one or more species. Anatomical studies reveal the main features of the system's structure and we may try to correlate them with our findings from functional studies in order to identify the system's circuitry. The dynamic properties of the system's elements we could study applying a technique commonly used by engineers (Papaikonomou *et al.*, in press). We should try to isolate each component from the rest of the system as gently as possible in order to minimize perturbation of its dynamics. Then we should stimulate it with signals of our own choice and measure its transient and steady-state response. In engineering jargon this is called input–output characteristics or transfer function discovery. After a little thought we see that this is an inverse form of the diagnostic process used in medical practice, where the physician wishes to discover the "input" to his patient (*i.e.*, the particular disease), from the symptoms (the "output") and his knowledge of normal human anatomy and physiology (the "transfer function").

At this stage, when the seven steps of our systems analysis algorithm have been made successfully, we possess enough experimental information about the system under study to enter the next phase in modern biological research, that of synthesis. This amounts to constructing a working model of the system, possibly and preferably simulated on a computer.

As an illustration of our strategy let us consider the neuroendocrine apparatus of mammals. We may distinguish three possible resolution levels of biological interest. First comes the distinction of different neuroendocrine subsystems such as, *e.g.*, the gonadal axis, the adrenal axis, the thyroid axis, etc. (first resolution level). These are the components of the neuroendocrine system at this level. The circuitry of the master system is just beginning to be investigated. Only little is known about the interactions between the different endocrine subsystems. Research has been mainly directed into the study of these subsystems in isolation. Let us now consider the adrenal subsystem. The adenohypophysis and the adrenal cortex were early recognized as elements of this subsystem; the hypothalamus and other parts of the brain followed (second resolution level). However, the exact circuitry of the adrenal system is not as yet completely defined. While research is continuing at this resolution level, investigation of the separate components is also being pursued. Consider now the adrenal cortex. Some features of its input–output characteristics are known from experiments by Urquhart and Li (1968). Our aim is to try to explain the overall dynamics of the adrenal component on the basis of its biochemical phenomena. However, the chain of reactions that, under stimulation by adrenocorticotropic hormone (ACTH), leads to the output of the adrenal element (which is for humans mainly cortisol), is presently only qualitatively known. In analyzing the adrenal component, we chose an intermediary resolution level consisting not of all the substances in the chain of internal biochemical reactions, but of only the main few of them. The functional interrelationships among them (laws of conversion of each substance to the next) could be described qualitatively and quantitatively using functional-integrative considerations. In this way we developed a computer model of adrenal function which satisfactorily simulates all known features of adrenal dynamics (Papaikonomou et al., in press; Papaikonomou, in press).

THEORETICAL REFLECTIONS ON THE GLUCOCORTICOID FEEDBACK: A SIMPLIFIED, CONTROL THEORETIC MODEL OF THE HYPOTHALAMO-PITUITARY/ADRENAL SYSTEM

The trouble with the adrenal system is that there is too much information available. The literature in this field is so complex and so controversial that, at the moment, any serious attempt to formulate a relatively sophisticated heuristic model of the system is doomed to be addressed by many investigators as a collection of well-meant but unfounded speculations. To avoid such a danger, we shall discuss only a simplified model of the adrenal system. This model we have been using as a starting point for the design of the experiments necessary in order to get the needed dynamic information for a synthesis of the system. It is shown in Fig. 1.

The blocks in this diagram stand for the transfer function properties of the different components of the adrenal system. These components are considered as information transducers receiving information coded in the form of a certain specific hormonal signal, which reaches them through the blood. They transform this information into another hormonal code, and transmit this hormonal output signal into the blood stream and through this to the next component in the diagram, always clock-wise. An

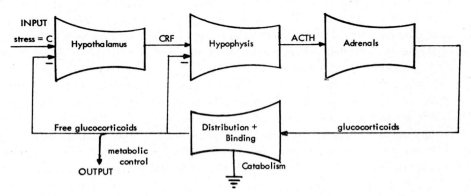

Fig. 1. A simplified model of the hypothalamo-pituitary/adrenal system.

important feature of the adrenal system is that it is of the closed-loop type. There is at least one closed informational loop in this system, namely its output, *i.e.*, the free glucocorticoid concentration of the blood is monitored by (or fed back to) the hypothalamus and/or pituitary.

It is evident that the adrenal system has the basic configuration of a regulating system. However, the hypothesis put forward by Yates *et al.* (1961) that this system may be considered as a linear negative feedback control system, with a set-point, has turned out to be unrealistic. It is now known that both static and dynamic characteristics of the different components of the system are softly non-linear, that there are delays in the information transduction (adrenal gland) and the information transmission (glucocorticoid feedback path), and that there is no clear set-point from which the feedback signal is subtracted. Such a subtraction indeed takes place in an actual set-point feedback control system, where the result of the subtraction (the error signal) is used to make the appropriate corrections on the output in order to keep it equal to a desired value (the set-point).

Strangely enough, the question whether the site of glucocorticoid feedback is in the hypothalamus or in the pituitary has not yet been settled. A few years ago there were two schools: the "pure hypothalamists", convinced that the feedback site is exclusively in the hypothalamus, and the "pure hypophysists" believing that the feedback site is solely in the hypophysis. Currently, the situation is somewhat obscure since a third school is gaining ground, that of the "impurists" who think that the feedback is primarily but not exclusively on either the hypothalamus or the pituitary.

Using a mixture of theoretical considerations and experimental data we were led to believe that the impurist's view of the glucocorticoid feedback is the right one. Our analysis is concerned with the steady-state function of the adrenal system under both resting conditions and stress. Transient phenomena and delays have been ignored, since on the one hand not all have as yet been experimentally discovered and on the other hand as Guyton *et al.* (1967) have remarked "Usually the human mind is capable of performing sufficient iteration to analyze the different steady-states of a system, but the transients are usually so elusive to the human mind that they can be demonstrated only by computer analysis".

We started from the fact, observed by many workers, that the adrenal system in steady-state behaves like a regulating system which is very sensitive to external changes in the feedback signal under resting conditions, but less sensitive when the system is under stress. We will show that only by assuming a feedback on both the hypothalamus and the pituitary, can this general property of the adrenal system be explained.

The input–output characteristics of the different components of the adrenal system at steady-state are shown from a pure hypothalamist's point of view in Figs. 2 and 3. Let us ignore the distribution element, since it does not influence the argument appreciably, and combine pituitary and adrenals in one block. Since this block and the hypothalamic one make up a single system in which the output of each block must be an input to the other, both their characteristics should hold simultaneously. Therefore, we may combine these characteristics. It is then obvious that the adrenal

References p. 301

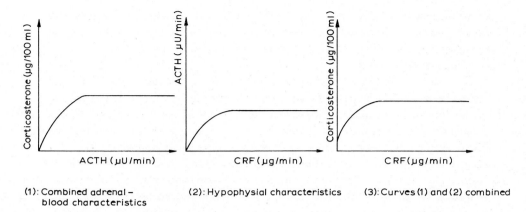

(1): Combined adrenal –
blood characteristics

(2): Hypophysial characteristics

(3): Curves (1) and (2) combined

Fig. 2. A "pure hypothalamist's" view of the adrenal system components input–output characteristics.

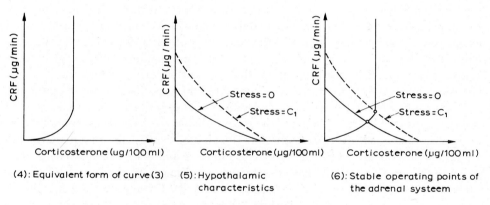

(4): Equivalent form of curve (3)

(5): Hypothalamic
characteristics

(6): Stable operating points of
the adrenal systeem

Fig. 3. Continuation of Fig. 2.

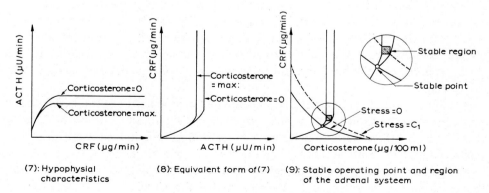

(7): Hypophysial
characteristics

(8): Equivalent form of (7)

(9): Stable operating point and region
of the adrenal systeem

Fig. 4. An "impurist's" view of Figs. 2 and 3.

system has different stable operating-points at rest and under stress, but it is equally sensitive in both cases (Fig. 3).

A pure hypophysist's view does not lead to a different conclusion. In an impurist's view, however, the hypophysial characteristics have a different form (Fig. 4). Here the glucocorticoid signal plays the role of a parameter. The feedback inhibition in this view is supposed to have the form of a mild modulation and it is basically different from that according to the pure hypophysist's view. Finally, in the characteristics of the complete system we see a stable operating-point for the system at rest but a stable operating-region under stress. After a little thought we can see that this justifies the experimental evidence about the great sensitivity of the adrenal system under normal conditions and its relative insensitivity under stress.

OPEN-LOOP TECHNIQUES FOR STUDYING THE ADRENAL SYSTEM DYNAMICS: A WAY FOR ASKING THE RIGHT QUESTIONS

We have said enough already about the why and how of experimentally studying the dynamics of the components of a system. Concerning the hypothalamo-pituitary/adrenal system, the adrenal component excepted, the rest is still awaiting such a study.

Cybernetic considerations indicate another line of investigation that might be also pursued. Since we are concerned with a closed-loop control system, we could try to quantitatively investigate different closed-loop properties of it such as, *e.g.*, stability, efficiency, etc., using open-loop techniques. These essentially amount to breaking the loop at one point, inserting on the one side a certain appropriate test-signal in the direction of signal flow in the loop, and measuring the resulting output on the other side. In this way we may get an idea about what dynamic changes the test-signal has undergone on traveling around the loop. From a quantitative point of view, we should try to estimate an important performance index, called, in engineering jargon, the open-loop gain (OLG) of the system. The assumption is, however, tacitly made, that the softly non-linear characteristics of the system's components can be considered approximately linear under the conditions of these particular experiments.

In an acute experiment, the experimental procedure itself produces a strong stress stimulus for the adrenocortical system. Since this stress input cannot be measured and, moreover, changes the parameters—as well as the transfer function properties—of at least one element of the system (namely the hypothalamus), we should preferably perform chronic experiments. The experimental procedure involved is, however, quite difficult to apply in small animals like the rat we are using. Therefore, it was important to see if we could derive some approximate information about the OLG of the adrenal system from an acute experiment. In this case, it would be necessary to adopt a linear view of the feedback and the component transfer functions. To simplify the calculation we also ignored the feedback on the hypophysis.

In Fig. 5 a possible experiment for acutely determining both steady-state and transient values of the OLG of the adrenal system is shown. The above mentioned assumptions about linearity are incorporated in the diagram and use is made of the

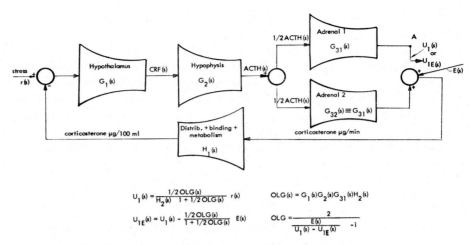

$$U_1(s) = \frac{1/2\,OLG(s)}{H_2(s)}\,\frac{}{1+1/2\,OLG(s)}\,r(s) \qquad OLG(s) = G_1(s)G_2(s)G_{31}(s)H_2(s)$$

$$U_{1E}(s) = U_1(s) - \frac{1/2\,OLG(s)}{1+1/2\,OLG(s)}\,E(s) \qquad OLG = \frac{2}{\frac{E(s)}{U_1(s)-U_{1E}(s)}-1}$$

Fig. 5. An open-loop technique for the adrenal system (see text).

important, simple—but not trivial—fact that the adrenal system has two adrenal components which, under acute conditions, may be assumed to have identical transfer functions.

In this figure the G's represent the linearized transfer functions of the different components, written in Laplace transform notation; r(s) represents the surgical stress signal, and E(s) is a disturbance signal equivalent to an infusion of glucocorticoid (corticosterone in the case of the rat). Using the output blood of the left adrenal gland we can estimate in 2-min intervals the value of the output of the right adrenal being a signal in the remaining closed loop. This output is equal to that of the left adrenal. When no disturbance is inserted, this signal can be calculated to be:

$$U_1(s) = \frac{1/2OLG(s)}{H_1\{1 + 1/2OLG(s)\}}$$

where, by definition:

$$OLG(s) = G_1(s)G_2(s)G_{31}(s)H_1(s)$$

while if a disturbance E(s) is interted, $U_1(s)$ becomes:

$$U_{1E}(s) = U_1(s) - \frac{1/2OLG(s)}{1 + 1/2OLG(s)}\,E(s)$$

We can easily see that:

$$OLG(s) = \frac{2}{\dfrac{E(s)}{U_1(s) - U_{1E}(s)} - 1}$$

E(t) is known, $U_1(t)$ and $U_{1E}(t)$ can be measured; their Laplace transforms can be estimated, when, by means of this beautiful formula the OLG(s) are calculated. Then, by transforming back to the time domain, we find an estimate for the OLG(t). This estimate is useful in studying stability, efficiency and other properties of the hypothalamo-pituitary-adrenal system.

EPILOGUE: AN EXAMPLE OF ANALYSIS WHERE THE PRINCIPLES DISCUSSED HERE HAVE NOT BEEN USED

What I have been trying to convey is essentially that a biological system's function cannot be discovered by analyzing only the system's anatomical topology. Only a systematic analysis of the information flow into, through and out of a system at its different dynamic states will enable us to gain more insight into its physiological significance.

I know no better way to show how beautifully one can be mistaken in trying to analyze a complex biological system using as a starting point only structural considerations, than to quote Thomas Wharton, a 17th century anatomist, who made a careful anatomical study of the thyroid gland and seriously believed it to have the following four purposes: "(1) To serve as a transfer point for the superfluous moisture from the nerves through the lymphatic ducts to the veins which run through the gland; (2) to keep the neck warm; (3) to lubricate the larynx, so making the voice lighter, more melodious, and sweeter; and (4) to round out and ornament the curve of the neck, especially in women".

REFERENCES

GUYTON, A. G., MILHORN, H. T. AND COLEMAN, T. G. (1967) Simulation of physiological mechanisms. *Simulation*, July-August.

PAPAIKONOMOU, E. (unpublished) Lectures on biomedical cybernetics. Lectures being given at the Department of Pharmacology, Free University, Amsterdam.

PAPAIKONOMOU, E. (1970) *Communication and Control Hierarchy in the Brain–Pituitary–Adrenal Axis*. M.Sc. Thesis, Dept. of Electrical Engineering, Technological University of Eindhoven.

PAPAIKONOMOU, E. (1972) *A Functional–Integrative Computer Model of the Adrenocortical Dynamics*. Proc. of the Third International Congress on Biocybernetics, Leipzig, August, 1971, in press.

PAPAIKONOMOU, E., SMITH, J. AND SCHADÉ, J. P. (1972) A computer simulation study of the adrenocortical dynamics. *Curr. Mod. Biol.*, in press.

URQUHART, J. AND LI, C. C. (1968) The dynamics of adrenocortical secretion. *Amer. J. Physiol.*, **214**, 73–85.

WIENER, N. (1961) *Cybernetics*. MIT Press, Cambridge, Mass.

YATES, F. E., LEEMAN, S. E., GLENISTER, D. W. AND DALLMAN, M. F. (1961) Interaction between plasma corticosterone concentration and adrenocorticotropin releasing stimuli in the rat: evidence for the reset of an endocrine feedback control. *Endocrinology*, **69**, 67.

DISCUSSION

DE WIED: Can I ask you one question: on one of your first slides you showed the characteristics of the model by increasing amounts of ACTH. Did the peak of the capacity of the system correspond with the data found in the literature? Did you use male or female rats?

PAPAIKONOMOU: I always use male rats. I suppose there would only be a difference in parameters and that the basic mechanism is exactly the same for male and female rats.

DE WIED: Would it be possible to predict how long the adrenal gland could maintain the high output of ACTH?

PAPAIKONOMOU: This particular feature has not been simulated in the computer; but it can be in the future of course.

MOLL: I have some problems concerning the idea of the setpoint in the system. Did I understand you correctly that the setpoint as such is not incorporated in the model?

PAPAIKONOMOU: It is a setpoint but it is not a linear one. By setpoint we mean a certain level from which the output is subtracted, and this is a linear operation.

The Pituitary–Thyroid Response to
Low Environmental Temperature

J. MOLL, M. W. RIBBE AND MIEKE A. HAGE

Department of Anatomy, Medical Faculty Rotterdam, Rotterdam (The Netherlands)

INTRODUCTION

Exposure of a mammal to a cold environment generally causes hyperactivity of the pituitary–thyroid system with increased secretion of thyroid stimulating hormone (TSH) and of thyroid hormones, thyroxine and tri-iodothyronine (TH) (see Yamada *et al.*, 1965, and Galton and Nisula, 1969, for recent papers discussing, respectively, the acute and chronic phases of the thyroidal response to cold; see D'Angelo, 1960c, for a brief general review). The stimulation by cold of the pituitary–thyroid system constitutes the most striking example of a pronounced and long lasting change in activity of this system, induced by a naturally occurring stimulus. However, it should be mentioned at this point that this response is possibly not present in all mammalian species. A species in which it is clearly present and in which it has been extensively studied is the rat. Therefore, whenever no species is mentioned in the following account, the rat is referred to.

The pituitary–thyroid cold response sets in nearly immediately after cold exposure (details and references below). This points to a neurally controlled mechanism. Also, a number of studies show that procedures such as heterotopic pituitary transplantation, which isolate the pituitary gland from the hypothalamus, may block the thyroidal cold response. Such data indicate that the cold response may be dependent on the well-documented hypothalamic control of pituitary–thyroid function (Greer, 1951; reviews by Brown–Grant, 1966, and Reichlin, 1966).

On the other hand, a body of data, obtained for the greater part after longer periods of cold exposure, indicates that the cold response may be due to the following chain of events: increased gastro-intestinal loss of TH in the cold, a tendency of the blood level of TH to fall, stimulation of TSH secretion by way of the well-known negative feedback between secretion of TH and TSH, increased TH secretion (see Galton and Nisula, 1969, for evidence supporting this view). If such a mechanism of the cold response should prove to be correct, hypothalamic involvement in the cold response can not be of crucial importance. It has been demonstrated that comparable responses, such as those caused by thyroidectomy and goitrogen treatment, are not dependent on hypothalamic TSH control. They are still present, albeit less pronounced, following isolation of the pituitary gland from the hypothalamus (Reichlin, 1966; Brown–

Grant, 1966; Van Rees and Moll, 1968; all with many references to other studies).

Therefore, one has to conclude that the total body of pertinent data points to different possible mechanisms of the pituitary-thyroid response to cold. In the next parts of this paper we will try to defend a concept of the cold response, reconciling the two possible types of mechanisms underlying this response.

CONCEPT OF A BIPHASIC COLD RESPONSE

In the thyroidal cold response an acute and a chronic phase with different physiological mechanisms could be present. In the acute phase stimulation of pituitary–thyroid activity could be caused by a change in neural input into the hypothalamus, leading to increased release of thyrotropin releasing factor (TRF). An increased release of TRF could lead to increased release of TSH, which, in turn, causes increased release of TH. This could be termed an open loop reaction, since a feedback mechanism, *i.e.*, an influence of the blood level of TH on TSH secretion, plays no role. In the second phase of the cold response the increased release of TSH could be dependent on a tendency of the blood level of TH to fall, a tendency caused by the already discussed increase in peripheral loss of TH in the cold. This second phase would fall under the category of closed-loop reactions.

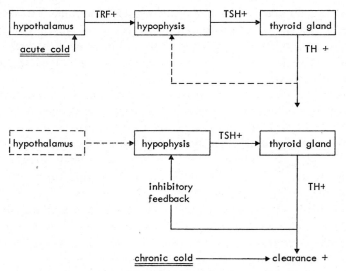

Fig. 1. Diagram of proposed biphasic mechanism of cold response. Upper half illustrates acute phase; lower half illustrates chronic phase. *Acute phase*: neural stimuli due to exposure to cold activate the hypothalamus and cause increased release of thyrotropin releasing factor (TRF+); in consequence, more thyroid stimulating hormone is secreted (TSH+) and this causes increased secretion of thyroid hormones (TH+). The inhibitory feedback of TH on TSH secretion is thought to be of little importance in acute cold (dashed line). *Chronic phase*: the main effect of chronic exposure to cold is increased clearance of TH. By way of the inhibitory feedback a compensatory increase in secretion of TSH (TSH+) and of TH (TH+) is brought about. The hypothalamic influence of TSH secretion is allegedly of little importance in this phase (dashed lines).

In the first phase, hypothalamic control of TSH secretion would be essential for the thyroidal cold response since the hypothalamus is an essential element of the proposed open-loop system. In the second phase, hypothalamic control would not be essential since the negative feedback control of TH secretion is largely independent of the hypothalamus, as has already been discussed. The question of the duration of the two phases can be tentatively answered by hypothesizing that the two phases overlap mainly during a period, extending from 24 h after initial cold exposure to possibly a week later. Evidence for this hypothesis will be forthcoming in the following sections of this paper in which we will try to adduce evidence for the suggested biphasic cold response of the pituitary–thyroid system. It should be emphasized that this concept is not new. Similar ideas have been brought forward previously by others (Brown–Grant, 1956; Cottle and Carlson, 1956; Knigge, 1960b, 1963; Van Beugen and Van der Werff ten Bosch, 1960).

Some questions which are not directly related to this concept will be considered also, since they seemed of interest from the points of view of thermoregulation or pituitary–thyroid function. However, no attempt will be made to deal with all aspects of the involvement of the pituitary–thyroid system in the complex of responses to environmental cold. Topics which will not be discussed are, *inter alia*, the complicated interplay between the pituitary–thyroid and pituitary–adrenal systems, the relation between hibernation and pituitary–thyroid function and the relative value of the various experimental methods of pituitary–thyroid physiology.

EVIDENCE FOR A NEURALLY INDUCED OPEN-LOOP REACTION AS FIRST PHASE OF THE COLD RESPONSE

The increased activity of the pituitary–thyroid system following cold exposure occurs very rapidly. This points to a neural mechanism, as has already been emphasized by Andersson *et al.* (1963b). In most studies on the interval between onset of cold exposure and increase in pituitary–thyroid activity, rise of TH secretion has been used as a parameter. In the interpretation of such studies it should be realized that there is an interval of about 1 h between a rise in TSH secretion and a rise in TH secretion (Brown–Grant *et al.*, 1954; Knigge, 1960a) and an interval of about 30 min between increased TRF release and rise in TSH secretion (Baugh *et al.*, 1970). A rise of TH secretion has been demonstrated in the goat and guinea pig 2 h after cold exposure (goat, Andersson *et al.*, 1962; guinea pig, Yamada *et al.*, 1965); 4 h after cold exposure in the hamster (Knigge, 1960a), the mouse (Melander and Rerup, 1968) and the rabbit (Brown–Grant *et al.*, 1954). For the rat the shortest recorded interval between cold exposure and the thyroidal response seems to be 8 h (Brown–Grant, 1956). Few studies have used other endpoints in the determination of the rapidity of the onset of the thyroidal response to cold. DelConte and Stux (1954), in the thyroid glands of cold-exposed guinea pigs, found cytological changes within 30 min; confirmation of this observation with the benefit of the electron microscope would be of great interest. A similar extremely rapid response was reported by Itoh *et al.* (1966) for the rat.

References p. 313

With bioassay methods, these authors found a rise of blood TSH even after 15 minutes. It should, however, be remarked that this study is somewhat out of line with other observations of TSH secretion in the cold since the rise in blood TSH was short-lived. In all other studies blood TSH remained elevated in the cold.

Although it has no immediate bearing on our present problem, it seems of interest to mention that the fall of pituitary–thyroid activity following transfer of rats from a cold to a warm environment may occur much slower than the cold response. Bauman and Turner (1967) observed a duration of this change of more than a week. This observation could be considered as indirect evidence for a specific mechanism underlying the acute pituitary–thyroidal cold response which is not the mirror-image of the response to transfer from a cold to warm environment.

Neural control of the first phase of the cold response is also clearly indicated by observations on TRF. Guillemin et al. (1969) found an increased hypothalamic TRF content after an exposure to cold for only 5 min; Redding and Schally (1969) observed in thyroidectomized–hypophysectomized rats a rise of the blood level of TRF after cold exposure of 2 h.

Further support for a neurally mediated acute cold response can be derived from the observations of Andersson et al. (1962, 1963a, 1965) in the goat and of McClure and Reichlin (1964) in the rat that hypothalamic cooling may induce pituitary–thyroid activation. This notwithstanding the doubt about the physiological occurrence of a fall of hypothalamic temperature following cold exposure (Hammel et al., 1963; Yamada et al., 1965).

Studies on the influence of procedures such as section of the pituitary stalk and destruction of the TSH area of the hypothalamus are of great interest for the proposed biphasic thyroidal response to cold. Conclusive support for this concept would be a body of data demonstrating absence of the acute cold response, but presence of a— possibly subnormal—chronic cold response in animals with hypothalamic lesions, stalk sections, etc. A summary of available data on the acute as well as on the chronic thyroidal cold response gives the following picture.

The acute cold response, i.e., increased pituitary–thyroid activity within the first 24 h after cold exposure, could be blocked in the hamster by ectopic transplantation of the pituitary gland and—in the same species—also by lesions in the median eminence and by reserpine treatment (Knigge and Bierman, 1958). The lesions used in these experiments can probably be considered as stalk sections. Lesions in the area of the paraventricular nuclei had the same blocking effect in the guinea pig (Yamada et al., 1965) as had also pituitary transplantation in the rabbit (Von Euler and Holmgren, 1956). These data, therefore, support the proposed concept of the acute cold response.

Data obtained after one to two weeks of cold exposure are not immediately relevant to our question, since it is uncertain whether this period should still be considered as part of the acute or already as part of the chronic phase of the cold response. In stalk-sectioned rats the cold response was found to be absent (Uotila, 1939a, b) as well as present but subnormal (László et al., 1966; Barnett and Greep, 1951) in this period of time. Similarly diverging results have been reported under these time conditions for rats with anterior hypothalamic lesions. Absence of the cold response in such animals has been reported by De Jong and Moll (1965), presence of the cold response by Van Beugen (1960) and Van Beugen and Van der Werff ten Bosch (1960, 1961).

As has been mentioned, data on animals with lesions, stalk sections, etc., and exposed to cold for long periods will be included here. Such data are few. Only Brolin (1946) and D'Angelo (1960a, b) have tested rats with pituitaries isolated from the hypothalamus after cold exposure of 2 weeks and more. Brolin (1946) found no signs of increased pituitary–thyroid activity in stalk-sectioned rats exposed to cold for 5–6 weeks, but his work lacked the benefit of the more sensitive present-day methods. D'Angelo (1960a, b) tested rats with anterior hypothalamic lesions after cold exposures of two weeks and longer. The data on his lesioned animals exposed to cold show a tendency of TSH levels to be lower than those of non-lesioned animals at standard temperature, no influence of cold on radio-iodine release, and presence in the cold of some thyroid hypertrophy. These latter observations constitute—at best— equivocal support for the presence, but at a subnormal level, of the chronic response. This was, as has been explained, requested by our hypothesis.

Evidence of still another type could support the concept of an acute cold response controlled by the hypothalamus. Release of TSH can be inhibited by administration of TH. If this inhibition is less pronounced in animals acutely exposed to cold, this would indicate increased release of TRF, induced by the exposure to cold. Competition of TH and TRF in the regulation of TSH release is well documented (Vale *et al.*, 1967). Experiments along this line have been performed in the hamster (Knigge, 1960a), goat (Andersson *et al.*, 1963b), guinea pig (Yamada *et al.*, 1965), rat (Héroux and Brauer, 1965) and mouse (Melander and Rerup, 1968). The experiments of Knigge (1960a) and of Héroux and Brauer (1965) point to an increased TRF release following acute cold exposure, but the work of the other authors does not. This does not constitute convincing counterevidence. In some experiments the doses of TH may have been too high to observe a difference between TSH release in the cold and at room temperature. In other experiments the effect of TH at room temperature, a necessary control, was not studied at all. Finally, the blood levels of TH have not been determined in any of these experiments. This seems highly desirable, since differences in peripheral loss of TH in the cold or at room temperature may cause unexpected variations of the TH levels at feedback receptors. It is of interest to remark that these experiments resemble those in which the adrenal response to stress is studied following exogenous corticosteroids. These experiments have raised many and in part still unanswered questions about the most correct type of experiment and about the interpretation of the results (Smelik, 1963a, b).

Finally, there is possibly negative evidence in favour of the proposed open-loop mechanism of the acute cold response, *i.e.*, the alternative explanation, a negative feedback response, is unlikely. Increased peripheral loss of TH, the only plausible cause of a negative feedback mechanism underlying the thyroidal response to cold in its acute phase, does occur, but later than the reported rise in pituitary–thyroid activity. In the next section we will discuss the temporal characteristics of increased peripheral TH loss in greater detail. Here it should be sufficient to state that increased peripheral loss of TH does not precede the cold response and can, therefore, not be its cause. In this context the time interval between a fall in blood TH and increased TH secretion is also of interest. The available pertinent data are conflicting. Suematsu *et al.* (1969) observed in the dog that it takes several days before TSH secretion rises in response to a fall in the blood level of TH, but Langer *et al.* (1971) reported an interval of less than an hour in the rat.

EVIDENCE FOR A NEGATIVE FEEDBACK REACTION AS SECOND PHASE OF THE COLD RESPONSE

It has already been remarked that the acute phase of the cold response, allegedly controlled by a neurally mediated open-loop reaction, is probably replaced over a period of 1–8 days after cold exposure by a purely hormonal negative feedback reaction, which constitutes the chronic phase. There is no evidence indicating a direct relationship between the transition from the acute to the chronic phase of the thyroidal cold response on the one hand and the acquisition of the so-called "acclimatization to cold" (Sellers *et al.*, 1951a), which in later years has been named "acclimation" (Steiner *et al.*, 1969), on the other. Acclima(tiza)tion occurs not earlier than about one month in the cold which is much later than the appearance of many features of the chronic phase of the thyroidal cold response, *e.g.*, the markedly increased peripheral TH loss (see next paragraphs). This point emphasizes that the thyroidal cold response is only one of a variety of physiological changes in the cold.

Indicative of a change with time in the nature of the thyroidal response to cold are observations of Andersson *et al.* (1962) suggesting that the effect of prolonged hypothalamic cooling on thyroid activity levels off after a period of 6 h, although other thermoregulatory responses persist.

Substantiation of the view that after longer periods of cold exposure increased pituitary–thyroid activity is due to a negative feedback reaction to increased peripheral loss of TH, can in principle be derived from data of various types: demonstration of increased peripheral loss of TH (1), demonstration of increased release of TH and of TSH (2), while demonstration of a normal blood level of TH would also constitute supporting evidence (3). A changed set-point of the "thyrostat" in the cold could, however, be imagined. In consequence, the proposed concept of the chronic phase could be reconciled with blood levels of TH above or below those at normal temperature. It is realized that data of only one of these three categories do not by themselves support the proposed concept. Moreover, data of some of these categories only provide definite support for the biphasic cold response if they can be obtained, as outlined above, only during the period suggested for the chronic phase and not immediately after cold exposure. In other words: two phases of the cold response with different physiological mechanisms can only be accepted if one or more characteristics of pituitary–thyroid function change during cold exposure.

It has already been mentioned that increased peripheral loss of TH occurs in the cold and that this cannot be the cause of the acute cold response. Increased peripheral loss of TH has been studied repeatedly in the rat. It has been observed after a cold exposure of 15 h (Bondy and Hagewood, 1952), of 24 h (Kassenaar *et al.*, 1956, 1959), of 3 days (Héroux and Petrovic, 1969), of 11 days (Intocia and Van Middlesworth, 1959), of 14 days (Rand *et al.*, 1952; Gregerman and Crowder, 1963), of 3 weeks (Harland and Orr, 1969), of 6 weeks (Héroux and Petrovic, 1969), and of 3 months (Galton and Nisula, 1969). Interestingly, these latter authors found increased peripheral TH loss still absent after 3 weeks, which is in marked contradiction to the other studies listed above. Possibly, this is related to the increase in food intake in the cold which in Galton and Nisula's experiments also occurred much later than has usually been found. Fewer data are available for species other than the rat. Yamada *et al.* (1965) observed an increased TH loss extremely rapidly in the guinea pig: after 2 h in the cold. Wills and Schindler (1970) found it in mice after 3 days, Freinkel and Lewis (1957) after 9–11 days in sheep. Most authors did not determine peripheral TH loss sooner or later than at the specified time. Although not directly relevant to our theme, the question as to the cause of the increased peripheral disappearance of TH may be discussed here. The answer to this question seems the following: there is no increased tissue consumption of TH, but increased peripheral loss of the hormones, primarily via the gastro-intestinal tract (Intocia and Van Middlesworth, 1959; Cottle, 1964; Héroux and Brauer, 1965; Galton and Nisula, 1969). This is of general physiological interest since it indicates that increased pituitary–thyroid activity in the cold is not immediately related to the increase in metabolism in the cold. The most plausible explanation for an increased gastro-intestinal loss of TH in the cold is a change in digestive function with, *inter alia*, increased food intake and increased bile secretion. At least in the rat, considerable amounts of TH can be found in the bile (see Galton and Nisula, 1969, for details on the above) and more TH may be conjugated and excreted by the liver in the cold (Cottle and Veress, 1966a). Net intestinal reabsorption of TH is absent in the rat according to Cottle (1964) and Galton and Nisula (1969), although this has not been thought so previously (Albert and Keating, 1952; Myant, 1957). A relationship between increased peripheral loss of TH and increased food intake is indicated by the temporal relationships: both have been noted already after 24 h of cold exposure (data on food intake in the cold of Cottle and Carlson, 1954, and of Baker and Sellers, 1957, for the rat; of Bauman *et al.*, 1968, for the hamster; data on TH loss quoted above). Similarly, Bauman *et al.*, (1968) in the hamster, observed a parallelism between decline of TH secretion and of food intake after long periods of cold exposure. Other similar indirect evidence is available. In the experiments of Galton and Nisula (1969) both, increased loss of TH and increased food intake, occurred much later than in other studies. Also, pituitary–thyroid activity is clearly subnormal in rats subjected to food restriction at various temperatures (Cottle, 1960; Yousef and Johnson, 1968). It should, however, also be remarked that in the cow no clear parallelism between thyroid function and food intake seems to exist (Yousef and Johnson, 1966). Both the quantity of material passing through the intestinal tract and other, not well defined changes in digestive function seem to contribute to the increased loss of TH in the cold (Van Middlesworth, 1957; Cottle, 1964). It should also be remarked that, besides biliary–faecal loss, other, as yet

References p. 313

unidentified, factors may add to peripheral loss of TH in the cold (Hillier, 1968; Straw, 1969). After this digression into allied topics we may summarize the above: increased peripheral loss of TH in the cold—a requirement for the proposed mechanism of the chronic phase of the cold response—has been convincingly demonstrated.

Another requirement for accepting the proposed feedback mechanism of the chronic thyroidal response to cold, is hypersecretion of TH in animals exposed to cold for periods longer than 48 h. This has already been demonstrated by Dempsey and Astwood (1943) in the rat with the goitre prevention technique and has been confirmed later in many species (hamster, Bauman et al., 1968; mouse, Wills and Schindler, 1970; sheep, Freinkel and Lewis, 1957; cow, Yousef and Johnson, 1966; guinea pig, Stevens et al., 1955; rat, D'Angelo, 1960c; Bauman and Turner, 1967; Galton and Nisula, 1969, and many others). Increased TSH secretion, which has the same bearing on our view on the chronic cold response, has also been demonstrated. It has been observed in guinea pigs after periods in the cold of one week and longer (Stevens et al., 1953, 1955; D'Angelo, 1960c), also in the rat after cold exposures of two weeks (Martin et al., 1970), of 4 weeks (Van Rees and Moll, unpublished), 5–6 weeks (Brolin, 1946) and of 7 weeks and longer (D'Angelo, 1960b).

Data on blood TH will be summarized next and will include those during the acute phase.

Many data indicate that during the first 48 h after cold exposure blood levels of TH are elevated. Duration of the period of elevated levels may vary from species to species. Elevated TH levels immediately after cold exposure have been reported for the goat (Andersson et al., 1962), mouse (Melander and Rerup, 1968), guinea pig (Yamada et al., 1965), and rat (Kassenaar et al., 1956). Only one study contradicts the data quoted above: Knigge (1960a) found in the hamster no elevation of blood TH in the first 4 h after cold exposure. The similar findings in the rat of Bondy and Hagewood (1952) can be dismissed, since they were obtained under the unphysiological condition of fasting.

As will be discussed now, normal blood levels of TH have generally been found after longer periods of cold exposure. The difference between the acute and chronic TH levels can, therefore, be considered strong evidence for a change from an open loop to a negative feedback control of pituitary–thyroid activity. Normal TH levels have been found in the rat after cold exposures of 3 days (Bondy and Hagewood, 1952), of two weeks (Gregerman and Crowder, 1963; Martin et al., 1970), of 6 weeks (Ershoff and Golub, 1951; Magwood and Héroux, 1968; Héroux and Petrovic, 1969), of 3 months (Héroux and Brauer, 1965; Galton and Nisula, 1969), of 2–52 days (Straw and Fregly, 1967). Also in other species, blood TH levels seem to be normal after cold exposure for more than 48 h: mouse (Wills and Schindler, 1970), sheep (Freinkel and Lewis, 1957), guinea pig (Stevens et al., 1953, 1955), hamster (Tashima, 1965). Here again a few conflicting results have been reported. Increased TH levels have been found in the cow (Yousef and Johnson, 1966) and in the rat (Harland and Orr, 1969). In the rat, subnormal levels have also been found (Rand et al., 1952; Cadot et al., 1969). The relation between total and free TH has received little attention in this work. Cottle and Veress (1966b) reported changes in binding in chronic cold-exposed rats, but Galton and Nisula (1969) and Martin *et al.* (1970) did not find such changes.

Evidence for the proposed concept of the chronic thyroidal response to cold from lesion studies, stalk sections, etc., has already been discussed in the section on the acute response. A general discussion of TSH/TH interplay can be found in Launay (1965).

MISCELLANEOUS ASPECTS OF THE COLD RESPONSE

The absence during chronic cold exposure of elevated blood levels of TH and of increased tissue consumption of the hormones indicates that the pituitary–thyroid response to cold is not a physiological requirement for adaptation to low environmental temperature, but a homeostatic response to the occurrence in the cold of increased peripheral loss of TH. One might expect, therefore, that the thyroidal cold response is not present without exceptions. This is indeed the case. The cold response seems to be dependent on temperature, with a diminution of the response at very low temperatures (1). The response may also be dependent on the duration of cold exposure, with a decrease of the response after long periods of cold exposure (2). Furthermore, the response may not be present in all mammals (3) and—if present— may be dependent on other environmental factors besides temperature (4); the diet may be one of these factors. These matters will be discussed now.

Data on the dependence of the thyroidal cold response on temperature have been reported by Brown–Grant *et al.* (1954) for the rabbit, by Brown–Grant (1956) for the rat and by Brown–Grant and Pethes (1960) for the guinea pig. In all instances a drop in temperature to about 0 °C no longer caused thyroid activation, but inhibition. Other factors must be involved, since Harland and Orr (1969) still found activation at −3 °C. In the guinea pig Yamada *et al.* (1965) observed that the thyroid response to a specific low temperature is dependent on the temperature condition before cold exposure.

The question whether thyroid activation by cold is a permanent condition has produced contradictory answers. A complete disappearance of the cold response after long periods has been reported for the hamster by Bauman *et al.* (1968) and for the rat by Leblond *et al.* (1944). A permanent cold response has been observed in the rat by Starr and Roskelley (1940) and by Woods and Carlson (1956). Possibly, the cold response becomes less pronounced, but does not disappear (rat: Schachner *et al.*, 1949; Woods and Carlson, 1956; hamster: Knigge, 1963; guinea pig: Pichotka, 1952). The dependence of cold response on the species is largely an unanswered question. In the preceding sections it has become apparent that this response is present in the mouse, the rat, the hamster (see also Knigge, 1957; Knigge *et al.*, 1957), the rabbit, the guinea pig, the cow and the sheep. The cold response may be absent in the cat (Knigge and Bierman, 1958). Data on man are conflicting (Ingbar *et al.*, 1954; Berg *et al.*, 1966; Suzuki *et al.*, 1967). In the baboon, Gale *et al.* (1970) found the response in only 50% of the animals. A possible explanation of these divergencies may be derived from the fact that faecal TH loss may vary from species to species.

References p. 313

It is much greater, *e.g.*, in the rat than in man (Gregerman and Crowder, 1963; Furth *et al.*, 1967).

Dependence of the cold response on other environmental conditions has been extensively studied by Héroux and collaborators. They found no cold response and even a tendency towards thyroid inhibition in rats under outdoor winter conditions, although other thermogenic reactions were clearly present (Héroux *et al.*, 1959b; Héroux and Brauer, 1965). These authors (Héroux and Brauer, 1965; Héroux and Petrovic, 1969) reviewed comparable findings obtained by others in other mammals (Delost and Naudy, 1956, and others). Dietary factors might well influence cold response, since they have a pronounced effect on pituitary–thyroid function (Van Middlesworth, 1957; Van Middlesworth *et al.*, 1959; Yamada, 1968). However, the findings on outdoor versus laboratory cold cannot be easily explained on the basis of diet, since the rats of Héroux and Brauer (1965) received the same food outdoors and in the laboratory. It seems possible that the fluctuating temperature outdoors affects the pituitary–thyroid system in another way than the thermostatically controlled temperature commonly used in the laboratory, but this has never been tested experimentally.

It should be remarked that not only the pituitary–thyroid system but also other physiological systems respond differently to laboratory cold and to outdoor cold (Héroux *et al.*, 1959a; Hart, 1964).

A possible influence of the diet on cold response is indicated by data showing a diminished thyroidal cold response, with other thermogenic responses clearly present, in rats on a high fat, low residue TH-free diet (Héroux, 1968; Magwood and Héroux, 1968; Héroux and Petrovic, 1969). As could be expected, the increase in faecal TH loss, which is normally seen in the cold, is less pronounced with this diet since increase in food intake contributes to increased faecal TH loss to a lesser extent, when the food does not contain TH. It remains to be seen, whether the special diet used by Héroux and co-workers affects the cold response mainly by way of absence of TH or by its other characteristics, high fat content and low residue. Additionally, in further analysis of the effect of such diets on the cold response the contribution of endogenous and dietary TH to faecal loss should be determined. The term "faecal clearance of thyroxine" (Magwood and Héroux, 1968) should probably not be used as a synonym for faecal thyroxine loss.

It would be of interest to investigate whether dietary changes influence only the chronic thyroidal cold response, as was the case in the experiments of Héroux *et al.*, or also the acute response. The question whether mammals in the cold change their diet, if they are allowed to do so, seems not to have been studied in relation to pituitary–thyroid function.

FUNCTIONAL SIGNIFICANCE OF THE THYROIDAL RESPONSE TO COLD

The simple interpretation of the cold response as an adaptation to increased tissue consumption of TH, which then could cause or contribute to the increased metabolism in the cold, seems incorrect. This is indicated, as has already been mentioned, by the absence of increased tissue consumption of TH in the cold. However, the observation that the blood level of TH is normal after longer periods of cold exposure, but increases immediately after cold exposure, indicates that the physiological significance of the thyroidal cold response may be different after short and longer periods of cold exposure.

The probable absence of a direct relationship between adaptation to cold and the thyroidal cold response does not negate a functional involvement of TH in adaptation to a cold environment. A detailed analysis of this subject is outside the scope of this paper, but some aspects may be mentioned. Thyroid involvement in the complex of adaptive reaction to cold is simply and convincingly demonstrated by the increase in mortality of thyroidectomized animals in the cold and its correction by TH treatment (rat: Leblond and Gross, 1943; Sellers and You, 1950; guinea pig: Stevens et al., 1955).

Interplay between thyroid function and the complex of other thermogenic responses is clearly demonstrated by the observation of Andersson et al. (1967) that other responses to cold are more pronounced in hypothyroid goats than in euthyroid animals. Of similar implication is the reverse experiment of Martin et al. (1970) in the rat. Here, the thyroidal cold response was supranormal after experimental blockade of other physiological responses to cold.

Brief general summaries of the total pattern of thermogenic responses to cold exposure can be found in Sellers et al. (1951a, b), Sellers (1957), Cottle (1960), Carlson (1960), Andersson et al. (1963a, 1967).

CONCLUSION

In this paper we have considered the following view on the pituitary–thyroid response to cold: the cold response starts as an open-loop reaction with the following elements: central nervous system, pituitary gland and thyroid gland; after longer periods of cold exposure thyroid function is controlled by the hormonal negative feedback system between pituitary TSH secretion and thyroid function, with only a minor modulatory influence of the hypothalamus. The available evidence indicates that this two-phase concept of the thyroidal cold response is highly likely. More evidence is required before it can be regarded as demonstrated conclusively. The timing and the interweaving of the two mechanisms (and phases) of the thyroidal response to cold are still uncertain.

REFERENCES

ALBERT, A. AND KEATING, F. R. (1952) The role of the gastro-intestinal tract, including the liver in the metabolism of radiothyroxine. *Endocrinology*, **51**, 427–443.

ANDERSSON, B., BROOK, A. H. AND EKMAN, L. (1965) Further studies of the thyroidal response to local cooling of the "heat loss center". *Acta physiol. scand.*, **63**, 186–192.

ANDERSSON, B., EKMAN, L., GALE, C. C. AND SUNDSTEN, J. W. (1962) Thyroidal response to local cooling of the preoptic "heat loss center". *Life Sci.*, **1**, 1–11.

ANDERSSON, B., EKMAN, L., GALE, C. C. AND SUNSTEN, J. W. (1963a) Control of thyrotrophic hormone (TSH) secretion by the "heat loss center". *Acta physiol. scand.*, **59**, 12–33.

ANDERSSON, B., EKMAN, L., HOKFELT, B., JOBIN, M., OLSSEN, K. AND ROBERTSHAW, D. (1967) Studies of the importance of the thyroid and the sympathetic system in the defence to cold in the goat. *Acta physiol. scand.*, **69**, 111–118.

ANDERSSON, B., GALE, C. C. AND OHGA, A. (1963b) Suppression by thyroxine of the thyroidal response to local cooling of the "heat loss center". *Acta physiol. scand.*, **59**, 67–73.

BAKER, D. G. AND SELLERS, E. A. (1957) Electrolyte metabolism in the rat exposed to low environmental temperatures. *Canad. J. Biochem.*, **35**, 631–636.

BARNETT, R. J. AND GREEP, R. O. (1951) Regulation of secretion of adrenotropic and thyrotropic hormones after stalk section. *Amer. J. Physiol.*, **167**, 569–575.

BAUGH, C. M., KRUMDIECK, C. L., HERSHMAN, J. M. AND PITMAN, J. A. (1970) Synthesis and biological activity of thyrotropin-releasing hormone. *Endocrinology*, **87**, 1015–1021.

BAUMAN, T. R., ANDERSON, R. R. AND TURNER, C. W. (1968) Thyroid hormone secretion rates and food consumption of the hamster *(Mesocricetus aureatus)* at 25.5° and 4.5°C. *Gen. comp. Endocr.*, **10**, 92–98.

BAUMAN, T. R. AND TURNER, C. W. (1967) The effect of varying temperatures on thyroid activity and the survival of rats exposed to cold and treated with L-thyroxine or corticosterone. *J. Endocr.*, **37**, 365–369.

BERG, G. R., UTIGER, R. D., SCHALCH, D. S. AND RETCHLIN, S. (1966) Effect of central cooling in man on pituitary-thyroid function and growth hormone secretion. *J. Appl. Physiol.*, **21**, 1791–1794.

BONDY, P. K. AND HAGEWOOD, M. A. (1952) Effect of stress and cortisone on plasma protein-bound iodine and thyroxine metabolism in rats. *Proc. Soc. exp. Biol. (N.Y.)*, **81**, 328–331.

BROLIN, S. E. (1946) A study of the structural and hormonal reactions of the pituitary body of rats exposed to cold. *Acta Anat. (Basel)*, **2**, Suppl. 3, 1–165.

BROWN–GRANT, K. (1956) Changes in the thyroid activity of rats exposed to cold. *J. Physiol. (Lond.)*, **131**, 52–57.

BROWN–GRANT, K. (1966) The control of thyroid-stimulating hormone secretion. In *The Pituitary Gland. Vol. 2*, G. W. HARRIS AND B. T. DONOVAN (Eds.), Butterworth, London, pp. 235–270.

BROWN–GRANT, K. AND PETHES, G. (1960) The response of the thyroid gland of the guinea pig to stress. *J. Physiol. (Lond.)*, **151**, 40–50.

BROWN–GRANT, K., VON EULER, C., HARRIS, G. W. AND REICHLIN, S. (1954) The measurement and experimental modification of thyroid activity in the rabbit. *J. Physiol. (Lond.)*, **126**, 1–28.

CADOT, M., JULIEN, M.-F. AND CEVILLARD, L. (1969) Estimation of thyroid function in rats exposed or adapted to environments at 5° or 30°C. *Fed. Proc.*, **28**, 1228–1233.

CARLSON, L. D. (1960) Non-shivering thermogenesis and its endocrine control. *Fed. Proc.*, **19**, 25–30.

COTTLE, W. H. (1960) Role of thyroid secretion in cold acclimation. *Fed. Proc.*, **19**, 59–63.

COTTLE, W. H. (1964) Biliary and faecal clearance of endogenous thyroid hormone in cold-acclimated rats. *Amer. J. Physiol.*, **207**, 1063–1066.

COTTLE, W. H. AND CARLSON, L. D. (1954) Adaptive changes in rats exposed to cold. Caloric exchange. *Amer. J. Physiol.*, **178**, 305–308.

COTTLE, W. H. AND CARLSON, L. D. (1956) Turn-over of thyroid hormone in cold-exposed rats as determined by radio-active iodine studies. *Endocrinology*, **59**, 1–11.

COTTLE, W. H. AND VERESS, A. T. (1966a) Urinary excretion of glucuronides by cold-acclimated rats. *Canad. J. Physiol. Pharmacol.*, **44**, 325–326.

COTTLE, W. H. AND VERESS, A. T. (1966b) Serum binding and biliary clearance of tri-iodothyronine in cold-acclimated rats. *Canad. J. Physiol. Pharmacol.*, **44**, 571–574.

D'ANGELO, S. A. (1960a) Endocrine function in hypothalamic-lesioned rats exposed to cold. *Acta Endocr. (Kbh.)*, Suppl. 50, 5–6.

D'ANGELO, S. A. (1960b) Hypothalamus and endocrine function in persistent estrous rats at low environmental temperature. *Amer. J. Physiol.*, **199**, 701–706.

D'ANGELO, S. A. (1960c) Adenohypophysial function in the guinea-pig at low environmental temperature. *Fed. Proc.*, **19**, 51–56.

DE JONG, W. AND MOLL, J. (1965) Differential effects of hypothalamic lesions on pituitary–thyroid activity in the rat. *Acta Endocr. (Kbh.)*, **48**, 522–535.

DELCONTE, E. AND STUX, M. (1954) Rapidity of thyroid reaction to cold. *Nature (Lond.)*, **173**, 83.

DELOST, P. ET NAUDY, J. (1956) Cycle saisonnier de la thyroïde chez les rongeurs sauvages non-hibernants. *C. R. Soc. Biol. (Paris)*, **150**, 906–909.

DEMPSEY, E. W. AND ASTWOOD, E. B. (1943) Determination of the rate of thyroid hormone secretion at various environmental temperatures. *Endocrinology*, **32**, 509–518.

ERSHOFF, B. H. AND GOLUB, O. J. (1951) Effects of prolonged exposure to cold on the serum protein-bound iodine of the rat. *Arch. Biochem.*, **30**, 202–206.

FREINKEL, N. AND LEWIS, D. (1957) The effect of lowered environmental temperature on the peripheral metabolism of labelled thyroxine in the sheep. *J. Physiol. (Lond.)*, **135**, 288–300.

FURTH, E., HURLEY, J., NUNEZ, E. AND BECKER, D. V. (1967) Comparative aspects of the entero-hepatic metabolism of thyroxine in rat, dog and man. *Fed. Proc.*, **26**, 258.

GALE, C. C., JOBIN, M., PROPPE, D. W., NOTTER, D. AND FOX, H. (1970) Endocrine thermoregulatory responses to local hypothalamic cooling in unanesthetized baboons. *Amer. J. Physiol.*, **219**, 193–201.

GALTON, V. A. AND NISULA, B. C. (1969) Thyroxine metabolism and thyroid function in the cold-adapted rat. *Endocrinology*, **85**, 79–86.

GREER, M. A. (1951) Evidence of hypothalamic control of the pituitary release of thyrotropin. *Proc. Soc. exp. Biol. (N.Y.)*, **77**, 603–608.

GREGERMAN, R. I. AND CROWDER, S. E. (1963) Estimation of thyroxine secretion rate in the rat by the radioactive thyroxine turn-over technique: influence of age, sex and exposure to cold. *Endocrinology*, **72**, 382–392.

GUILLEMIN, R., BURGUS, R. AND VALE, W. (1969) TSH-releasing factor: an RF model study. *Progress in Endocrinology, Proc. 3rd. Int. Congress of Endocrinology, 1968.* Excerpta Medica, Amsterdam.

HAMMEL, H. T., JACKSON, D. S., STOLWIJK, J. A. J., HARDY, J. D. AND STRØMME, S. B. (1963) Temperature regulation by hypothalamic proportional control with adjustable set point. *J. Appl. Physiol.*, **18**, 1146–1154.

HARLAND, W. A. AND ORR, J. S. (1969) A model of thyroxine metabolism based on the effects of environmental temperature. *J. Physiol. (Lond.)*, **200**, 297–310.

HART, J. S. (1964) Insulative and metabolic adaptations to cold in vertebrates. *Symp. Soc. exp. Biol.*, **18**, 31–48.

HÉROUX, O. (1968) Thyroid parameters and metabolic adaptation to cold in rats fed a low-bulk thyroxine-free diet. *Canad. J. Physiol. Pharmacol.*, **46**, 843–846.

HÉROUX, O. AND BRAUER, R. (1965) Critical studies on determination of thyroid secretion rate in cold-adapted animals. *J. Appl. Physiol.*, **20**, 597–606.

HÉROUX, O., DEPOCAS, F. AND HART, J. S. (1959a) Comparison between seasonal and thermal acclimation in white rats. *Canad. J. Biochem.*, **37**, 473–478.

HÉROUX, O. AND PETROVIC, V. M. (1969) Effect of high- and low-bulk diets on the thyroxine turn-over rate in rats with acute and chronic exposure to different temperatures. *Canad. J. Physiol. Pharmacol.* **47**, 963–968.

HÉROUX, O., SCHÖNBAUM, E. AND DES MARAIS, A. (1959b) Adrenal and thyroid adjustments in white rats during seasonal and thermal acclimation. *Fed. Proc.*, **18**, 67.

HILLIER, A. P. (1968) The biliary-faecal excretion of thyroxine during cold exposure in the rat. *J. Physiol. (Lond.)*, **197**, 123–134.

INGBAR, S. H., KLEEMAN, C. R., QUINN, M. AND BASS, D. E. (1954) The effect of prolonged exposure to cold on thyroid function in man. *Clin. Res. Proc.*, **2**, 86.

INTOCIA, A. AND VAN MIDDLESWORTH, L. (1959) Thyroxine excretion increase by cold exposure. *Endocrinology*, **64**, 462–464.

ITOH, S., HIROSHIGE, T., KOSEKI, T. AND NAGATSUGAWA, T. (1966) Release of thyrotropin in relation to cold exposure. *Fed. Proc.*, **25**, 1187–1192.

KASSENAAR, A. A. H., LAMEIJER, L. D. F. AND QUERIDO, A. (1956) The effect of environmental temperature on the blood protein-bound iodine content of thyroxine maintained thyroidectomized rats. *Acta Endocr. (Kbh.)*, **21**, 37–40.

KASSENAAR, A., LAMEIJER, L. D. F. AND QUERIDO, A. (1959) Studies on the peripheral disappearance of thyroid hormone, VI. The effect of environmental temperature on the distribution of ^{131}I in thyroidectomized, L-thyroxine maintained rats after the injection of ^{131}I-labeled L-thyroxine. *Acta Endocr. (Kbh.)*, **32**, 575–578.

KNIGGE, K. M. (1957) Influence of cold exposure upon the endocrine glands of the hamster, with an apparent dichotomy between morphological and functional response of the thyroid. *Anat. Rec.*, **127**, 75–79.

KNIGGE, K. M. (1960a) Time study of acute cold-induced acceleration of thyroidal I^{131} release in the hamster. *Proc. Soc. exp. Biol. (N.Y.)*, **104**, 368–371.

KNIGGE, K. M. (1960b) Neuro-endocrine mechanisms influencing ACTH and TSH secretion and their role in cold acclimation. *Fed. Proc.*, **19**, 45–51.

KNIGGE, K. M. (1963) Thyroid function and plasma binding during cold exposure of the hamster. *Fed. Proc.*, **22**, 755–760.

KNIGGE, K. M. AND BIERMAN, S. M. (1958) Evidence of central nervous system influence upon cold-induced acceleration of thyroidal I^{131} release. *Amer. J. Physiol.*, **192**, 625–630.

KNIGGE, K. M., GOODMAN, R. S. AND SOLOMON, D. H. (1957) Role of pituitary, adrenal and kidney in several thyroid responses of cold-exposed hamsters. *Amer. J. Physiol.* **189**, 415–419.

LANGER, P., PONEC, J., CVEČKOVÁ, L. AND LICHARDUS, B. (1971) Short-term regulation of blood thyroxine level following the acute removal of circulating hormone by isorolemic exchange transfusion. *Neuroendocrinology*, **8**, 59–69.

LÁSZLÓ, F. A., CSERNAY, L. UND KOVÁCS, K. (1966) Untersuchung der Schilddrüsenfunktion bei hypophysenstiellädierten Ratten. *Endokrinologie*, **50**, 72–78.

LAUNAY, M. P. (1965) The effect of thiouracil derivates on the pituitary–thyroid axis: a paradox in search of a solution. *Rev. Canad. Biol.*, **24**, 299–304.

LEBLOND, C. P. AND GROSS, J. (1943) Effect of thyroidectomy on resistance to low environmental temperature. *Endocrinology*, **33**, 155–160.

LEBLOND, C. P., GROSS, J., PEACOCK, W. AND EVANS, R. D. (1944) Metabolism of radio-iodine in the thyroids of rats exposed to high or low temperatures. *Amer. J. Physiol.*, **140**, 671–676.

MAGWOOD, S. G. A. AND HÉROUX, O. (1968) Fecal excretion of thyroxine in warm- and cold-acclimated rats. *Canad. J. Physiol. Pharmacol.*, **46**, 601–607.

MARTIN, J. B., BOLLINGER, J. A. AND REICHLIN, S. (1970) Pituitary–thyroid regulation in immuno-sympathectomized cold-exposed rats. *Fed. Proc.*, **29**, 581 (Abstract).

McCLURE, J. N. AND REICHLIN, S. (1964) Thermosensitive hypothalamic areas regulating thyroid function and body temperature. *Fed. Proc.*, **23**, 109.

MELANDER, A. AND RERUP, C. (1968) Studies on thyroid activity in the mouse. I. The effect of thyroxine, corticosteroids and change in environmental temperature. *Acta Endocr. (Kbh.)*, **58**, 202–214.

MYANT, N. B. (1957) Faecal clearance rate of endogenous thyroid in rats. *J. Physiol. (Lond.)*, **136**, 198–202.

PICHOTKA, J. (1952) Das Verhalten der Schilddrüse und der Körpertemperatur bei der Adaption an niedere Umgebungstemperaturen. *Arch. exp. Pathol. Pharmakol.*, **215**, 299–316.

RAND, C. G., RIGGS, D. S. AND TALBOT, N. B. (1952) The influence of environmental temperature on the metabolism of the thyroid hormone in the rat. *Endocrinology*, **51**, 562–569.

REDDING, T. W. AND SCHALLY, A. V. (1969) Studies on the thyrotropin-releasing hormone (TRH) activity in peripheral blood. *Proc. Soc. exp. Biol. (N.Y.)*, **131**, 420–425.

REICHLIN, S. (1966) Control of thyrotropic hormone secretion. In *Neuro-Endocrinology*, *Vol. I*, L. MARTINI AND W. F. GANONG, (Eds.), Academic Press, London, pp. 445–536.

SCHACHNER, H. G., GERLACH, Z. S. AND KREBS, A. T. (1949) Project No. 6-64-12-02-(6), Med. Dep. Field Res. Lab., Fort Knox, Ky. (quoted by Cottle and Carlson, 1954).

SELLERS, E. A. (1957) Adaptive and related phenomena in rats exposed to cold. *Rev. Canad. Biol.*, **16**, 175–188.

SELLERS, E. A., REICHMAN, S. AND THOMAS, N. (1951a) Acclimatization to cold: Natural and artificial. *Amer. J. Physiol.*, **167**, 644–650.

SELLERS, E. A., REICHMAN, S., THOMAS, N. AND YOU, S. S. (1951b) Acclimatization to cold in rats: metabolic rates. *Amer. J. Physiol.*, **167**, 651–655.

SELLERS, E. A. AND YOU, S. S. (1950) Role of the thyroid in metabolic responses to a cold environment. *Amer. J. Physiol.*, **163**, 81–91.

SMELIK, P. G. (1963a) Failure to inhibit corticotrophin secretion by experimentally induced increases in corticoid levels. *Acta Endocr. (Kbh.)*, **44**, 36–46.

SMELIK, P. G. (1963b) Relation between the blood level of corticoids and their inhibiting effects of the hypophyseal stress response. *Proc. Soc. exp. Biol. (N.Y.)*, **113**, 606–609.

STARR, P. AND ROSKELLEY, R. (1940) A comparison of the effects of cold and thyrotropic hormone on the thyroid gland. *Amer. J. Physiol.*, **130**, 549–556.

STEINER, G., JOHNSON, G. E., SELLERS, E. A. AND SCHÖNBAUM, E. (1969) Nervous control of brown adipose tissue metabolism in normal and cold-acclimated rats. *Fed. Proc.*, **28**, 1017–1021.

STEVENS, C. E., D'ANGELO, S. A., PASCHKIS, K. E., CANTAROW, A. AND SUNDERMAN, F. W. (1953) Effect of cold on pituitary–thyroid–adrenal relationships in the guinea-pig. *J. clin. Endocr.*, **13**, 872.

STEVENS, C. E., D'ANGELO, S. A., PASCHKIS, K. E., CANTAROW, A. AND SUNDERMAN, F. W. (1955) The response of the pituitary–thyroid system of the guinea pig to low environmental temperature. *Endocrinology*, **56**, 143–156.

STRAW, J. A. (1969) Effects of fecal weight on thyroid function in cold-exposed rats. *J. Appl. Physiol.*, **27**, 630–633.

STRAW, J. A. AND FREGLY, M. J. (1967) Evaluation of thyroid and adrenal–pituitary function during cold acclimation. *J. Appl. Physiol.*, **23**, 825–830.

SUEMATSU, H., MATSUDA, K., SHIZUME, K. AND NAKAO, K. (1969) Thyroid response to acute reduction of circulating thyroid hormone level. *Endocrinology*, **84**, 1161–1165.

SUZUKI, M., TONOUE, T., MATSUZAKI, S. AND YAMAMOTO, K. (1967) Initial response of human thyroid, adrenal cortex and adrenal medulla to acute cold exposure. *Canad. J. Physiol. Pharmacol.*, **45**, 423–432.

TASHIMA, L. S. (1965) The effects of cold exposure and hibernation on the thyroidal activity of *Mesocricetus aureatus. Gen. comp. Endocr.*, **5**, 267–277.

UOTILA, U. U. (1939a) On the role of the pituitary stalk in the regulation of the anterior pituitary, with special reference to the thyrotrophic hormone. *Endocrinology*, **25**, 605–614.

UOTILA, U. U. (1939b) Role of pituitary stalk in regulation of thyrotropic and thyroid activity. *Proc. Soc. exp. Biol. (N.Y.)*, **41**, 106–108.

VALE, W., BURGUS, R. AND GUILLEMIN, R. (1967) Competition between thyroxine and TRF at the pituitary level in the release of TSH. *Proc. Soc. exp. Biol. (N.Y.)*, **125**, 210–213.

VAN BEUGEN, L. (1960) *Studies Concerning the Central Nervous Control of Thyroid Activity.* Doctoral Thesis, Leiden (The Netherlands), in Dutch with summary in English.

VAN BEUGEN, L. AND VAN DER WERFF TEN BOSCH, J. J. (1960) Cerebral lesions and thyroid response to cold in the rat. *Acta Endocr. (Kbh.)*, Suppl. 50, 95–96.

VAN BEUGEN, L. AND VAN DER WERFF TEN BOSCH, J. J. (1961) Effects of hypothalamic lesions and of cold on thyroid activity in the rat. *Acta Endocr. (Kbh.)*, **38**, 585–597.

VAN MIDDLESWORTH, L. (1957) Thyroxine secretion, a possible cause of goiter. *Endocrinology*, **61**, 570–573.

VAN MIDDLESWORTH, L., JAGIELLO, G. AND VAN DER LAAN, W. P. (1959) Observations on production of goiter in rats with propylthiouracil and goiter prevention. *Endocrinology*, **64**, 186–190.

VAN REES, G. P. AND MOLL, J. (1968) Influence of thyroidectomy with and without thyroxine treatment on thyrotrophin secretion in gonadectomized rats with anterior hypothalamic lesions. *Neuroendocrinology*, **3**, 115–126.

VON EULER, C. AND HOLMGREN, B. (1956) The role of the hypothalamo-hypophysial connexions in thyroid secretion. *J. Physiol. (Lond.)*, **131**, 137–146.

WILLS, P. I. AND SCHINDLER, W. J. (1970) Radiothyroxine turn-over studies in mice; effects of temperature, diet, sex and pregnancy. *Endocrinology*, **86**, 1272–1280.

WOODS, R. AND CARLSON, L. D. (1956) Thyroxine secretion in rats exposed to cold. *Endocrinology*, **59**, 323–330.

YAMADA, T. (1968) Effect of fecal loss of thyroxine on pituitary-thyroid feedback control in the rat. *Endocrinology*, **82**, 327–332.

YAMADA, T., KAJIHARA, A., ONAYA, T., KOBAYASHI, I., TAKEMURA, Y. AND SHICHYO, K. (1965) Studies on the acute stimulatory effect of cold on thyroid activity and its mechanism in the guinea pig. *Endocrinology*, **77**, 968–976.

YOUSEF, M. K. AND JOHNSON, H. D. (1966) Blood thyroxine degradation rate of cattle as influenced by temperature and feed intake. *Life Sci.*, **5**, 1349–1363.

YOUSEF, M. K. AND JOHNSON, H. D. (1968) Effects of heat and feed restriction during growth on thyroxine secretion of male rats. *Endocrinology*, **82**, 353–358.

DISCUSSION

TER HAAR: I am not too surprised about the response from the hypothalamic area. When the temperature gets low then also the biochemical wheels are slowed down by the enzyme reaction.

MOLL: There are some other factors that come into play, *e.g.*, I have left out the very conflicting and

(control), one neonatally p-estradiol-treated rat (p-estradiol), one 14-day ovariecto-mized (ovariectomized), and of one ovariectomized rat given early replacement therapy (replacement therapy).

The rats were anaesthetized before ovariectomy or sham operation using one intraperitoneal injection of Nembutal (10 γ/g body weight). Ovariectomy was per-formed using a small ventral incision which was closed with sutures. The sham operation consisted of anaesthesia, incision, sighting the ovaries and suturing.

References p. 326

difficult aspect of the cold response. There is also an interaction between the pituitary–thyroid system and the pituitary–adrenal system. The explanation of Grant is that the stress component is predominant in severe cold. The stress effect may, and this holds for other conditions also, inhibit the pituitary–thyroid system. You can say that the whole biochemical machinery works slower at very low temperatures, but the animals are able to tolerate also temperatures of zero degrees centigrade. The machinery itself is, I would say, not slowing down, it may be even increasing. There are quite a number of biochemical changes in the cold but I have now been concentrating on the pituitary–thyroid response.

BATTA: I have just two small questions: I would be interested to know whether in rabbits, which have a lot of brown fat, you also find a cold response. The second one: what effect d...

β-estradiol treatment was performed by a subcutaneous injection of β-estradiol valerianate (1 γ/g body weight) dissolved in 1 mg/ml sesame oil every three days. Controls were injected with 0.1 ml of the vehicle exclusively. Rats surviving treatment were kept with their lactating mothers until weaning at 28 days of age.

Electrical activity of the brain

An electroencephalogram was obtained from normal and experimental rats at 8, 16, 21 and 28 days of age. In many experiments recording of spontaneous electrical waves was done with insulated stainless steel wires (100 μm diameter), inserted through small holes in the skull. In other cases the skull was partially removed and golden wires (100 μm diameter), chloridized at the tip, were placed on the pial surface.

These variations in recording technique did not produce either significant amplitude or frequency differences among preparations at a given stage of development. Both monopolar and bipolar recordings were obtained. In addition, an electrode was placed on the trunk for the purpose of monitoring body movements, including respiration, and the electrocardiogram. The rats used for EEG recording were discharged from all behavioural tests.

Behaviour tests

All tests were conducted when the animals were 30 days old. First the "Home Cage" test was performed, secondly the "Open Field" test and lastly the "Shuttle Box" test.

Running motility in Home Cage

This test was performed by placing a rat in a "Home Cage" slightly modified for studying its running activity. The parameters recorded were: a) the total number of movements in 6 min (total activity); b) the number of movements during the first 3 min; c) the number of movements during the last 3 min. Each rat was tested under each hormonal condition at least three times at different days.

Motility in Open Field

The "Open Field" consisted of an area of 80 × 80 cm surrounded by a wall 30 cm high and divided by strips into one hundred squares, ten on each side. Each rat was placed in the middle squares and its behaviour observed for 3 min. Its locomotion was recorded and scored for the following: a) the total number of squares crossed (total activity); b) the time elapsed from the moment when the rat was placed on the middle squares to the moment at which the rat left them; c) the number of faecal boluses dropped per test. Each rat was tested three times on different days under each hormonal condition.

Shuttle-box

Each rat was tested individually under each hormonal condition at least 5 times on different days for conditioning in an automatic reflex conditioner (U. Basile model). The effect of 20 stimuli during 10 min was recorded: conditioning light stimulus (3 sec); additional electrical stimulus (3 sec); rest (24 sec). The intensity of the additional electrical stimulus was 60 V. The "Shuttle-box" test was repeated, in the same manner, 10 and 20 days after conditioning, in order to test the rat's memory. The parameters recorded were: a) number of electric shocks avoided; b) number of electric shocks received before learning to avoid 3, 4, 5 or 8 shocks.

Statistical analysis of data

All measurements relating to the effects of the several treatments were subjected to statistical analysis and a highly significant correlation has been accepted at $P < 0.01$.

Results

Fig. 1 shows the electroencephalograms recorded from developing rat brain in all experimental hormonal conditions. During the first week after birth, in normal rats the electrical activity detectable from the cerebral cortex was irregular, intermittent and characterized by a theta rhythm of a relatively low amplitude (Fig. $1A_1$). Between the 8th and 16th day of age, a marked trend towards regularity, rhythmicity and continuous activity was observed. EEG activity was at 7–8 Hz, 40–50 μV of amplitude and showed theta frequency (Fig. $1B_1$).

The patterns observed at 21–28 days of age were basically similar to those of the adult rat. The frequency varied from several up to about 20 Hz/sec, while the amplitudes were several tenths of a millivolt (Fig. $1C_1$ and D_1).

Treatment with β-estradiol modified the spontaneous EEG recorded during rat brain development. For example, at 8 days of age it was more regular at 8–9 Hz, showing a 15 μV amplitude with irregular theta frequency of 20–40 μV amplitude (Fig. $1A_2$). At 16 days of age, EEG activity was at 9–11 Hz irregular with a theta frequency of 40–60 μV of amplitude (Fig. $1B_2$).

The EEG recorded from 21 day-old rat after β-estradiol treatment showed a regular fast theta rhythm of 80–90 μV amplitude (Fig. $1C_2$). At 28 days of age it was at 9–11 Hz irregular and 60–70 μV in amplitude.

A progressive decrease in frequency of spindles finally disappearing completely was the most striking feature observed after ovariectomy.

EEG activity, recorded at 21 days of age from ovariectomized rat, showed a regular slow theta rhythm of 25–30 μV amplitude (Fig. $1C_3$). At 28 days of age and 14 days after castration, EEG activity showed an irregular theta rhythm of 30–40 μV amplitude (Fig. $1D_3$). Replacement therapy with β-estradiol in ovariectomized rat restored EEG activity to the normal level; *i.e.*, at 21 days of age EEG activity was irregular at 8–12

References p. 326

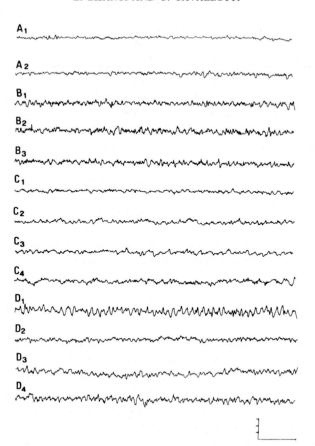

Fig. 1. Effect of β-estradiol on spontaneous EEG during rat brain development. A, 8; B, 16; C, 21; D, 28 days old. 1, control; 2, β-estradiol; 3, ovariectomized; 4, replacement therapy. Calibrations: horizontal, 1 sec except in A where it is 2 sec; vertical, 75 μV per division in A, 100 μV in B, 150 μV in C and D_1, 50 μV in D_2, D_3, D_4.

Hz and 70–80 μV in amplitude (Fig. $1C_4$) and at 28 days of age the recording was irregular at 8–10 Hz and of 90–100 μV amplitude (Fig. $1D_4$).

Moreover, three aspects of rat behaviour were studied under each hormonal condition. The data of running activity of rat in its natural habitat, *i.e.*, its motility in the "Home Cage", are reported in Table I. As can be seen statistically significant differences between the four experimental groups did not exist.

Table II shows the data related to the rat's emotionality in the "Open Field". The differences between the 4 experimental groups were not statistically significant and the behaviour of the treated animals was indistinguishable from that of normal rats.

The "Shuttle-Box" test shows that both ovariectomy and β-estradiol treatment induce greater modifications of behaviour by learning or memory preserving (Table III). Learning to avoid a noxious stimulus, *i.e.*, shock, by responding appropriately to a warning signal and the changes in responsiveness to repeated stimulation were